HEALTH SERVICES MANAGEMENT

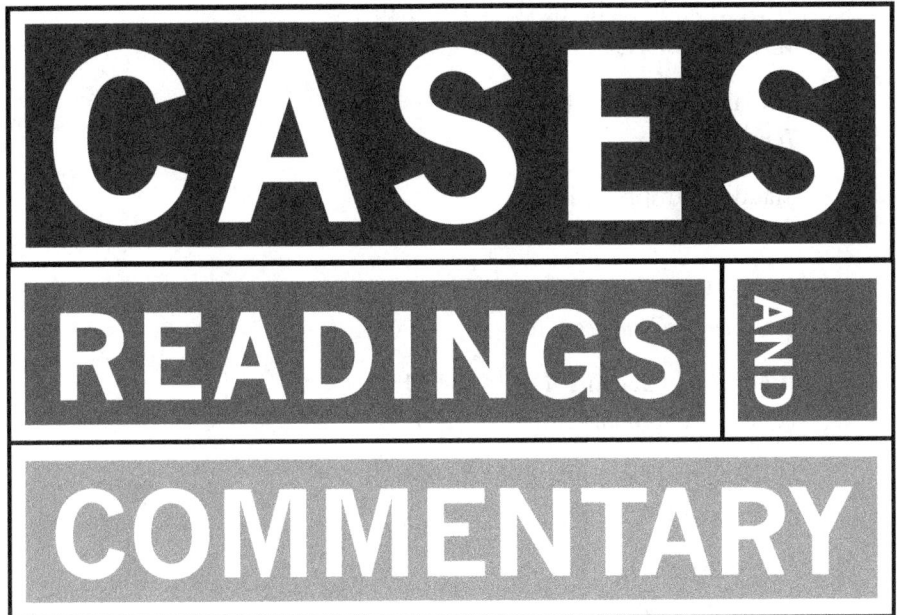

CASES
READINGS AND
COMMENTARY

TENTH EDITION

HEALTH SERVICES MANAGEMENT

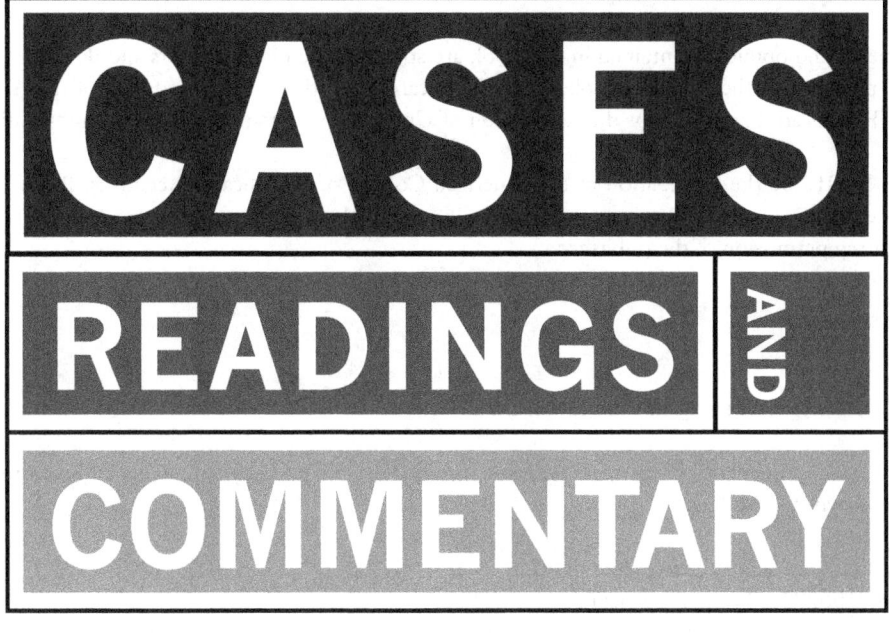

CASES

READINGS AND

COMMENTARY

TENTH EDITION

Ann Scheck McAlearney • Anthony R. Kovner

AUPHA

Health Administration Press, Chicago, Illinois

Association of University Programs in Health Administration,
Arlington, Virginia

Your board, staff, or clients may also benefit from this book's insight. For more information on quantity discounts, contact the Health Administration Press Marketing Manager at (312) 424–9470.

17   16   15   14   13   5   4   3   2   1

Library of Congress Cataloging-in-Publication Data

Health services management : cases, readings, and commentary / edited by Ann Scheck McAlearney and Anthony R. Kovner. -- 10th ed.
    p. cm.
 Includes bibliographical references and index.
 ISBN 978-1-56793-490-8 (alk. paper)
 1. Health services administration--Case studies. I. McAlearney, Ann Scheck. II. Kovner, Anthony R.
 RA971.H434 2012
 362.1068--dc23
                            2012029500

The paper used in this publication meets the minimum requirements of American National Standard for Information Sciences—Permanence of Paper for Printed Library Materials, ANSI Z39.48-1984. ∞ ™

Acquisitions editor: Carrie McDonald; Project manager: Amy Carlton; Cover designer: Scott Miller; Layout: Scott Miller

Found an error or a typo? We want to know! Please e-mail it to hapbooks@ache.org, and put "Book Error" in the subject line.

For photocopying and copyright information, please contact Copyright Clearance Center at www.copyright.com or at (978) 750–8400.

Health Administration Press
A division of the Foundation of the American
   College of Healthcare Executives
One North Franklin Street, Suite 1700
Chicago, IL 60606–3529
(312) 424–2800

Association of University Programs
in Health Administration
2000 North 14th Street
Suite 780
Arlington, VA 22201
(703) 894–0940

To our students, past, present, and future, who have to make sense out of the healthcare organizational predicament, find their own way, and take ownership of their own careers.

Ann Scheck McAlearney
Tony Kovner

CONTENTS

Part II: CONTROL

Part III: ORGANIZATIONAL DESIGN

Part IV: PROFESSIONAL INTEGRATION

Part V: ADAPTATION

Part VI: ACCOUNTABILITY

PREFACE TO THE TENTH EDITION

*H*ealth Services Management: Readings, Cases, and Commentary is distinctive in its overview of management and organizational behavior theory. The book is organized in a framework that begins with those parts of work over which managers have the greatest control—the manager herself and control systems—then extends to cover parts of the work over which managers have a good deal of control (at least over the short run)—organizational design and professional integration—and concludes with those parts of the work over which managers have less control—adaptation, including implementation of strategy, and accountability to interests that supply the organization with resources. Throughout, there is an emphasis on the case method approach to teaching healthcare management.

The cases take place in a variety of organizations, including a faculty practice, a neighborhood health center, a small rural hospital, an HMO, a multihospital health system, a medical group, an academic medical center, a home health organization, an ambulatory care center, and a number of community hospitals.

An instructor's manual is available online that includes suggested syllabi, approaches for discussing several topics in each part—for example, on the role of the manager, suggested topics include history of the manager's role in healthcare, organizational settings here and abroad, and career planning for managers in healthcare—and teaching notes for the case studies, the great majority of which have been classroom-tested. For information about the online instructor's materials, please e-mail hap1@ache.org.

We wrote and edited *Health Services Management: Readings, Cases, and Commentary* with the idea that it will be used as a stand-alone textbook, but it can also be used as a complement to other textbooks. For this edition, we have again presented a single textbook of readings, cases, and commentary, for the following reasons: (1) less expense for the student, (2) facilitation of course use of other textbooks, and (3) availability of the readings on the Internet, which means they do not have to be included in the textbook (although we include at least one reading for each of the text's six parts). A note for students on how to retrieve journal articles through the Internet is included in the text. This book can still be viewed as a casebook, but also includes suggested readings.

Some things have not changed through the ten editions of this text (this is now the thirty-fifth year of writing these books). The first has been the desire to have readings that build on good evidence rather than just opinion. At first, this goal was hard to achieve because of the lack of literature. Now it is hard to choose among many good papers. Second has been our goal to link theory with practice—to build a bridge between the social science literature and the actual work of improvement. Third, the text has always been divided into six sections—the role of the manager, control, organizational design, professional integration, adaptability, and accountability—each with a commentary.

We welcome dialogue with our readers and can be reached via e-mail at:

Ann Scheck McAlearney   mcalearney.1@osu.edu
Anthony R. Kovner   anthony.kovner@nyu.edu

STABILITY AND CHANGE: REFLECTIONS ON 35 YEARS AND TEN EDITIONS

Duncan Neuhauser and Anthony R. Kovner

Health Services Management: Cases, Readings, and Commentary, published by Health Administration Press, appears in its tenth edition in 2012. The first edition was published in 1978, and thousands of copies have been sold since then. How has the field of healthcare management changed over the past 40 years? What has remained unchanged? Why should one care about the past? What predictions can be made about the future?

The content of this textbook can be seen as one way to observe the evolution of health services management ideas. The origin of this textbook goes back to a task force on organization and management of the Association of University Programs in Health Administration (AUPHA) that met from 1971 to 1974. The task force's assignment was to review current course reading lists and to recommend readings for graduate students (AUPHA 1972). The need for a book of preferred readings became obvious.

Since 1978 the editors' goal has been to bring forth essential readings and ideas for students of health services management. Kovner and Neuhauser have each accumulated more than 30 years of teaching and consulting experience and board memberships, and Kovner has 12 years of operating management experience (Kovner 2000). The editors have reviewed hundreds of articles to select the few included as readings. New cases and readings and new words in the index reflect changes in the field.

Continuity of ideas is as interesting as change. The organizing structure of this textbook has remained unchanged for 35 years. It has always been divided into six sections: role of the manager, organizational design, control, professional integration, adaptation, and accountability. The section on professional integration is an important difference from a general management textbook. The need for companion cases led to the first book of case studies in 1981. Readings and cases have now been merged into one book.

1850 to 1975: From Matron to Superintendent to Administrator

The history of thinking about health services management goes back to the 1800s (ACHE 2008). At that time, this literature was largely about architecture (Thompson and Goldin 1975). The goal was to build the hospital so as to let the sunlight in and to locate it in a salubrious place. This would protect against bad air, miasmas, and mortality from hospital infections (hospitalism). Florence Nightingale's *Notes on Hospitals* (1863) can be seen as the first modern text on hospital management and was way ahead of its time.

From the 1930s to 1950s in America, the textbook by Malcolm MacEachern, MD, went through three editions and exceeded 1,000 pages (MacEachern 1957). In the 1930s, the superintendent of a cottage hospital needed to know all the details of the work involved, and these are reflected in this monumental text. It was organized by department (e.g., medical records and admitting) and included sample forms to be used in the work of the hospital.

By the 1950s and 1960s, hospitals had become larger and more complex: more technologies, specialties in medicine and nursing, medical record librarians, housekeepers, physical therapists, accountants, personnel directors, and more. The administrator had to get work done through a team of experts. The administrator's job was to hire qualified specialists and get them to work together. Interpersonal skills came to the foreground.

With the launch of Medicare and Medicaid in 1966, costs and prices began their steady rise, leading third-party payers to impose constraints on care, and the chief executive increasingly had to focus on external relations.

1975 to 2012: Administrator to Executive Director to President, COO, and CEO

The past 35 years have seen notable changes in healthcare. Fewer hospitals exist, and other types of organizations—such as home care agencies, surgicenters, and hospices—have emerged. Freestanding hospitals have closed or entered into larger systems in part to manage referral patterns and in part to meet complex environmental demands. A less-than-superhuman manager of a freestanding 25-bed hospital would find today's regulatory and reimbursement environment overwhelming. The amount of information about costs and quality has increased tremendously. The process of care is more standardized. That ventilator infection and handwashing rates are being compared worldwide would have been inconceivable in 1975. The growth in numbers and proportion of practitioners other than physicians has made teamwork and coordination more important. The rise in healthcare costs has made the field central to national politics. These system changes affect health services managers.

Terms that occurred in the first edition index—such as "medical staff," "long-range planning," "informal organization," "Hill-Burton Act," and "unity of command"—have been replaced in this edition with "strategic planning," "contingency planning," and "strategic cycling," reflecting a more flexible approach. A major change since the first edition has been the new language and ideas related to quality improvement, including benchmarking, CQI, errors, Baldrige Criteria, system thinking, pay-for-performance, and the Toyota production system. Evidence-based medicine and management are new concepts. The term "computers" first appears in the 1978 index; this edition has a guide to the Internet.

The Six Components of Health Services Management

1. The Role of the Manager

Stability: Managerial functions remain the same. Every edition of these casebooks, starting in 1981, includes Kovner's case study "The Assistant Director and the Controllers." It is about the conflict between line and functional accountability in an ambulatory satellite of a larger health system. The case raises issues of hierarchy, managerial specialization, performance measurement, hiring, and coordination. The manager's focus on mission, vision, and values remains unchanged. Managers must still obey trustees and work cooperatively with physicians.

Change: The book has increasingly emphasized teamwork and coordination across institutions. By the 1980s, medicine was expected to be practice-based on evidence of efficacy. Evidence-based nursing joined this movement. These ideas then filtered to management. How do managers know they are making decisions on the basis of evidence that these policies really accomplish what they are supposed to achieve? Healthcare managers are being paid more but are expected to be more accountable for meeting quality and financial performance objectives.

2. Control

Stability: Managers still need to guide their organizations toward objectives using control mechanisms. Governance, goal clarity, and information are constants. Cost analysis and managerial cost accounting remain essential. The need to generate information for third-party reimbursement is necessary for survival. Finance still drives operations and resource allocation more than a focus on community-added value does. The composition of boards of trustees has changed little, and they operate similarly to the way they did 35 years ago.

Change: The growth in information and in standards for compiling this information so that comparisons can be made has been tremendous. These controls from outside the organization come from third parties, regulators, competitive purchasers, and accrediting agencies. Quality measurement is joining cost analysis as equally important. The computerization of medical records has made available an overwhelming amount of quality information that can be compared across providers, such as www.hospitalcompare.hhs .gov. Quality information has gone from practically nonexistent in 1975 to overwhelming in 2010. The quality improvement movement has represented a massive change in thinking.

3. Organizational Design

Stability: The underlying logic of care—one patient's complaint, diagnosis, treatment, and follow-up—remains. The centrality of physicians and nurses, beds, tests, surgery, and infection control is worldwide. Larger and more complex organizations call for a balance between decentralization and integration. The period from 1975 to 2012 has been one of relentless growth in costs, new technologies, and percent of gross national product spent on health. Design is still organized by professions and not by service lines. Physicians continue to be organized separately from hospitals.

Change: Large systems have developed ways of linking the periphery to the center. New kinds of organizations have come into prominence, including matrix organizations, HMOs, PPOs, "focused factories," urgent care clinics, and accountable care organizations. There is an increased emphasis on teamwork at the bedside, in the clinic, and across large systems. Fragmentation of care is now accepted as a major challenge.

4. Professional Integration

Stability: The distinctive semiautonomous role of physicians remains, combined with the need to create relationships with physicians who will support the organization's mission. Physicians and hospitals still have their own goals that do not totally overlap. Nursing continues its cycles of supply shortage and sufficiency. Allied health professionals continue to seek more autonomy. Interdisciplinary cooperation is necessary for high-quality care.

Change: The expanding role of nurses, the emergence of hospitalist physicians, the increasing number of women in medicine, the decline of solo practice, the introduction of boutique medicine, the continuing further division of labor, the enhanced potential for self-care (through websites such as www.patientslikeme.com), and the direct marketing of drugs to the public are all changing practice. Pharmacy-based, nurse-run clinics and the option of lower-cost high-quality care abroad are seen as possible disruptive changes. Patients are increasingly being asked to evaluate provider care, and third parties are asking more questions about high cost variation in care. Posting patient opinions about their care and publicly available outcome measures will make or break individual practices. Now more than ever, surgeons and dentists who have rave reviews on the Internet may earn very large incomes, but they face the risk that online reputations can now collapse overnight.

5. Adaptation

Stability: Adjusting to ever-shifting environments is a constant. Managers realize they must adapt to external change. Hospitals are remarkable organizations in their ability to adopt new diagnostic and treatment technologies, procedures, and drugs that are the result of continuing scientific advances.

Change: Small institutions can no longer go it alone and find it essential to become parts of large systems of care and form strategic partnerships. The separation of CEO and COO is one response to the need for full-time attention to the environment. Planning is becoming more sophisticated, and large consulting firms often provide this expertise. Larger organizations are growing more complex, and the role of government has been expanding.

6. Accountability

Stability: The centrality of the patient and the patient's needs remains paramount. This all too often is more talk than action. The accountability mechanisms of trustee governance, annual reports, and meetings have not changed. Seeing the care experience through the patient's eyes remains underused. A century ago, the successful doctor knew each of his patients and understood each patient's wishes and needs (Cathell 1913).

Change: Now patient satisfaction is not evaluated just one patient at a time, but also for whole groups of patients cared for by one organization through surveys, focus groups, complaint reports, and the application of a marketing perspective that was almost unknown to patient care in 1975. Patient satisfaction has joined costs and outcomes as a legitimate end result of care. At the organizational level, profits are evaluated in bond prospectuses, the Guidestar website for nonprofits (www.guidestar.org), and new government requirements that nonprofits justify their tax-exempt status by demonstrating community benefit.

The Future

Reading history can be an entertaining and instructive hobby. History can also be used to test our theories about how the world works by giving examples of other relevant experiences. We can extrapolate and forecast from the past into the future. Knickman and Kovner (2011) predict that within five years, the healthcare reform law will change considerably; growth of healthcare costs will slow; a two- or three-tier health system will continue to develop; electronic medical records will be implemented widely; more resources will go into prevention, public health, and primary care; and fewer hospital beds will exist. What will happen in the next 25 years?

Florence Nightingale assumed the correctness of the miasmatic theory of disease. What if our present theory of disease drastically changed? It has, with the understanding of molecular biology. This advance of knowledge has been extraordinary, but has not yet had that great an impact on care. This may change. For example, we may be able to control the aging process rather than merely treating the many symptoms of aging, as we now do.

There have been a lot of changes that we did not predict, such as the quality improvement movement. Perhaps with hindsight we will realize that the most important driver for change in the last 35 years has been computerization. This technology, even more influential than Gutenberg's printing press, is changing all healthcare, and this change is far from over.

Some changes that should happen probably will not, such as the merger of medicine and nursing into a single but diverse healing profession. Here is the power of historical inertia at work.

On an optimistic note, in the last century, US health services management has not had to face the kind of major disruptions that we worry about today—new infectious diseases such as Ebola virus, asteroids, earthquakes, global warming, or nuclear winter, to name a few possible calamities.

In his preface to the 1978 first edition of *Health Services Management*, Jerry Katz wrote of the "unprecedented challenges, demands, and opportunities" for health services managers "in organizations of increasing size, complexity, and visibility." Health services management has been an exciting and challenging profession, and we doubt that this will change.

References

American College of Healthcare Executives (ACHE). 2008. *Coming of Age: The 75-Year History of the American College of Healthcare Executives.* Chicago: Health Administration Press.

Association of University Programs in Health Administration (AUPHA). 1972. *Report of the Task Force on Organization and Administration.* Washington, DC: AUPHA.

Cathell, D. W. 1913. *The Physician Himself,* 12th ed. Baltimore: Cushings and Bailey.

Knickman, J. R., and A. R. Kovner. 2011. "The Future of Health Care Delivery in the United States." In *Jonas and Kovner's Health Care Delivery in the United*

States, 10th ed., ed. by J. R. Knickman, A. R. Kovner, and V. D. Weisfeld, 353–64. New York: Springer.

Kovner, A. 2000. *Health Care Management in Mind.* New York: Springer.

MacEachern, M. T. 1957. *Hospital Organization and Management.* Chicago: Physicians Record Company.

Nightingale, F. 1863. *Notes on Hospitals,* 3rd ed. London: Longmans Green.

Thompson, J. D., and G. Goldin. 1975. *The Hospital: A Social and Architectural History.* New Haven, CT: Yale University Press.

Acknowledgments

The authors would like to express thanks to Lucy McPhail and John Donnellan for their comments.

A SHORT HISTORY OF THE CASE METHOD OF TEACHING

Karen Schachter Weingrod and Duncan Neuhauser

Teaching by example is no doubt as old as the first parent and child. In medicine it surely started with a healer, the first apprentice, and a patient. University education in medicine started about 800 years ago, focused on abstract principles and scholastic reasoning, and was removed from practicality. In the late 1700s in France, medical education moved into hospitals or "the clinic," where patients in large numbers could be observed, autopsies performed, and the physiological state linked back to the patients' signs and symptoms (Foucault 1973). This was one step in the departure from the abstract medical theorizing in universities (often about the "four humours"), which may have had no bearing on actual disease processes.

Education in law also became increasingly abstract, conveyed through the erudite lecture. It built theoretical constructs and was logically well reasoned. The professor spoke and the student memorized and recited without much opportunity for practical experience or discussion. This had become the standard by the late 1850s.

It is only by comparison with what went on before in universities that the case method of teaching represented such a striking change. The historical development of the case method can be traced to Harvard University. Perhaps it is not surprising that this change occurred in the United States rather than in Europe, with the American inclinations toward democratic equality, practicality, and positivism, and the lack of interest in classic abstract theorizing.

The change started in 1870 when the president of Harvard University, Charles William Eliot, appointed the obscure lawyer Christopher Columbus Langdell as dean of the Harvard Law School.

Langdell believed law to be a science. In his own words: "Law considered as a science, consists of certain principles or doctrines. To have such a mastery of these as to be able to apply them with constant faculty and certainty to the ever-tangled skein of human affairs, is what constitutes a good lawyer; and hence to acquire that mastery should be the business of every earnest student of the law" (Langdell 1967).

The specimens needed for the study of Langdell's science of law were judicial opinions as recorded in books and stored in libraries. He accepted the science of law, but he turned the learning process back to front. Instead of giving a lecture that would define a principle of law and give supporting examples of judicial opinions, he gave the students the judicial opinions without the principle and by use of a Socratic dialogue extracted from the students in the classroom the principles that would make sense out of the cases. The student role was now active rather than passive. Students were subjected to rigorous questioning of the case material. They were asked to defend their judgments and to confess to error when their judgments were illogical. Although this dialectic was carried on by the professor and one or two students at a time, all of the students learned and were on the edge of their seats, fearing or hoping they would be called on next. The law school style that evolved has put the student under public pressure to reason quickly, clearly, and coherently in a way that is valuable in the courtroom or during negotiation. After a discouraging start, Langdell attracted such able instructors as Oliver Wendell Holmes, Jr. They carried the day, and now the case method of teaching is nearly universal in American law schools.

The introduction of the case method of teaching to medicine is also known. A Harvard medical student of the class of 1901, Walter B. Cannon, shared a room with Harry Bigelow, a third-year law student. The excitement with which Bigelow and his classmates debated the issues within the cases they were reading for class contrasted sharply with the passivity of medical school lectures.

In 1900, discussing the value of the case method in medicine, Harvard president Charles Eliot (1900) described the earlier medical education as follows:

> I think it was thirty-five years ago that I was a lecturer at the Harvard Medical School for one winter; at that time lectures began in the school at eight o'clock in the morning and went on steadily till two o'clock—six mortal hours, one after the other of lectures, without a question from the professor, without the possibility of an observation by the student, none whatever, just the lecture to be listened to, and possibly taken notes of. Some of the students could hardly write.

In December 1899, Cannon persuaded one of his instructors, G. L. Walton, to present one of the cases in written form from his private practice as an experiment. Walton printed a sheet with the patient's history and allowed the students a week to study it. The lively discussion that ensued in class made Walton an immediate convert (Benison, Barger, and Wolfe 1987). Other faculty soon followed, including Richard C. Cabot.

Through the case method, medical students would learn to judge and interpret clinical data, to estimate the value of evidence, and to recognize the gaps in their knowledge—something that straight lecturing could never reveal. The case method of teaching allowed students to throw off passivity in the lecture hall and integrate their knowledge of anatomy, physiology, pathology, and therapeutics into a unified mode of thought.

As a student, Cannon (1900) wrote two articles about the case method in 1900 for the *Boston Medical and Surgical Journal* (later to become *The New England Journal of Medicine*). He sent a copy of one of these papers to the famous clinician professor Dr. William Osler of Johns Hopkins University. Osler replied, "I have long held that the only possible way of teaching students the subject of medicine is by personal daily contact with cases, which they study not only once or twice, but follow systematically" (Benison, Barger, and Wolfe 1987). If a written medical case was interesting, a real live patient in the classroom could be memorable. Osler regularly introduced patients to his class and asked students to interview and examine the patient and discuss the medical problems involved. He would regularly send students to the library and laboratory to seek answers and report back to the rest of the class (Chesney 1958). This is ideal teaching. Osler's students worshipped him, but with today's division of labor in medicine between basic science and clinical medicine, such a synthesis is close to impossible.

The May 24, 1900, issue of the *Boston Medical and Surgical Journal* was devoted to articles and comments by Eliot, Cannon, Cabot, and others about the case method of teaching. In some ways this journal issue remains the best general discussion of the case method. This approach was adopted rapidly at other medical schools, and books of written cases quickly followed in neurology (1902), surgery (1904), and orthopedic surgery (1905) (Benison, Barger, and Wolfe 1987).

Cannon went on to a distinguished career in medical research. Cabot joined the medical staff of the Massachusetts General Hospital, and in 1906 published his first book of cases. (He also introduced the first social worker into a hospital[1] [Benison, Barger, and Wolfe 1987].) He was concerned about the undesirable separation of clinical physicians and pathologists; too many diagnoses were turning out to be false at autopsy. To remedy this, Cabot began to hold his case exercises with students, house officers, and visitors.

Cabot's clinical/pathological conferences took on a stereotypical style and eventually were adopted in teaching hospitals throughout the world. First, the patient's history, symptoms, and test results would be described. Then an invited specialist would discuss the case, suggest an explanation, and give a diagnosis. Finally, the pathologist would present the autopsy or pathological diagnosis and questions would follow to elaborate points.

In 1915, Cabot sent written copies of his cases to interested physicians as "at home case method exercises." These became so popular that in 1923 the *Boston Medical and Surgical Journal* began to publish one per issue, starting with the October 1923 issue. This journal has since changed its name to

The New England Journal of Medicine, but the "Cabot Case Records" still appear with each issue.

A look at a current *New England Journal of Medicine* case will show how much the case method has changed since Langdell's original concept. The student or house officer is no longer asked to discuss the case; rather, it is the expert who puts her reputation on the line. She has the opportunity to demonstrate wisdom, but can also be refuted in front of a large audience. Although every physician in the audience probably makes mental diagnoses, the case presentation has become a passive affair, like a lecture.

Cabot left the Massachusetts General Hospital to head the Social Relations (sociology, psychology, cultural anthropology) department at Harvard. He brought the case method with him, but it disappeared from use there by the time of his death in 1939 (Buck 1965). The social science disciplines were concerned with theory building, hypothesis testing, and research methodology, and to such "unapplied" pure scientists perhaps the case method was considered primitive. Further, the use of the case method of teaching also diminished in the first two preclinical years of medical school as clinical scientists came more and more to the fore with their laboratory work and research on physiology, pharmacology, biochemistry, and molecular biology. Today problem-solving learning in medical schools is widespread and replacing the passive learning of traditional lectures.

In 1908, the Harvard Business School was created as a department of the Graduate School of Arts and Sciences. It was initially criticized as merely a school for "successful money-making." Early on, an effort was made to teach through the use of written problems involving situations faced by actual business executives, presented in sufficient factual detail to enable students to develop their own decisions. The school's first book of cases, on marketing, was published in 1922 by Melvin T. Copeland.[2] Today nearly every class in the Harvard Business School is taught by the case method.

Unlike the law school, where cases come directly from judicial decisions (sometimes abbreviated by the instructor) and the medical school, where the patient is the basis for the case, the business faculty and their aides must enter organizations to collect and compile their material. This latter mode of selection offers substantial editorial latitude. Here more than elsewhere the case writer's vision, or lack of it, defines the content of the case.

Unlike a pathologist's autopsy diagnosis, a business case is not designed to have a right answer. In fact, one usually never knows whether the business in question lives or dies. Rather, the cases are written in a way that splits a large class (up to 80 students) into factions. The best cases are those that create divergent opinions; the professor becomes more an orchestra leader than a source of truth. The professor's opinion or answer may never be made explicit. Following a discussion, a student's question related to what really happened or what should have been done may be answered, "I don't know" or "I think the key issues were picked up in the case discussion." Such hesitancy on the part of the instructor is often desirable. To praise or condemn a particular faction in the classroom can discourage future discussions.

William Ellet (2007) defines a business school case as describing a real situation with three characteristics: "A significant business issue or issues, significant information on which to base conclusions, and having no stated conclusions." A good case allows the reader to construct conclusions, filter out irrelevant information, furnish missing information through inference, and combine evidence from different parts of the case to support the conclusions.

The class atmosphere in a business school is likely to be less pressured than in a law school. Like a good surgeon, a good lawyer must often think very quickly, but unlike the surgeon his thinking is demonstrated verbally and publicly. He must persuade by the power of his logic rather than by force of authority. Business and management are different. Key managerial decisions—What business are we in? Who are our customers? Where should we be ten years from now?—may take months or even years to answer.

The fact that the business manager's time frame reduces the pressure for immediate answers makes management education different from physician education in other ways. Physicians are required to absorb countless facts on anatomy, disease symptoms, and drug side effects. Confronted with 20 patients a day, the physician often has no time, even over the Internet, to consult references. The manager has a longer time horizon for decision making in business. Therefore, managerial education focuses more on problem-solving techniques than does standard medical education.

Not all business schools have endorsed the case method of teaching. Some schools focus on teaching the "science" of economics, human behavior, and operations research. The faculty are concerned with theory building, hypothesis testing, statistical methodology, and the social sciences. Some business schools use about half social sciences and half case method. Each school is convinced that its teaching philosophy is best. Conceptually, the debate can be broken into two aspects: science versus professionalism, and active versus passive learning.

There is little question that active student involvement in learning is better than passive listening to lectures. The case method is one of many approaches to increasing student participation. Student-written reports are another form of active learning.

Academic science is not overly concerned with the practical problems of the world, but professionals are and professional education should be. The lawyer, physician, and manager cannot wait for perfect knowledge; they have to make decisions in the face of uncertainty. Science can help with these decisions to varying degrees. To the extent that scientific theories have the power to predict and explain, they can be used by professionals. In the jargon of statistics: The higher the percentage of variance explained, the more useful the scientific theory, the smaller the role for clinical or professional judgment, and the lesser the role for case method teaching as opposed to, for example, mathematical problem solving.

It can be argued that the professional will always be working at the frontier of the limits of scientific prediction. When science is the perfect predictor, then often the problem is solved, or the application is delegated to computers or technicians, or, as in some branches of engineering, professional skills focus on the manipulation of accurate but complex mathematical equations.

Scientific medicine now understands smallpox so well that it no longer exists. Physicians spend most of their time on problems that are not solved: cancer, heart disease, or the common complaints of living that bring most people to doctors. In management, the budget cycle, personnel position control, sterile operating room environment, and maintenance of the business office ledgers are handled routinely by organizational members and usually do not consume the attention of the chief executive officer. In law, the known formulations become the "boilerplate" of contracts.

The debate between business schools over the use of cases illustrates the difference in belief in the power of the social sciences in the business environment. Teaching modes related to science and judgment will always be in uneasy balance with each other, shifting with time and place. Innovative medical schools have moved away from the scientific lectures of the preclinical years and toward a case problem-solving mode. On the other side of the coin, a quiet revolution is being waged in clinical reasoning. The principles of statistics, epidemiology, and economics, filtered through the techniques of decision analysis, cost-effectiveness analysis, computer modeling, and artificial intelligence, are making the Cabot Case Record approach obsolete for clinical reasoning. Scientific methods of clinical reasoning are beginning to replace aspects of professional or clinical judgment in medicine (Barnes, Christensen, and Hansen 1994).

This does not mean that the professional aspect of medicine will be eliminated by computer-based science. Rather, the frontiers, the unknown areas calling for professional judgment, will shift to new areas, such as the development of socioemotional rapport with patients—what used to be called "the bedside manner."[3]

The cases that make up this book are derived from the business school style of case teaching. As such, they do not have answers. The cases can be used to apply management concepts to practical problems; however, these concepts (scientific theory seems too strong a term to apply to them) may help solve these case problems but will not yield the one "right" answer. They all leave much room for debate.

Notes

1. Although not the first hospital-based social worker to work with Cabot, his best-known social worker colleague was Walter Cannon's sister, Ida Cannon.
2. For more on the history of the case method of teaching managers, see Roy Penchansky, *Health Services Administration: Policy Cases and the Case Method* (Boston: Harvard University Press, 1968), 395–453.
3. A proposal to increase the problem-solving content of medical education is found in Association of American Medical Colleges, *Graduate Medical Education: Proposals for the Eighties* (Washington, DC: AAMC, 1980). This is also reprinted as a supplement in *Journal of Medical Education* 56, no. 9 (September 1981), part 2.

References

Barnes, L. B., C. R. Christensen, and A. J. Hansen. 1994. *Teaching and the Case Method*, 3rd ed. Boston: Harvard Business School Press.

Benison, S., A. C. Barger, and E. L. Wolfe. 1987. *Walter B. Cannon: The Life and Times of a Young Scientist*, 65–75, 417–18. Cambridge, MA: Harvard University Press.

Buck, P. (ed.). 1965. *The Social Sciences at Harvard*. Boston: Harvard University Press.

Cannon, W. B. 1900. "The Case Method of Teaching Systematic Medicare." *Boston Medical and Surgical Journal* 142 (2): 31–36; and "The Case System in Medicine." *Boston Medical and Surgical Journal* 142 (22): 563–64.

Chesney, A. M. 1958. *The Johns Hopkins Hospital and the Johns Hopkins University School of Medicine*, vol. 11, *1893–1905*, 125–28. Baltimore, MD: The Johns Hopkins Press.

Eliot, C. 1900. "The Inductive Method Applied to Medicine." *Boston Medical and Surgical Journal* 142 (22): 557.

Ellet, W. 2007. *The Case Study Handbook*. Boston: Harvard Business School Press.

Foucault, M. 1973. *The Birth of the Clinic*. New York: Vintage.

Langdell, C. C. 1967. *Cases and Contracts (1871)*. Cited in *The Law at Harvard*, 174. Cambridge, MA: Harvard University Press.

LEARNING THROUGH THE CASE METHOD

Anthony R. Kovner

A "case" is a description of a situation or problem facing a manager that requires analysis, decision, and planning a course of action. A decision may be to delay a decision, and a planned course of action may be to take no action. A case takes place in time. A case must have an issue. As McNair says, "there must be a question of what somebody should do, what somebody should have done, who is to blame for the situation, what is the best decision to be made under the circumstances" (Towl 1969). A case represents selected details about a situation; it represents selection by the case writer.

The case method involves class discussion that is guided by a teacher so that students can diagnose and define important problems in a situation, acquire competence in developing useful alternatives to respond to such problems, and improve judgment in selecting action alternatives. Students learn to diagnose constraints and opportunities faced by the manager in implementation and to overcome constraints such as limited time and dollars.

As Ellet (2007) points out, "You have to read a case actively and construct your own meaning." Students should consider what the situation is, what the manager has to know about the situation, and what the manager's working hypothesis is. Can the problem be defined differently? What's the biggest downside of the recommended decision? Has the student been objective and thorough about the evaluative findings that do not jibe with the overall assessment?

Students often have difficulty adjusting to a classroom without an authority figure, without lectures from which to take notes, and in which little information is offered by the teacher, at least until the class discussion has ended. Some students find it irritating to have to listen to their peers when they are paying to learn what the teacher has to say.

Students must learn to take responsibility for their own view of a case, to develop an argument that they can explain, and to listen to others who disagree. Students should speak up early. To learn to be a good participant, students must participate. When students go to the classroom, they should be familiar with the information in the case, have a conclusion about the main issue, have evidence explaining why their conclusion is reasonable, and show they have thought about other conclusions. It is suggested that students spend at least two hours preparing for case discussion.

In a case course, students are often asked to adopt the perspectives of certain characters in the case, to play certain roles. To deny someone or persuade someone requires an understanding of the needs and perceptions of others. Role-playing can promote a better understanding of viewpoints that otherwise may seem irrational. Students can better understand their own values and underlying assumptions when their opinions are challenged by peers and teachers.

To conclude, understanding what a case is not and what case method cannot teach is important. Cases are not real life—they present only part of a situation. Writing or communicating a case may be as difficult as or more difficult than evaluating someone else's written case. Like many a consultant, the student can never see the results—what would have happened if the case participants had followed his advice.

Some aspects of management can be learned only by managing. How else can one understand when someone says one thing but means another? How else can one judge whether to confront or oppose a member of the ruling coalition when that member's behavior appears to threaten the long-range interests of the organization? Students and managers have to form and adopt their own value systems and make their own decisions. A case course can give students a better understanding of the nature of the role they will be playing as managers—an understanding that can help them to manage better, if not well.

References

Ellet, W. 2007. *The Case Study Handbook*. Boston: Harvard Business School Press.
Towl, R. 1969. *To Study Administration, 67*. Boston: Graduate School of Business Administration, Harvard University.

HOW TO RETRIEVE JOURNAL ARTICLES FROM THE INTERNET—A GUIDE FOR STUDENTS

Many of the journal articles referenced in this text may be easily accessed and printed from the Internet free of charge, presupposing the publisher has granted your school library access to its electronic archives. The following steps are intended to guide one through the process of locating, viewing, and printing journal articles from the Internet.

1. Access your school library homepage. If you do not know the web address of your school library homepage, you can probably find a link to it on your school's homepage.
2. Locate the directory of electronic journals to which your school library subscribes. Many library homepages display a link to "Electronic Journals and Texts" or "E-Journals and Texts" or the like. If so, click on this link. If the link is not on the homepage, try searching for the directory in areas such as "research," "databases and catalogs," or "journals."
3. Locate the directory that is likely to contain the journal you are looking for. The journal directories are often stratified according to broad subject areas. For instance, if you are looking for an article in the *Harvard Business Review*, click on the "Business" directory heading. Likewise, an article in *Health Care Management Review* would be found by clicking on the "Medicine and Health" directory heading.
4. Locate and click on the journal title in the directory. Some directories offer an option to search for the journal using a key word in the title. Otherwise, find the journal title according to the first letter in the title. If you do not see the journal title you are looking for, either the publisher has not made an electronic version of the journal available or your school's library does not subscribe to the journal. (However, this does not mean that the paper version is not available in the library.)
5. Choose and click on the volume and issue number of the journal that contains the article. A table of contents of that issue will appear. Occasionally, issues may not be included in the archive because they are either too old or too new.

6. Choose and click on the article you wish to print. The article will appear.
7. Print the article by clicking on your web browser's Print button or by choosing "Print" from the File menu.

OVERVIEW

Why do we do what we do?
How do we know it works?
How can we do it better?
—*John Bingham, Twin Falls, Idaho*

Throughout the tenth edition of this casebook, we discuss management in health services organizations. Yet the boundaries of management are not clear. As managers, we bring our full selves to work. We manage relationships with family, friends, and significant others as well as our feelings about subordinates, bosses, and peers.

In this text, we view managers in four ways: (1) by the extent to which managers control their work; (2) by the processes by which managers make decisions; (3) by managerial performance relative to norms and positive outliers; and (4) by aspects of organizational performance to which managers make contributions, including financial performance.

We focus on the work managers do and how they talk about management. Thinking about how managers function, what they want, and how they achieve their goals is critical to improving performance. A key to success at work is being able to think reflectively in the present. This does not mean that managers cannot learn from the past or from planning creatively for the future. Managers learn by doing, not by talking about what they are going to do. If managers reflect too long about what they are going to be doing, they will often be too late. People want answers. Reflecting before doing or saying something, to ask, "Is what I am going to do or say going to be good for me?" takes only a moment. We define "good for me" as the right action, which can mean something quite different with the benefit of hindsight. Managers do not always act based on what is good for them or for the organization, but they can often reflect in advance about how what they are going to do or say will affect themselves and others. Helping another person, not taking the credit, being charitable, or being grateful may or may not be the right action depending on the managerial context. The right action will involve achieving their own and organizational goals, subject to situational and other constraints.

The Healthcare Sector

Healthcare is a unique sector of the American economy. Part of healthcare deals with life-or-death matters. Patients and their families have strong feelings about many of the services they receive. Many health services are not measureable in terms of their outcomes. Most Americans do not pay most health expenses themselves. Rather, these expenses are paid for by private and public insurance.

The healthcare sector is large, one-sixth of the gross national product. The health sector has its own language, cultures, and history. The context of healthcare organizations (HCOs) is different from the context of banking, education, manufacturing, or farming enterprises. For example, central to healthcare are core services provided by independent physician contractors.

The Institute for Healthcare Improvement (IHI) describes the "Triple Aim" of HCOs as providing the best care (improving the patient experience) for the whole population at the lowest cost (IHI 2010). Yet any one of these goals is controversial at the organizational level. What does "improving the patient experience" mean if somebody isn't going to pay for it? Why should we "contain costs," if by increasing costs this enables us to increase profits and thereby retain earnings so we can then expand services and take care of more patients? Similarly, what does "improve the health of the population" mean, if this would involve penalizing people for bad health behavior, such as smoking, poor diet, lack of sleep and exercise, and so forth? These goals are not the job of managers in organizations. But these issues can be framed so that they represent more acceptable organizational aims for managers: to improve patient experiences that people are willing to pay for, only to increase costs where the organization is adequately paid, and to help people who wish to change their health behavior so that their health may be improved.

There are numerous stakeholders in HCOs: owners, managers, clinicians, consumers and taxpayers, pharmaceutical and insurance companies, payers, and organizations that regulate or accredit organizations. Managers have to operate in contexts where powerful stakeholders do not agree with each other. In a sense, there is no such thing for the manager as "the organization"—only powerful groups within and without whose leaders seek to control organizational decision making.

Levels and Issues

Prospective employers examine a manager's track record. What individuals have done in the past is the best guide to what they will do in the future. Assessing the skills that managers have is relevant to learning what skills managers need to carry out the demands of a new job. Each job has its demands, its constraints (what the job occupant cannot do), and a range of choices associated with the position. Managers generally have more choices in their work than other workers.

We have organized this text into six parts that parallel the levels of work over which managers have influence. These six levels range from greater to lesser, as managers have the greatest influence over themselves and the least influence over the external environment. We describe the least controllable level as *accountability*, in which managers influence those who supply the organization with inputs to which the organization adds value and influences them and other organizations and people to buy back the value-added goods and services. Levels, issues, and the degree to which the manager can influence activities are shown in Exhibit 1.

EXHIBIT 1

Examples of Issues and Problems Associated with Different Levels of the Organization

Degree to which manager can influence activities

	Manager can influence	Manager cannot influence

I Role of the Manager	Leadership style
	  How the manager spends his or her time
	  What the manager does
	  Whom the manager talks to
	
	The management team
	  Who they are
	  What they do
		Manager's personality and previous experience
		Limits of the manager's capacity
		Authority of office
		Actions of trustees

II, III Control, Organizational Design	Structure of organization Procedures Resources Information systems Incentive systems Scope of services provided	Resource limits Technological imperatives Information overload Delays, distortions
IV Professional Integration	Labor relations Morale Skill mix of staff Personnel policies Level of conflict	Values of staff Historical organizational structure Professional organizations, unions Informal groups
V Adaptation	Community perception Funding Workforce supply	Social history Competition Government regulations
IV General Environment (accountability)	Health behavior	Socioeconomics Prevalence of illness Value systems

Degree to which manager cannot influence activities

Part I, "The Role of the Manager," is concerned with the immediate context within which managers work, how they spend their time, the importance of judgment, the kinds of problems managers face, and the opportunities and constraints managers respond to in implementing change and sustaining the organization. In Level I, managers have greater influence on whom they work with, on what activities they perform (and in what order), and on how they spend their time.

In Parts II and III, "Control" and "Organizational Design," managers rely on other managers to get things done, using formal rules and hierarchy, budgets, information systems, and other impersonal techniques of control and evaluation. Managers attempt to structure and monitor activities of others to varying extents to achieve organizational objectives. Managers are limited in these efforts by resource availability and political acceptability. Structural changes and control systems are not error-free, need to be changed over time, and can be expensive, both in money and in managerial time spent in implementation and system maintenance.

Organizational stakeholders respond to managerial initiatives by independent action, resistance, or cooperation. A distinctive element in HCOs addressed in Part IV, "Professional Integration," is the degree to which the activities of clinicians can be aligned with organizational goals. Clinicians and others are subject to varying degrees to external reference and representing bodies, such as professional associations and labor unions. Their buy-in is often essential to organizational goal achievement and managerial effectiveness.

Managers must adapt to changes in the organization's internal circumstances and to the organization's specific external environment, as discussed in Part V, "Adaptation." Finally, managers must be accountable to the communities or publics served, as discussed in Part VI, "Accountability." The environments that organizations face are constantly changing, and the pace of change is increasing. Managers must adapt to change or their organizations will not survive at current levels of effectiveness. Managers may have modest influence on legislation, regulation, third-party financing, and community perceptions, particularly when they are constituents of effective lobbying and public relations organizations, such as trade associations. Many of the activities of external stakeholders cannot be effectively controlled by managers and health organizations and those representing them, nor should they be in a democratic society.

Evidence-Based Management

Evidence-based management aims to do the right things right. It has been defined by Blumenthal and Thier (2003) as "systematic application of the best available evidence to the evaluation of management strategies for improving organizational performance." The evidence-based approach has six steps: framing a question that can be answered, obtaining the evidence, validating the evidence, adapting the evidence to local organizational circumstances, determining whether the organization can act based on the evidence, and determining whether the evidence is adequate to take appropriate action.

For example, in attempting to reduce wait time in the emergency department (ED), managers have often intervened by increasing the size of the ED, which has led unexpectedly to increased waiting times, as patients are unable to be admitted into beds that are not available until the existing patients are first discharged.

Rather than looking for evidence to justify action that the manager has already decided on, managers using evidence-based tactics take three approaches to discover evidence: searching the available literature, locating best managerial practice in similar organizations, and conducting their own local research (e.g., surveying night and day nurses separately if it is believed that the nurses who work different shifts stay and leave the organization for different reasons).

Skills and Competencies

During the past ten years, professional education has moved toward requiring students to demonstrate specific competencies rather than simply requiring them to learn about topics or areas. Programs in healthcare management are required to specify competencies and show how these competencies are met to be accredited. The process occurs whether the program is located in a school of business, public health or other school, and these other schools typically have their own accreditation requirements. Programs are required to cover the following content areas in healthcare management: population health, policy formulation, implementation and evaluation, organizational behavior, management, operations management, human resources management, information management, governance, leadership, communications skills, statistics, economics, marketing, financial management, ethics, strategy, quality improvement, and professional skills development.

In addition, to become accredited, programs must specify competencies and how they will be met in the various courses offered. New York University's (NYU) program specifies five competencies for managers: leadership; process and quality management; health policy; critical decision making; and communication, networking and continuous learning. Competencies addressed in the basic management course at NYU include the following:

- The ability to examine and synthesize data used in information systems and apply evidence-based management principles for use in organizational analysis, problem solving, and strategic decision making
- The ability to measure, monitor, and improve safety, quality, access, and system and care delivery processes in HCOs

Scientific data that relate how students demonstrate competencies to success on the job are lacking, and vast differences exist in competency sets required for different management jobs in HCOs. Jobs range from managing community advocacy to managing information systems to managing operations and quality improvement.

Competencies can also be used to analyze organizations as well as managers. Management theory has shown that having a distinctive competency pays off for organizations more than trying to be all things to all people. Ways that organizations are shown to be distinctive include providing the lowest cost service, providing the most comprehensive services, and providing niche services (e.g., "Our hospital provides the highest-quality eye care on the Eastern Seaboard").

Performance Requirements

Organizations can also be viewed in terms of performance requirements (Mouzelis 1971). Organizations have to attain goals to receive resources from the environment. They have to maintain themselves as systems to achieve the goals. They have to change and adapt to new circumstances. And they have to align or integrate the values of those who work in the organization to achieve goals, maintain systems, and adapt to change.

Kaplan and Norton (1992) use a similar scheme, examining organizational performance from different perspectives: financial and customer (goals in Mouzelis's terms), internal operations (system maintenance and values integration), and learning and growth (adaptation). Kaplan and Norton argue that to sustain themselves and grow, organizations must operate profitably, satisfy customers, run internal operations smoothly, and adapt to change by learning and growing. The value of this perspective is in the importance of looking beyond financial success to other important aspects of performance, which affect financial performance as well as market share and growth or stagnation.

Conclusion

This overview classifies organizations and their management in several ways. The first is by degree of influence of the manager over a level of operations (from greater to lesser influence): the role of the manager, control (of operations), organizational design, professional integration, adaptation, and accountability. Of these, professional integration is a key concern for healthcare managers because of the prominent, semiautonomous nature of the many highly skilled professionals who play important roles in care. Another way of looking at managers in organizations is the extent to which managers make critical decisions using an evidence-based management approach. This means making management interventions based on higher-quality evidence than would likely be otherwise obtained using traditional approaches.

A third way to view organizations and their managers is to evaluate how their performance compares with industry norms and benchmark performance of similar organizations and their managers. A fourth way of looking at organizations and managers focuses on aspects of performance in terms of goal attainment, system maintenance, adaptive capability, and values integration (or finance, customer perception, internal operations, and learning and growth).

This overview has introduced four ways of looking at HCOs and managers and linked them to the various parts of our text. Using these perspectives, the reader is more ready to form his or her own views on the readings, cases, and commentaries that follow.

References

Blumenthal, D., and S. O. Thier. 2003. "Improving the Generation, Dissemination, and Use of Management Research." *Health Care Management Review* 28 (4): 366–75.

Institute for Healthcare Improvement (IHI). 2010. "IHI Triple Aim Initiative." Accessed June 28, 2012. www.ihi.org/offerings/Initiatives/TripleAim/Pages/default.aspx.

Kaplan, R. S., and D. P. Norton. 1992. "The Balanced Scorecard—Measures That Drive Performance." *Harvard Business Review*, January–February 1992, 71–79.

Mouzelis, N. 1971. *Organization and Bureaucracy.* Chicago: Aldine.

Selected Bibliography

Berry, L. L. and K. D. Seltman. 2008. *Management Lessons from the Mayo Clinic*. New York: McGraw-Hill.

Bohmer, R. M. J. 2009. *Designing Care*. Boston: Harvard Business Press.

Boyatzis, R. E., S. S. Cowen, D. A. Kolb, and Associates. 1990. *Innovation in Professional Education*. San Francisco: Jossey-Bass.

Institute of Medicine (IOM). 2001. *Crossing the Quality Chasm*. Washington, DC: National Academies Press.

Lee, T. H., and J. J. Mongan. 2009. *Chaos and Organization in Health Care*. Cambridge, MA: MIT Press.

Reid, T. R. 2009. *The Healing of America: A Global Search for Better, Cheaper, and Fairer Health Care*. New York: The Penguin Press.

White, K. R., and J. R. Griffith. 2011. *The Well-Managed Healthcare Organization*, 7th ed. Chicago: Health Administration Press.

THE ROLE OF THE MANAGER

A leader is best
When people barely know that he exists
Not so good when people obey
And acclaim him,
Worst when they despise him.
Fail to honor people,
They fail to honor you;
But of a good leader, who talks little,
When his work is done, his aim fulfilled,
They will say, 'we did this ourselves.'
—Lao Tzu

COMMENTARY

What's different about managing healthcare organizations (HCOs)? The goals of HCOs—including patient care, research, teaching, and community service—are more complex than those of car manufacturers or police forces. Translating such goals into measurable objectives is difficult, as the objectives of most HCOs cannot be reduced to greater profits or reduced budgets. Healthcare is labor intensive, the work is often complex, and it involves professionals with different occupational training working together. The health services manager must gain buy-in from a variety of stakeholders—including board members, patients, the community, doctors, nurses, other workers, payers, and regulators—some of whom may not agree with the organization's goals and often vague and conflicting objectives.

What Do Healthcare Managers Do?

Managers do what they are supposed to do, what they want to do, and what they can do. Managers confront reality, develop agendas and networks, think strategically, and manage themselves to accomplish organizational goals. Because they generally lack ownership of the firm, healthcare managers are often risk averse. They worry about their own survival as well as goal attainment. They make trade-offs between improving patient care, breaking even financially, and keeping clinicians content.

Key internal stakeholders may not want or see the need for strategic interventions, yet external stakeholders who supply the organization with necessary resources may be demanding change. Healthcare managers must help their organizations respond to the demands of those external stakeholders while mobilizing the support of, or placating, internal interest groups.

Purchasers of healthcare are demanding lower prices, documented quality, and responsive services. Competition from existing or new organizations is increasing. HCOs provide primarily medical care, which is only one factor affecting patient or population health. Sometimes more medical care may not even be good for the patient, either because a treatment is unnecessary or because the patient is injured as a result of the treatment.

Doctors and nurses may see managers primarily as support staff for their work. This image may vary with a manager's view of herself as "relating the organization to its environment" or "coordinating processes of care to achieve measurable objectives." Managerial work is accomplished in part through e-mails and meetings that some clinicians may regard largely as a waste of their time; they feel they could be more usefully involved in providing patient care.

Financing is complex for many HCOs. Managers must understand and generate sources of funds from varied payers and contributors. Healthcare is difficult to measure; therefore, managers must have patience and show creativity in applying quantitative measures, which are often more relevant to process than to outcomes of care. Change is frequently resisted because it can be measured against any standardized output. This is changing, though, as best practices have been developed and disseminated and as payers have begun to implement pay-for-performance incentives.

Other than financing, no organizational factor is unique to health services. Yet while the features of HCOs can be found elsewhere, the combination of such features make HCOs distinctive. In addition, healthcare is a large part of the US economy: one in ten Americans is employed in healthcare, and $1 out of every $6 is spent on healthcare.

The role of the health services manager has changed substantially over time. Medicare and Medicaid, introduced in 1965, fostered the growing complexity and increasing costs of healthcare. New organizations have appeared, with medical homes and accountable care organizations following health maintenance organizations, preferred provider organizations, skilled nursing homes, ambulatory surgery centers, neighborhood health centers, and minute clinics. Healthcare management is no longer primarily inpatient acute care management, and many hospitals now provide a range of services extending far beyond acute care.

Different Organizational Settings

The work of healthcare managers varies by the type of organization. HCOs include academic medical centers, neighborhood health centers, small rural community hospitals, Medicaid-focused health maintenance organizations, large public hospitals, visiting nurse services, Veterans Administration hospital networks, and health departments, among others. These organizations can be for-profit, not-for-profit, or governmental; large or small; rural, suburban, or urban; financially well endowed or struggling. They face different challenges and can respond to different opportunities.

Expectations for Managerial Performance

The healthcare manager's work is being transformed by revolutions in information and performance expectations. Healthcare managers are expected to support quality improvement, lead revenue generation, contain costs, and manage relationships with important stakeholder groups. Many managers are challenged by having inadequate resources to provide high-quality care. Greater performance expectations are being placed on managers in the face of limitations on what HCOs can charge for their services, while costs increase at a faster rate.

Top management gets excellent performance by hiring great people, creating a performance culture that links rewards with results, demands shared values, and believes that everyone counts. This is how General Electric does it. GE wants managers with high energy who can energize the people around them, who have an "edge" so they can make tough decisions, and who can execute those decisions (Hogan 2001).

Ullian (2001) says that being a successful manager means picking the right boss. Further, effective managers can communicate the "bad" news, are accountable for performance, respect others, have the courage to take action, and can learn from their mistakes and weaknesses. Successful managers are self-confident and cheerful (Ullian 2001).

Managers should ask themselves: Who are the key stakeholders impacting goal achievement? What do these stakeholders expect? How satisfied are they with current performance? Managerial interventions should always be financially and politically feasible. The manager should know where the money is coming from before he suggests an initiative and where the buy-in is going to come from for successful implementation.

Managers should reflect on what they intend to accomplish over the next 12 months, and determine whose support they need to achieve these goals. Every manager should consider her resume as her lifeline and keep it current. She should ask herself: What results did I achieve last year? Will I achieve results this year that make for a convincing track record of accomplishment?

Managers average six years in any position and should consider themselves independent contractors in charge of their own careers. Managers should take ownership of their careers and never accept a position without an exit strategy. This means determining in advance the conditions under which they would no longer be willing to work in a position and what steps they would take once they had made that decision.

Thinking Strategically About the Job

Managers should understand the flexibility of their positions. Each managerial job has three characteristics: (1) the demands of the job that the manager must actively carry out; (2) the constraints on the position, or those activities that the manager is not allowed to carry out; and (3) the options or choices that the manager can make concerning how she is going to spend her time and presence (Steward and Fondas 1992). The manager should reflect on how she can strengthen relationships with those on whom she depends for goal achievement; managing herself is essential for this to happen.

Goleman (1998) stresses the importance of emotional intelligence for management success, suggesting that it is more important than a high IQ and great technical skills, and that it can be learned. The five components of emotional intelligence are:

1. Self-awareness (how managers see themselves being seen by others)
2. Self-regulation (thinking before speaking)
3. Motivation (the drive to achieve results)
4. Empathy (seeing others as they see themselves)
5. Social skills (in listening and responding)

All managers make decisions based on evidence. How can they obtain better evidence to make more effective decisions? Managers should be able to do the following (Kovner, Elton, and Billings 2000):

- Identify emerging opportunities.
- Precisely define management challenges or opportunities.
- Collect data.
- Find and critically appraise relevant information from published and nonpublished sources.
- Understand the process of change, including stakeholder expectations and capacity.
- Be able to conduct and evaluate experiments in which new methods are piloted.

McCall, Lombardo, and Morrison (1988) have suggested the following framework for management development:

- Find out about shortcomings.
- Accept responsibility for any shortcomings that result because of a lack of knowledge, skills, or experience, or because of personality, limited ability, or being a situational misfit.
- Decide what to do about it accordingly. Either build new strengths, such as finding ways to get help and support while learning; anticipate situations, such as seeking advice or counsel; compensate, for example, by avoiding certain situations; or change yourself (which is very difficult to do), either through intensive counseling and coaching or through personal change efforts.

Summary

Increasingly, the work of HCOs is being standardized because of external pressures and improved results as work processes are continuously measured against benchmarks. The world of large HCOs of broad scope has more specialized managers, in areas such as operations, marketing, strategy, knowledge management, internal auditing, public relations, and human resources, among others. Many of these functional specialists have not been trained in healthcare before being employed in HCOs. Physician organizations are also growing in size and employing a greater number of managers. Interdisciplinary teams are the order of the day, working in a culture of putting the patient first. Managers must justify higher salaries in terms of quality, cost, and access results, as they are held accountable by owners and regulators, and as managerial contributions become increasingly transparent.

References

Goleman, D. 1998. "What Makes a Leader?" *Harvard Business Review* 76 (6): 93–102.

Hogan, J. 2001. "Thriving in Healthcare—Learning Every Day." *Journal of Healthcare Administration Education* (Spec. No.): 63–67.

Kovner, A. R., J. Elton, and J. Billings. 2000. "Transforming Health Management: An Evidence-Based Approach." *Frontiers of Health Services Management* 16 (4): 3–24.

McCall, M. W., M. M. Lombardo, and A. M. Morrison. 1988. *The Lessons of Experience: How Successful Executives Develop on the Job.* Lexington, MA: Lexington Books.

Steward, R., and N. Fondas. 1992. "How Managers Can Think Strategically About Their Jobs." *Journal of Management Development* 11 (7): 10–17.

Ullian, E. 2001. Presentation at the National Summit on the Future of Education and Practice in Health Management and Policy. Orlando, FL, February 8–9.

THE READINGS

The authors of "Evidence-Based Management Reconsidered" suggest that the sense of urgency associated with improving the quality of medical care does not exist with respect to improving the quality of management decision making. Managers often seek evidence to validate decisions they have already made rather than seeking the highest-quality evidence available before they evaluate alternative approaches to a management challenge. To aid the manager in understanding and applying an evidence-based approach to decision making, the authors provide practical tools, techniques, and resources for immediate use.

The required supplementary readings provide interesting perspectives on effective managers; Arndt and Bigelow look to the past to examine visions for the future of hospital administrators in the early 1900s, and Clayton Christensen looks to the future to forecast innovations that disrupt models of hospital care, physician practice, and chronic care. Similarly, Kovner discusses what made CEOs of large HCOs effective 25 years ago, while Griffith and White focus on the need now and in the future to build a culture of excellence—a first priority for every excellent HCO, as the expression "culture eats strategy" emphasizes.

Evidence-Based Management Reconsidered

Anthony R. Kovner and Thomas G. Rundall
From *Frontiers of Health Services Management* 22 (Spring 2006): 3–46

"What we do for and with patients and *how we organize* those efforts should, to the extent possible, be based on knowledge of what works. Put differently, both the application of clinical medicine and the application of organizational behavior should be evidence based."

Stephen M. Shortell, PhD, FACHE (Shortell 2001)

"What discourages our use of research is something that is typical of all health systems. That is, we are on a rapid cycle....We don't have two years to study something. Sometimes having 40 percent of the information on something may be enough. We make a decision and change it if it doesn't work."

Health system manager (Kovner 2005)

The numerous developments in evidence-based decision making over the past decade should influence health organization leaders and managers to explicitly incorporate such decision making in their management processes. For example, the considerable use of evidence-based decision making by physicians has resulted in the proliferation of patient care guidelines and related decision-support materials for physicians (AHRQ 2006a; Eddy 2005; Friedland 1998; Geyman, Deyo, and Ramsey 2000; Sackett et al. 2000, 1996). Acceptance of the evidence-based approach has been growing in nursing, public health, health policymaking, and other specialty areas in the health sciences (Brownson et al. 2003; Donaldson, Mugford, and Vale 2002; Fox 2005; Hatcher and Oakley-Browne 2005; Lavis et al. 2003; Muir Gray 2004; Lavis et al. 2002; Lomas 2000; Shojania and Grimshaw 2005; Stewart 2002). As Muir Gray suggests (2004), an evidence-based approach would improve the competence of decision makers and their motivation to use more scientific methods when making a decision. In their book *Management Mistakes in Healthcare*, Paul Hofmann and Frankie Perry (2005) call for the identification, correction, and prevention of management mistakes in healthcare. Moreover, articles have appeared in health management and health services research journals urging health services managers to examine the nature of decision making in their organizations and to consider adopting an evidence-based approach (Axelson 1998; Clancy and Cronin 2005; Davies and Nutley 1999; Greenhalgh et al. 2004; Kovner, Elton, and Billings 2000; Muir Gray 2004; Walshe and Rundall 2001). Web-based sources of evidence for managers have emerged, including compendiums of primary research studies and research syntheses developed by the Agency for Healthcare Research and Quality, or AHRQ (www.ahrq.gov/research/), the Cochrane Effective Practice and Organization of Care Group (http://epoc.cochrane.org/) and others. Federal agencies have supported research to improve quality, safety, and efficiency in the organization and delivery of health services (AHRQ 2006b). For example, since 2000 the AHRQ has funded the Integrated Delivery System Research Network, now Accelerating Change and Transformation in Organizations and Networks (ACTION), which was explicitly designed to create, support, and disseminate scientific evidence about what works and what does not work. Since 1991, the Center for Health Management Research (www.nsf.gov/eng/iip/iucrc/directory/chmr.jsp), a National Science Foundation–funded Industry-University Research Collaborative, has been facilitating collaborative research among university-based health services researchers and health system managers. Finally, evidence-based decision making has been increasingly incorporated into lists of competencies necessary for effective management of modern health services organizations. The management competencies proposed by the Healthcare Leadership Alliance (2005) include acquiring, appraising, and applying research findings to management decisions.[1] Similarly, the Health Leadership Competency Model, developed by the National Center for Healthcare Leadership (2006), incorporates competencies supporting evidence-based decision making, most notably the competency referred to as "analytical thinking":

> The ability to understand a situation, issue, or problem by breaking it into smaller pieces or tracing its implications in a step-by-step way. It includes organizing the parts of a situation, issues, or problem systematically; making systematic comparisons of different features or aspects; setting priorities on a rational basis; and identifying time sequences, causal relationships, or if-then relationships.

Similar developments are unfolding in the health systems of other developed countries. Indeed, if anything, countries with national health insurance or a public delivery system have developed more resources than the United States for evidence-based health services management. For example, the United Kingdom National Institute for Health Research has established the NIHR Health Services and Delivery Research Programme (www.netscc .ac.uk/hsdr/), the UK National Health Service (NHS) Evidence in Health and Social Care program (www.evidence.nhs.uk/), and the Health Management Online resource within the NHS in Scotland (http://www.health managementonline.co.uk/); the Canadian government has established the Canadian Health Services Research Foundation (http://www.chsrf.ca/).

Research in the United Kingdom and in Canada suggests that health services managers and policy-makers make little use of the evidence-based approach to decision making and, indeed, reveals a wide gap between the health services research and health policy and management communities (Canadian Health Services Research Foundation 2004, 2000; Lavis et al. 2002). In those countries, a number of steps have been identified that could increase the uptake of evidence-based health services management (EBHSM). For example, the Canadian Health Services Research Foundation (2000, 7) suggests:

> [D]ecision makers need to find more effective ways to organize and communicate their priorities and problems, while researchers and research funders must develop mechanisms to access information on these priorities and problems and turn them into research activity. . . . Researchers need to learn how to simplify their findings and demonstrate their application to the health system to communicate better with decision makers and knowledge purveyors. . . . The knowledge purveyors have to improve their ability to screen and appraise information—to sort the facts from the stories. . . . Decision makers and their organizations need to improve their capacity to receive such appraised and screened information and to act on it.

Moreover, studies in Canada and the United Kingdom have noted the substantial differences between health services managers and health services researchers in their understandings of what is considered evidence, what type of systematic review of evidence is helpful to decision makers, and the extent to which management and policy decision making can and should be evidence based (Canadian Health Services Research Foundation 2005; Lavis et al. 2005; Mays, Pope, and Popay 2005; Pawson et al. 2005; Sheldon 2005).

No study of US health services managers' perspectives on evidence-based decision making exists; hence we have little evidence to guide us in developing strategies to strengthen understanding and use of EBHSM among health services managers. The purpose of this article is fourfold: (1) to briefly describe the evidence-based management approach; (2) to describe the questions to which EBHSM can be applied; (3) to report on a study conducted by one of the authors (Kovner 2005) to understand better the use of evidence in decision making by health services managers; and (4) to suggest a number of practical strategies that US health services organizations can use to implement or strengthen an evidence-based approach to decision making in their organization.

What Is Evidence-Based Health Services Management?

Evidence-based health services management applies the idea of evidence-based decision making to business process, operational, and strategic decisions in health services organizations. Simply put, EBHSM is the systematic application of the best available evidence to the evaluation of managerial strategies for improving the performance of health services organizations. What distinguishes EBHSM from other approaches to decision making is the notion that whenever possible, health services managers should incorporate into their decision making evidence from well-conducted management research. It must be emphasized that other sources of information and knowledge, such as personal experience, experiences of others in similar situations, expert opinion, and simple inspection of data trends and patterns, can and should be used if such information is the best available evidence for a given decision. As is the case with evidence-based medicine, the research evidence one uses in EBHSM does not replace but rather complements other types of knowledge and information.

The EBHSM approach recognizes that decision making is a process rather than a simple act of choosing among alternatives. Under ideal circumstances, this process involves a number of steps. Exhibits I.1 and I.2 depict the contribution of the EBHSM approach to two frequently used decision-making processes in health organizations.

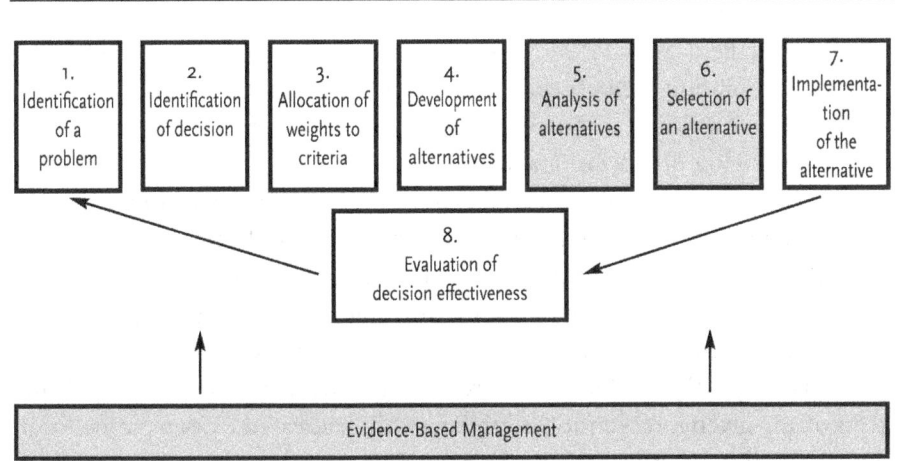

EXHIBIT I.1
The Eight-
Step Decision-
Making Process

Source: Adapted from Robbins and DeCenzo (2004, 106).

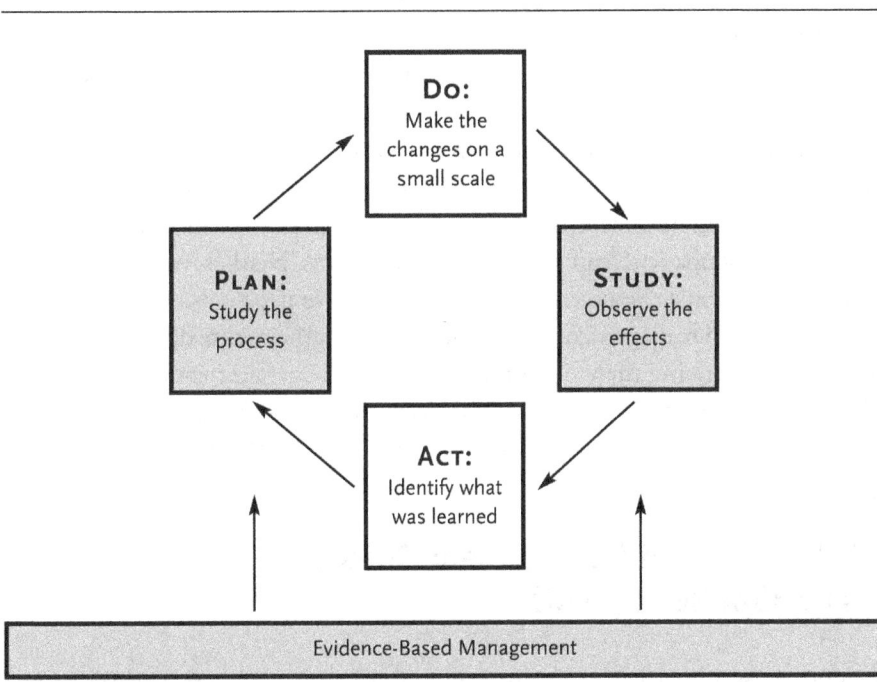

EXHIBIT I.2
The Shewhart
PDSA Quality
Improvement
Cycle

Source: Adapted from Kelly (2003, 32).

The decision-making process begins with the identification of a problem (step 1), or more specifically, identification of the discrepancy between an existing and a desired state of affairs. The decision maker(s) uses various techniques, types of information, analyses, and actions to complete the cycle, with information gained from an evaluation of the decision (step 8) helping to determine whether the problem continues to exist in the future. Of special interest to the field of EBHSM are steps 5 and 6. The promise of EBHSM is that by incorporating the best evidence available at the time, alternatives must be assessed and a decision must be made that will result in better decisions, thereby improving organizational performance.

Exhibit I.2 depicts the familiar Shewhart PDSA (plan-do-study-act) cycle frequently used in quality improvement efforts in health organizations (Kelly 2011; Institute for Healthcare Improvement 2003; Juran 1989). Although research evidence can be useful in making decisions throughout this cycle, the knowledge base created by the Plan and Study steps—understanding the nature of the problem, the process in which it is embedded, and the effects of any given intervention—can be greatly increased by comparing local data with studies of other organizations.

The generic eight-step decision-making model and the PDSA decision-making approach for improving quality share several strengths. The models help managers systematically identify causes of problems. They provide insights necessary for designing and implementing interventions to improve performance. Each encourages monitoring and evaluation of decisions to continually improve performance over time.

These models also share some important weaknesses. They tend to make improvement processes "inward looking," focusing on information and data that are available or can be generated within the organization. The models place little emphasis on systematic research in other organizations. Neither model makes use of modern electronic resources to help managers solve problems. Hence, the use of evidence-based management techniques can strengthen these decision-making processes by extending the vision of decision makers beyond their organization's walls, bringing existing evidence into the decision-making process and providing managers access to the entire spectrum of evidence available on the Internet.

To What Types of Management Questions Can EBHSM Be Applied?

Evidence-based health services management can be applied to three types of management issues: core business transaction management, operational management, and strategic management. Management questions include those that directly influence the way in which patient care is financed, organized, and delivered, as well as those that are supportive to patient care and those that involve external arrangements among nonclinical personnel (see Exhibit I.3).

Although EBHSM techniques can be applied to management decisions regarding core business transactions, research on these issues is not easily available to health services managers. Management decisions regarding core business transactions may be made by trial and error, copying successful processes in other organizations, or seeking technical consultation. On the other hand, considerable research is available to address many (but not all) operational and strategic issues confronting health services managers. Indeed, systematic reviews exist that summarize research evidence on each of the operational and strategic management questions listed in Exhibit I.3 at the Agency for Healthcare Research and Quality (www.ahrq.gov/research/), the Cochrane Collaboration Effective Practice and Organization of Care Group (www.epoc.cochrane.org), and the Cochrane Consumers and Communication Review Group (www.latrobe.edu.au/chcp/cochrane/) websites. These sites also provide a considerable amount of research regarding organizational structures and processes that may influence patient care processes and patient outcomes.

EXHIBIT I.3

Examples of Management Questions to Which EBHSM Can Be Applied

Type of Management Issue	Management Questions
Core Business Transactions	• How can the payer process MD claims for payment more quickly? • How can the health system's information on patient eligibility for benefits be made more accurate? • What methods for paying physician claims achieve speed, convenience, and accuracy requirements?
Operational Management	• How can nurse absenteeism be reduced? • Will decreasing the patient/nurse ratio improve patient outcomes? • Does hospital discharge planning and follow up improve patients' outcomes? • Does hand washing among healthcare workers reduce hospital-acquired infections? • Does basing part of employees' compensation on achievement of unit or team goals improve teamwork and coordination?
Strategic Management	• How do hospital mergers affect administrative costs? • Do hospital-physician joint ventures, such as orthopedic surgery centers, have negative effects on in-hospital surgery? • Does the implementation of an electronic medical record improve the quality of patient care? • Do pay-for-performance incentives substantially improve targeted care processes?

Applying evidence to the assessment of alternatives and the selection of a "best" alternative is itself a five-step process:

1. Formulating the research question
2. Acquiring the relevant research findings and other types of evidence
3. Assessing the validity, quality, and applicability of the evidence
4. Presenting the evidence in a way that will make it likely it will be used in the decision process
5. Applying the evidence in decision making

The brief exposition of each step will illuminate the main features of the approach. (For other more detailed discussions of evidence-based decision making, see Mack, Crawford, and Reed 2004; Mays, Pope, and Popay 2005; and Muir Gray 2004).

Formulating the Research Question

The first step is to turn the management question into a research question, framing the issue in a way that will increase the probability of locating useful research studies. This task requires more thought than one may first believe. Often, a specific management question will have to be broadened to find relevant research, but overly broad, vague, or highly abstract research questions must be avoided. For example, if a manager is interested in knowing the likely effect of implementing a hospitalist program on the cost and quality of care for patients treated for cardiac problems in a suburban Arizona hospital, finding even one study that meets all the inclusion criteria implied by such a narrow, specific question is unlikely. Broadening the management question somewhat (e.g., What is the impact of a hospitalist program on the cost and quality of inpatient care in US community hospitals?) makes it more likely that studies will be found that will be of some value to the hospitalist program implementation decision. However, broadening the question too much (e.g., What is the impact of hospitalists on the healthcare delivery system?) makes it likely that many studies included will not be relevant to the specific issue of interest to the manager. A good guideline for formulating the research question is to incorporate into the question statements that clarify the technique, the setting, and the outcome of interest (see "Guidelines in Formulating an Appropriate Research Question").

Guidelines in Formulating an Appropriate Research Question

1. What management tool or technique is being considered?
2. What is the setting in which the technique would be applied?
3. What is the desired managerial process or outcome?

Acquiring Research Evidence

Evidence relevant to the management research question can be obtained from a wide array of sources; colleagues, consultants, and known experts are frequent sources of evidence. Many managers will find it helpful to use the Internet to locate research articles. Health organizations that have made significant investments in knowledge management may have libraries, trained librarians and webmasters, intranet information resources, or an in-house management decision-support system. The vast majority of managers will not have such resources and will be limited to what they can find on the open Internet.

Two general approaches can be used to acquire research evidence via the open Internet:

1. Searching websites that provide access to systematic reviews or meta-analyses. For example, the Effective Practice and Organization of Care (EPOC) group within the Cochrane Library as mentioned previously may provide insight.
2. Searching bibliographic databases such as MEDLINE, PubMed, or Google Scholar for published and unpublished primary studies of relevance to the research question (see "Resources for Health Services Management Research"). For example, using the search terms "hospitalist," "cost," and "quality" to search the Google Scholar database produces more than 7,400 citations, many of which appeared to be qualitative or quantitative research studies. One of those articles was coauthored by one of us (Coffman and Rundall 2005).

A research synthesis of a large number of primary research articles is especially useful to decision makers because the authors of the synthesis have already made an attempt to assess the quality of the evidence and to draw out the conclusions that are supported by the evidence. Once relevant articles have been found, they may be electronically stored and, if desired, printed out to make them easier to read and assess.

What types of evidence can be incorporated in evidence-based management? This issue has caused considerable debate in the EBHSM literature. Some analysts have argued that EBHSM should follow the lead of evidence-based medicine and rely on evidence syntheses, which are systematic reviews of the evidence from studies of the effects of a particular policy or managerial intervention.

Critics of this rather restrictive definition of evidence point out that relatively few evidence syntheses are available on issues of concern to health services managers, that the standard procedures for carrying out systematic reviews dismiss many useful studies as methodologically weak, and that from a managerial

Resources for Health Services Management Research

Agency for Healthcare Research and Quality:
   www.ahrq.gov/research/
Effective Practice and Organization of Care Group:
   www.epoc.cochrane.org
Consumers and Communication Review Group:
   www.latrobe.edu.au/chcp/cochrane/
Center for Health Management Research:
   www.nsf.gov/eng/iip/iucrc/directory/chmr.jsp
PubMed: www.ncbi.nlm.nih.gov/pubmed/
Google Scholar: http://scholar.google.com

perspective the knowledge and insights gained from qualitative case studies, expert opinion, and personal experience should be considered evidence (Bero and Jadad 1997; Davies and Nutley 1999; Mays, Pope, and Popay 2005; Pawson et al. 2005). This issue is far from resolved as it involves the age-old debate over the need for balance between rigor and relevance in applied research.

As Ham (2005) pointed out, dismissing the relevance of systematic reviews and giving personal experience and other kinds of intelligence equal standing with the evidence generated by formal research studies runs the risk of "throwing the baby out with the bath water." A compromise approach may be to relax the criteria for the inclusion of studies and extend search strategies beyond established databases (Ham 2005). Moreover, researchers and managers must remember that the principles of EBHSM as described at the outset of this article explicitly incorporate both rigorous research as well as experiential judgment and research studies conducted with smaller samples and weaker designs than would be desirable. The point of the EBHSM approach is to create an expectation that managers will seek the best research evidence available at the time a decision is made and to incorporate this evidence with other sources of information, such as expert opinion and personal experience in the decision-making process.

Assessing the Quality of the Evidence

Managers must have some minimal competency in assessing management research, critical appraisal skills that will enable them to judge the quality of the evidence available. Ideally, managers should have, or have available to them, competency to assess the following:

- Strength of the research design
- Study context and setting

- Sample sizes of the study groups
- Control for confounding factors
- Reliability and validity of the measurements
- Methods and procedures used
- Justification of the conclusions
- Study sponsorship
- Consistency of the findings with other studies

In many cases, these issues will be addressed in the research report itself. For example, in the Coffman and Rundall (2005) evidence synthesis of studies of the effect of hospitalists on hospital costs and quality of care, 21 studies were identified that met minimal inclusion and exclusion search criteria. Still, these studies varied significantly in their overall research designs (e.g., experimental design with randomized control group versus quasi-experimental designs without randomization); types of comparison groups used in the quasi-experimental studies (e.g., concurrent versus historical); the size of the intervention and control or comparison groups; the statistical control for confounding factors; and the length of time over which the intervention was operative before evaluation data were collected. To understand the findings from these studies, these important differences in the strengths of the studies, and hence in the quality of the evidence, were incorporated in the synthesis. At a minimum, managers should be aware of the importance of assessing these aspects of research studies and be able to evaluate the extent to which they have been addressed in any given primary research study or research synthesis.

Presenting the Evidence

Managers and researchers should present evidence to the decision-making process in a way that is timely, brief, avoids technical jargon, provides clear descriptions of the questions addressed, incorporates the context of the research and findings, offers an assessment of the strength of the evidence, gives the results and implications for practice, and is easy to access (see "Guidelines for Presentation of Evidence"). The Coffman and Rundall (2005) synthesis attempted to present the evidence found in multiple studies in a way that would be understandable to managers and other nonspecialists in the field. The 21 studies were organized into groups based on strength of research design and methods. Simple tables were used showing how many of the 21 studies in each group demonstrated reduction in resource use (e.g., lower total costs or charges), improvement in measures of quality of care (e.g., lower readmission rate), and increase in patient satisfaction (e.g., self-reported satisfaction with patient care experience).

Guidelines for Presentation of Evidence

Present timely evidence.
Be brief.
Avoid technical jargon.
Provide clear descriptions of the questions addressed.
Incorporate the context of the research and findings.
Offer an assessment of the strength of the evidence.
Give the results and implications for practice.
Make the presentation easy to access.

The Coffman and Rundall article is not offered as a "best practice" of how to present evidence to health services managers. Indeed, publishing a briefer version in a journal explicitly marketed to managers would have increased its reach. However, we believe that managers, clinicians, and patients who searched for and found this article would have understood the findings. Managers and clinicians in hospitals and physician organizations could have easily incorporated these findings, including the qualifications proposed by the authors, into their assessment of the likely effects of adopting a hospitalist program.

Applying the Evidence to the Decision

Getting health services organization decision makers to use evidence may be the most challenging step. Most organizations today do not have the incentives or capabilities necessary for routinely using evidence in decision making. Substantial staff time is often required to ensure an adequate deliberative process. Opportunity costs are associated with disseminating and discussing the implications of research findings for a particular decision in a given organization. Ego costs to managers and others who feel their preferences are challenged by the evidence might be incurred.

The multiple ways in which research evidence assists the decision-making process are poorly understood. Many users demand that the available evidence have immediate, instrumental use for a particular decision, but often the available research evidence cannot be used in that way. Rather, the evidence is better used to increase the decision maker's enlightenment regarding the decision issue by increasing the manager's understanding of the nature of a problem; opening up communication among managers and other stakeholders; enabling the manager to generate creative solutions; and enhancing the manager's ability to estimate the likely effects of each alternative solution to a problem. These are important, but underappreciated, contributions of the evidence-based approach to decision making.

In fact, the same body of evidence can be used for instrumental and enlightenment purposes by organizations in different stages of a decision process. For example, the Coffman and Rundall evidence synthesis on the effects of hospitalists on hospital costs and quality of care was presented to representatives of several health systems that are members of the Center for Health Management Research (CHMR). This presentation increased the representatives' awareness of the availability of the various studies and their findings. More instrumental use was made of the synthesis by one of the CHMR member health systems who invited a coauthor of the study to present the results to more than 60 middle- and senior-level managers as part of a seminar on evidence-based management. The findings from the synthesis were incorporated in ongoing discussions about whether and how to implement hospitalist programs in the system's hospitals. At another CHMR health system, the results of the synthesis were presented at a board of directors' meeting and contributed directly to the system's decision to implement hospitalist programs in two of its hospitals.

A Study of the Use of Evidence in Decision Making by Health Services Managers in the United States

Kovner (2005) conducted a study designed to identify and explore factors associated with knowledge transfer between researchers and managers of health systems. The research focused on managers of five health systems and four types of decisions. The decision issues were: selecting the indicators for assessing the success of diabetes management programs; strengthening the relationship between budgeting procedures and strategic priorities; selecting the operational metrics to include in managerial dashboards; and adapting compensation systems for managers of physician performance. The study methodology included 68 interviews of managers of 17 nonprofit health systems located in regions throughout the United States. Of these interviews, 56 were with managers of five health systems that were members of the CHMR. The other 12 interviews were with managers in 12 health systems similar in size and sponsorship to one or more of the five CHMR health systems. In each interview, each manager was asked a series of questions to gain an understanding of whether they used evidence in decision making about each of the four issues described above, and how evidence was used to make decisions in their organization. Specifically, the managers were asked:

- Can you tell us about a recent decision that you are or were part of making?
- What process did the team working on the decision use to find evidence?
- In what respect was this a typical process, or not, for this type of decision?

- How do you assess if the evidence is of high quality, relevant, and applicable?
- What are three professional journals, websites, or other publications you find most useful in making decisions?

As in the Canadian and United Kingdom studies of evidence use by health services managers, US managers reported little use of this evidence-based approach for decision making. None of the 68 managers interviewed mentioned using evidence from management research to make strategic decisions. The journals that managers found useful were not research journals, or if they were research journals, they were not management journals. Journals cited included the *Harvard Business Review, Modern Healthcare, Health Affairs,* and *The New England Journal of Medicine.* Twenty-two websites were mentioned as useful, including those of the Agency for Health Care Research and Quality (www.ahrq.gov), Centers for Medicare & Medicaid Services (cms.hhs.gov), the Institute for Healthcare Improvement (www.ihi.org), and The Joint Commission (www.jcaho.org). The data from this study suggest a good deal of similarity between US health services managers and their Canadian and British counterparts.

Interestingly, when asked, "How do you feel that your organization's culture promotes your use of evidence in decision making?" respondents gave generally positive comments. All 15 of the respondents in the five health systems that were specifically asked this question spoke positively that their system's culture promoted the use of evidence in decision making. The apparent contradiction between the reported nonuse of EBHSM and organizational cultures favorable to the use of evidence in decision making is rooted in the managers' working definition of "evidence." As in Canada and the United Kingdom, the definition of evidence among health services managers differs from that used by most health services researchers (Canadian Health Services Research Foundation 2004). Many respondents indicated that they used evidence in making decisions, but what they referred to as evidence was frequently their own experience, anecdotes that had been communicated to them, information from Internet sites, and advice from consultants and advisory organizations such as the Health Care Advisory Board. None of the managers interviewed reported that in their organizations the evidentiary process for strategic decision making was regularly reviewed or that there was formal oversight of the deliberative process.

In further analyzing the data to identify ideas and strategies that might be used to increase the use of EBHSM, Kovner (2005) identified four factors that respondents suggested may influence use of management research in health systems:

1. External demands for performance accountability
2. An accountability structure for knowledge transfer
3. A questioning organizational culture
4. Participation in management research

From these findings, we recommend strategies for increasing the use of evidence-based decision making among health services managers.

Strategies to Increase the Use of EBHSM

External Demands for Performance Accountability

The increasing demands for accountability by external organizations have conflicting effects on the use of evidence-based management. Managers reported that their systems were increasingly expected or required to meet process and outcome performance targets set by purchasers, quality improvement organizations, and public and private regulatory groups. These external organizations—such as The Joint Commission, the Centers for Medicare & Medicaid Services, the National Quality Forum, the Leapfrog Group, and national and regional pay-for-performance programs—are increasingly identifying healthcare patient care process and outcome criteria and setting performance standards for health systems. Health system managers clearly recognize the strategic importance of the recognition and rewards offered by these external organizations, and in many cases such external pressures for accountability increase the use of evidence-based management. However, in other cases managers are concerned that motivation to search for and use research evidence in their quality improvement efforts is undermined by the focus on quality improvement processes, outcomes, and performance targets set by external agencies. One health system manager expressed this concern in the following way:

> In the past, before there were so many requirements for data reporting, we had a different process for setting performance indicators. We looked at the literature for the right thing to do, and then we met with committees of physicians and nurses and asked them what was important. . . . Today, however, there is so much demand for publicly reported data that we don't choose which areas to try to develop and improve dashboards and scorecards. We respond to demand.

In environments where external stakeholders are setting health systems' performance criteria and standards, we suggest that managers clearly link evidence searching and application to the development of organizational structures and processes that improve organizational performance on the externally set criteria, in effect marrying evidence-based medicine and evidence-based management to deliver the right treatment to the right patient, for the right condition, at the right time. In this way the strategic importance of evidence-based management can be established and enhanced over time as the use of research evidence is seen to contribute to the design of more effective processes for delivering care that meets externally set performance targets. If evidence-based management is not perceived to be strategically important to a health system, few resources will be devoted to it.

An Accountability Structure for Knowledge Transfer

Formalizing the responsibility structure for dissemination and use of evidence focuses and increases the impact of knowledge transfer. If no one is responsible for a function, it is unlikely that the function will be performed effectively in a complex, large HCO. To be a priority goal, dissemination and use of management research must be seen as consistent with and as contributing to the organizational goals of the leadership. On the other hand, the lack of an accountability structure contributes to a casual approach to searching for evidence that typically relies on convenient sources and minimal effort. For example, one health system manager reported:

> I get evidence from two sources: conversations with other people in the healthcare industry and my past professional experience.

Unfortunately, health systems do not designate managers as being responsible and accountable for knowledge transfer or for assessing research evidence as part of their decision-making process. Moreover, metrics are lacking to assess the benefits of obtaining better evidence for management decision making. Clearly, the use of evidence-based management would increase if health systems assigned responsibility for knowledge management to individuals or teams within the organization. A parallel strategy is to fix management responsibility for review of deliberative processes as part of the regular process of strategic decision making.

A Questioning Organizational Culture

A questioning culture affects the amount and speed of knowledge transfer between producers, disseminators, and targets of evidence-based management research. Health systems that support evidence-based decision making have cultures that recognize that encouraging questioning behavior among managers can lessen future problems that arise out of hasty and insufficiently considered decisions. However, challenging decisions and introducing research evidence into problem-solving discussions can cause anxiety among managers, creating a sense that managerial judgment and expertise are perceived by colleagues as inadequate or not trustworthy. As a health system respondent put it:

> On a philosophical basis, people tend to agree [about the desirability of evidence-based management]. When it comes to actually doing the work though, you start getting push back.

We suggest several strategies for building a questioning culture (see sidebar). Managers can participate in research "rounds," management research journal clubs, or research seminars led by internal managers or researchers from academic or other research institutions. Managers can routinely be asked by senior leaders to analyze the results of past operational and strategic decisions, including comparing their systems' performance with findings from research on other organizations. Staff development programs can be conducted to help institutionalize evidence-based decision making and enhance managers' abilities to find, assess, and apply research findings. Managers' compensation can be linked to metrics related to obtaining and using relevant evidence in decision making and sharing evidence with key stakeholders. Finally, we suggest that health systems develop organizational guidelines for decision making that require an assessment of available research evidence.

Participation in Management Research

Research dissemination, use, and impact will be affected by the level of participation of health system management in knowledge transfer. Lavis

---

Building a Questioning Culture

- Organize research rounds, management research journal clubs, and research seminars.
- Analyze the results of past operational and strategic decisions, including comparing the system's performance with findings from research on other organizations.
- Conduct staff development programs to enhance managers' abilities to find, assess, and apply research findings.
- Link compensation to metrics related to obtaining and using relevant evidence in decision making and sharing evidence with key stakeholders.
- Develop guidelines for decision making that require an assessment of research evidence.

and colleagues (2003) found that research transfer often required interactive engagement, as it is a very time-consuming and skill-intensive process. They stress the importance of developing uptake skills for research among target audiences. In the Kovner study, managers who conducted their own studies, focus groups, or market assessments were more supportive of evidence-based decision making. However, these managers had limited evidence-searching and appraisal skills. None of the health systems employed specialists in knowledge management. Access to resources such as the Cochrane Collaboration website or even management journals was limited. Clearly, familiarity with research and with the skills and technologic apparatus associated with health services research are important factors driving the use of evidence in decision making. In some cases, these shortcomings can be overcome through the use of consulting or specialized research services. In the case of one health system:

> We developed a strategic plan for our heart services. Part of that was gaining an understanding of the minds of consumers in the local market. . . . We used a national company to do a random study. . . . This was an empirical work; it was a conjoint study. It gave us longitudinal ideas and information about our primary market. The national company asked questions that were our questions. We hired a company that does consumer research and we told them what we wanted to know.

Several strategies can increase health systems managers' research capability and actual participation in management research:

- Management training in evidence-based management
- Investing internal funds in management research projects
- Partnering with research organizations, such as survey firms and academic research centers
- Implementing information technology and knowledge management systems

To put in perspective the findings reported above, we introduce some key ideas from the work of Shortell and his colleagues (2000) on the key success factors for clinical integration in health services. Shortell and his colleagues identified four organizational dimensions (strategic, structural, cultural, and technical) that influence delivery systems' ability to achieve significant organizational change, such as clinical integration. We adapted their framework and have applied it to our findings about the use of evidence-based management in health systems.

The Strategic Dimension

The strategic dimension emphasizes that significant organizational change—such as the adoption of evidence-based management practices—must focus on strategically important issues facing the health system. The implication is that to be widely used in health systems, evidence-based management must be seen by health system managers as a core strategic priority of the system. Our finding regarding the influence of external demands for performance accountability—a key strategic issue for health systems—on managers' support for evidence-based management is consistent with this dimension.

The Structural Dimension

The structural dimension refers to the overall structure of the system to support evidence-based management, including the use of designated committees, task forces, and individuals identified as responsible for implementing and diffusing evidence-based management practices. Our finding about the need for an accountability structure for knowledge transfer fits well within this dimension.

The Cultural Dimension

The cultural dimension refers to the beliefs, norms, values, and behaviors of people in the health system who may either support or oppose evidence-based management. Our findings regarding the importance of having a questioning culture as a precondition for evidence-based management are consistent with this dimension.

The Technical Dimension

The technical dimension refers to the extent to which people have the necessary knowledge, training, and skills to practice evidence-based management and the extent to which they have access to information technology and other technological assets. Again, our findings with regard to the importance of managers' having research skills, experience in performing research, and the critical appraisal skills necessary to assess research evidence performed by others is consistent with this dimension.

As Shortell and colleagues (2000) argue, to achieve a high degree of organizational change in core processes—such as the integration of clinical services or the use of research evidence in management decision making—health systems "must attend to all four dimensions simultaneously and attempt to align them with each other" (p. 140). In Exhibit I.4, we have suggested what happens when one or another dimension is missing.

When the strategic dimension is missing, no important decisions are made using research evidence. When efforts are made to practice evidence-based management, they have little effect because they are not directed at the strategic priorities of the system.

When the structural dimension is missing, sporadic, isolated efforts to incorporate research evidence in decision making may occur, but little system-wide use of evidence-based decision making is present. This is because no one

EXHIBIT 1.4

Effect of
Organizational
Components
on Use of
EBHSM

EXTERNAL DEMANDS FOR PERFORMANCE ACCOUNTABILITY (STRATEGIC DIMENSION)	ACCOUNTABILITY STRUCTURE FOR KNOWLEDGE TRANSFER (STRUCTURAL DIMENSION)	QUESTIONING CULTURE (CULTURAL DIMENSION)	PARTICIPATION IN MANAGEMENT RESEARCH (TECHNICAL DIMENSION)	RESULT
	✔	✔	✔	No significant use of research evidence on anything really important
✔		✔	✔	Inability to acquire research evidence and disseminate it throughout the system
✔	✔		✔	Small, intermittent use of evidence in decision making; no lasting impact
✔	✔	✔		Frustration and false starts in attempts to incorporate evidence in decision making
✔	✔	✔	✔	Lasting systemwide adoption of evidence-based management

✔ = PRESENT   ☐ = ABSENT

Source: Adapted from Shortell et al. (2000).

is accountable for diffusing these practices throughout the system, and few appropriate committees or task forces train and disseminate the concepts and techniques of evidence-based decision making.

When the cultural component is missing, efforts to introduce evidence-based decision making quickly wither and fade away because the organizational culture does not support evidence-based management. People do not believe evidence-based decision making will produce better decisions, and it is not rewarded by the organization.

Absence of the technical dimension results in frustration and false starts in attempts to implement evidence-based management because managers do not have the necessary training in the principles of evidence-based decision making, evidence searching, and research appraisal, and they may not have access to needed Internet and other resources.

This interpretation of the findings may indicate why evidence-based management is so little used, and suggests that a concerted effort will be required to change the situation. Only when all four dimensions are simultaneously made more supportive of evidence-based management and aligned with each other will sustainable progress occur.

Conclusion

The extent to which evidence-based decision making remains outside the repertoire of many health services managers is reflected in the way management mistakes are handled in most organizations and by instances of major decisions being made without regard to existing evidence that bears on the issue.

The rationale for using an evidence-based approach to managing health services organizations mirrors the rationale for evidence-based medicine. The movement toward evidence-based clinical practice was prompted by the observation of unexplained wide variations in clinical practice patterns, by the poor uptake of therapies of known effectiveness, and by the persistent use of treatments and technologies known to be ineffective. These problems are also common in managerial practice in HCOs.

The sense of urgency associated with improving the quality of medical care does not exist with respect to improving the quality of management decision making. One reason for this complacency is that instances of overuse, underuse, and misuse of management tactics and strategies receive far less attention and are much more difficult to document than their clinical equivalents. Surely, mistakes of judgment that result in irrefutable harm to people, significant financial loss, or profound organizational change may motivate public and private inquiries into how could this have happened. For example, the failed merger of the hospitals owned by Stanford University and the University of California at San Francisco cost both institutions a combined $176 million over a 29-month period and stimulated considerable public discussion of the reasons for the failure of the merger (Russell 2000). However, the visibility of the Stanford–UCSF hospital fiasco stands in stark contrast to the way most management mistakes are handled. Relatively few ineffective or harmful management decisions are acknowledged, examined, and used as the source of organizational learning (Hofmann 2005; Jones 2005; Russell and Greenspan 2005). Moreover, the fact that a merger of two highly rated hospitals with close ties to world-renowned universities could proceed in spite of a substantial body of research that was available at the time that raised serious concerns about that type of merger (Alexander, Halpern, and Lee 1996; Bogue et al. 1995; Brooks and Jones 1997; Conner et al. 1997) serves as a vivid and painful reminder of a management quality chasm in health services organizations. A substantial gap exists between what is known about many management questions and what health managers do. We *must* close this gap.

Note

1. The Healthcare Leadership Alliance comprises the American College of Healthcare Executives, American College of Physician Executives, American Organization of Nurse Executives, Healthcare Financial Management Association, Healthcare Information and Management Systems Society, Medical Group Management Association, and American College of Medical Practice Executives.

Acknowledgment

The authors gratefully acknowledge the assistance of Chris Kovner, Juliana Tilemma, and Erica Foldy, and of course the managers whom Kovner interviewed in the collection of information used in the preparation of this article. We would also like to acknowledge the financial support of the Center for Health Management Research in conducting the research reported here.

References

Agency for Healthcare Research and Quality (AHRQ). 2006a. "National Guideline Clearinghouse." Accessed July 5, 2012. www.guideline.gov.

———. 2006b. "Research Findings." Accessed July 5, 2012. www.ahrq.gov/research/.

Alexander, J. A., M. T. Halpern, and S-Y. D. Lee. 1996. "The Short-Term Effects of Merger on Hospital Operations." *Health Services Research* 30 (6): 827–47.

Axelson, R. 1998. "Towards an Evidence-Based Health Care Management." *International Journal of Health Planning and Management* 13: 307–17.

Bero, L. A., and A. R. Jadad. 1997. "How Consumers and Policymakers Can Use Systematic Reviews for Decision Making." *Annals of Internal Medicine* 127 (1): 37–42.

Bogue, R. J., S. M. Shortell, M.-W. Sohn, L. M. Manheim, G. Bazzoli, and C. Chan. 1995. "Hospital Reorganization After Merger." *Medical Care* 33 (7): 676–86.

Brooks, G. R., and V. G. Jones. 1997. "Hospital Mergers and Market Overlap." *Health Services Research* 31 (6): 701–22.

Brownson, R. C., E. A. Baker, T. L. Leet, and K. N. Gillespie. 2003. *Evidence-Based Public Health*. Oxford, UK: Oxford University Press.

Canadian Health Services Research Foundation. 2005. *Conceptualizing and Combining Evidence for Health System Guidance.* Ottawa, Canada: Health Services Research Foundation.

———. 2004. *What Counts? Interpreting Evidence-Based Decision-Making for Management and Policy.* Ottawa, Canada: Health Services Research Foundation.

———. 2000. *Health Services Research and Evidence-Based Decision Making.* Ottawa, Canada: Health Services Research Foundation.

Clancy, C., and K. Cronin. 2005. "Evidence-Based Decision Making: Global Evidence, Local Decisions." *Health Affairs* 24 (1): 151–62.

Cochrane Consumers and Communication Review Group. 2006. Accessed July 5, 2012. www.latrobe.edu.au/chcp/cochrane/.

Cochrane Effective Practice and Organization of Care Group. 2006. Accessed July 5, 2012. www.epoc.cochrane.org.

Coffman, J., and T. G. Rundall. 2005. "The Impact of Hospitalists on the Cost and Quality of Inpatient Care in the United States: A Research Synthesis." *Medical Care Research and Review* 62 (4): 379–406.

Conner, R. A., R. D. Feldman, B. E. Dowd, and T. A. Radcliff. 1997. "Which Types of Hospital Mergers Save Money?" *Health Affairs* 16 (6): 62–74.

Davies, H. T. O., and S. M. Nutley. 1999. "The Rise and Rise of Evidence in Health Care." *Public Money and Management* (Jan–Mar): 9–16.

Donaldson, C., M. Mugford, and L. Vale. 2002. *Evidence-Based Health Economics.* London: BMJ Books.

Eddy, D. M. 2005. "Evidence-Based Medicine: A Unified Approach." *Health Affairs* 24 (1): 9–17.

Friedland, D. J., ed. 1998. *Evidence-Based Medicine: A Framework for Clinical Practice.* Stamford, CT: Appleton & Lange.

Fox, D. 2005. "Evidence of Evidence-Based Health Policy: The Politics of Systematic Reviews in Coverage Decisions." *Health Affairs* 24 (1): 114–22.

Geyman, J. P., R. A. Deyo, and S. D. Ramsey. 2000. *Evidence-Based Clinical Practice: Concepts and Approaches.* Boston: Butterworth and Heinemann.

Greenhalgh, T., G. Robert, F. Macfarlane, P. Bate, and O. Kyriakidou. 2004. "Diffusion of Innovations in Service Organizations: Systematic Review and Recommendations." *Milbank Quarterly* 82 (4): 581–629.

Ham, C. 2005. "Don't Throw the Baby Out with the Bath Water" (commentary). *Journal of Health Services Research and Policy* 10 (S1): 51–52.

Hatcher, S., and M. Oakley-Browne. 2005. *Evidence-Based Mental Health.* London: Churchill Livingston.

Healthcare Leadership Alliance. 2005. "Competency Directory." Accessed July 30, 2012. www.healthcareleadershipalliance.org/directory.htm.

Hofmann, P. B. 2005. "Acknowledging and Examining Management Mistakes." In *Management Mistakes in Healthcare: Identification, Correction, and Prevention,* ed. P. B. Hofmann and F. Perry, 3–27. Cambridge, UK: Cambridge University Press.

Hofmann, P. B., and F. Perry. 2005. *Management Mistakes in Healthcare: Identification, Correction, and Prevention.* Cambridge, UK: Cambridge University Press.

Institute for Healthcare Improvement. 2003. "Breakthrough Series Collaboratives." Accessed August 27, 2012. www.ihi.org/knowledge/Pages/IHIWhitePapers/TheBreakthroughSeriesIHIsCollaborativeModelforAchievingBreakthroughImprovement.aspx.

Jones, W. J. 2005. "Identifying, Classifying and Disclosing Mistakes." In *Management Mistakes in Healthcare: Identification, Correction, and Prevention,* ed. P. B. Hofmann and F. Perry, 40–73. Cambridge, UK: Cambridge University Press.

Juran, J. M. 1989. *Juran on Leadership for Quality: An Executive Handbook.* New York: The Free Press.

Kelly, D. L. 2003. *Applying Quality Management in Healthcare: A Systems Approach.* Chicago: Health Administration Press.

Kovner, A. R. 2005. "Factors Associated with Use of Management Research by Health Systems." Unpublished report for the Center for Health Management Research, University of Washington, Seattle.

Kovner, A. R., J. J. Elton, and J. Billings. 2000. "Transforming Health Management: An Evidence-Based Approach." *Frontiers of Health Services Management* 16 (4): 3–25.

Lavis, J., H. Davies, A. Oxman, J.-L. Denis, K. Golden-Biddle, and E. Ferlie. 2005. "Towards Systematic Reviews That Inform Health Care Management and Policy-Making." *Journal of Health Services Research and Policy* 10 (S1): 35–48.

Lavis, J. N., D. Robertson, J. M. Woodside, C. B. McLeod, J. Abelson, and The Knowledge Transfer Group. 2003. "How Can Research Organizations More Effectively Transfer Research Knowledge to Decision Makers?" *Milbank Quarterly* 81 (2): 221–48.

Lavis, J. N., S. E. Ross, J. E. Hurley, J. M. Hohenadel, G. L. Stoddart, C. A. Woodward, and J. Abelson. 2002. "Examining the Role of Health Services Research in Public Policy Making." *Milbank Quarterly* 80 (1): 125–53.

Lomas, J. 2000. "Using 'Linkage and Exchange' to Move Research into Policy at a Canadian Foundation." *Health Affairs* 19 (3): 236–40.

Mack, K. E., M. A. Crawford, and M. C. Reed. 2004. *Decision Making for Improved Performance.* Chicago: Health Administration Press.

Mays, N., C. Pope, and J. Popay. 2005. "Systematically Reviewing Qualitative and Quantitative Evidence to Inform Management and Policy-Making in the Health Field." *Journal of Health Services Research and Policy* 10 (S1): 6–20.

Muir Gray, J. A. 2004. *Evidence-Based Health Care: How to Make Health Policy and Management Decisions.* New York: Churchill Livingston.

National Center for Healthcare Leadership. 2004. *Health Leadership Competency Model,* version 2.1, 1–9. Chicago: National Center for Healthcare Leadership.

Pawson, R., T. Greenhalgh, G. Harvey, and K. Walshe. 2005. "Realist Review—A New Method of Systematic Review Designed for Complex Policy Interventions." *Journal of Health Services Research and Policy* 10 (S1): 21–34.

Robbins, S. P., and D. A. DeCenzo. 2004. *Fundamentals of Management: Essential Concepts and Applications,* 4th ed. Upper Saddle River, NJ: Pearson Prentice Hall.

Russell, J. A., and B. Greenspan. 2005. "Correcting and Preventing Management Mistakes." In *Management Mistakes in Healthcare: Identification, Correction and Prevention*, ed. P. B. Hofmann and F. Perry, 84–102. Cambridge, UK: Cambridge University Press.

Russell, S. 2000. "$176 Million Tab on Failed Hospital Merger." *San Francisco Chronicle*, December 14.

Sackett, D. L., W. M. Rosenberg, J. A. Gray, R. B. Haynes, and W. S. Richardson. 1996. "Evidence-Based Medicine: What It Is and What It Isn't." *British Medical Journal* 312 (7023): 71–72.

Sackett, D. L., S. E. Straus, W. S. Richardson, W. Rosenberg, and R. B. Haynes. 2000. *Evidence-Based Medicine: How to Practice and Teach EBM,* 2nd ed. New York: Churchill Livingston.

Sheldon, T. 2005. "Making Evidence Synthesis More Useful for Management and Policy-Making." *Journal of Health Services Research and Policy* 10 (S1): 1–4.

Shojania, K. G., and J. M. Grimshaw. 2005. "Evidence-Based Quality Improvement: The State of the Science." *Health Affairs* 24 (1): 138–50.

Shortell, S. 2001. "A Time for Concerted Action." *Frontiers of Health Services Management* 18 (1): 33–46.

Shortell, S. M., R. R. Gillies, D. A. Anderson, K. M. Erickson, and J. B. Mitchell. 2000. *Remaking Health Care in America*, 2nd ed. San Francisco: Jossey-Bass.

Stewart, R. 2002. *Evidence-Based Management: A Practical Guide for Health Professionals*. Abingdon, UK: Radcliffe Medical Press.

Walshe, K., and T. Rundall. 2001. "Evidence-Based Management: From Theory to Practice in Health Care." *Milbank Quarterly* 79 (3): 429–47.

Discussion Questions on Required Reading

1. How can you tell whether a major medical center is or is not using evidence-based management?
2. Develop an action plan for implementing evidence-based management in a large academic medical center.
3. Make the business case for using evidence-based management.
4. How do the incentives under which healthcare managers function constrain the implementation of evidence-based management?

Required Supplementary Readings

Arndt, M., and B. Bigelow. 2007. "Hospital Administration in the Early 1900s: Visions for the Future and the Reality of Daily Practice." *Journal of Healthcare Management,* January–February: 34–48.

Christensen, C., R. Bohmer, and J. Kenagy. 2000. "Will Disruptive Innovations Cure Healthcare?" *Harvard Business Review,* September–October: 102–12.

Griffith, J. R., and K. R. White. 2005. "The Revolution in Hospital Management." *Journal of Healthcare Management* 50 (3): 170–90.

Kovner, A. R. 1987. "The Work of Effective CEOs in Four Large Health Organizations." *Hospital & Health Services Administration,* August: 285–305.

Discussion Questions for Required Supplementary Readings

1. What are the risks and rewards to healthcare managers considering implementing "disruptive innovations"?
2. How can effective leaders get buy-in from their clinicians and other associates who work in the HCO?
3. How would you estimate the value that healthcare managers contribute to their organizations in relation to the compensation they are paid?
4. How would you examine how effective an entry-level healthcare manager is?

Recommended Supplementary Readings

Berry, L. L., and K. D. Seltman. 2008. *Management Lessons from Mayo Clinic.* New York: McGraw-Hill.

Gilmartin, M. J., and T. A. D'Aunno. 2007. "Leadership Research in Healthcare: A Review and a Roadmap." *Academy of Management Annals,* April 9: 387–438.

Griffith, J. R. 1993. *The Moral Challenges of Healthcare Management.* Chicago: Health Administration Press.

Institute of Medicine. 2001. *Crossing the Quality Chasm.* Washington, DC: National Academies Press.

Kovner, A. R. 2000. *Healthcare Management in Mind: Eight Careers.* New York: Springer.

Lee, T. H., and J. J. Mongan. 2009. *Chaos and Organization in Health Care.* Cambridge, MA: MIT Press.

McAlearney, A. S. 2008. "Using Leadership Development Programs to Improve Quality and Efficiency in Healthcare." *Journal of Healthcare Management* 53 (5): 319–31.

———. 2006. "Leadership Development in Healthcare Organizations: A Qualitative Study." *Journal of Organizational Behavior* 27 (7): 967–82.

Studer, Q. 2003. *Hardwiring Excellence.* Gulf Breeze, FL: Fire Starter Publishing.

THE CASES

Personnel decisions, critical to managerial effectiveness, are often postponed by managers or not handled with sufficient care. For example, considerably more time may be spent on the decision to purchase or lease a piece of valuable equipment costing $900,000 with a useful life of seven years than on hiring a registered nurse who will earn $75,000 a year and who may work for the organization for 12 years.

Even more important than the hiring decision is the continuous evaluation and motivation of subordinates and colleagues, many of whom may have been hired by a manager's predecessors. If associates do not perform at an expected level of competence, what are the supervisor's options? What are the manager's options if she disagrees with her own boss's expectations or evaluation? If the boss does not fire or transfer the manager being evaluated, her own effectiveness may suffer because she may not be supported in her efforts to implement strategy or negotiate organizational politics. Taking such actions may be difficult because ineffective managers may be loyal, searching for and training a new manager costs time and money, and managers know that a new hire's performance may not be as anticipated.

Managerial personnel decisions become even more complicated when, as in "The Associate Director and the Controllers," the manager is dealing with a functional specialist who has line responsibility to the top manager and staff responsibility to the chief controller in a multi-unit medical center. In this case, the straight and dotted lines of authority on the organizational chart become fuzzy and difficult to manage, especially when the associate director's boss and the medical center director of finance distrust each other. Here, key staff of two recently merged units have different value orientations—the hospital primarily serves attending physicians in their private practices, while the ambulatory health services program focuses on providing respectful patient care to low-income patients residing in the local community.

The manager's job is often a lonely one. Important decisions are seldom made on an either-or basis, and often involve personal as well as organizational risks and benefits. In "A New Faculty Practice Administrator for the Department of Surgery" the weighing of risks and benefits is different for Sam Francis, the chair of surgery, than it is for Donald Matthews, the faculty practice administrator, or for Matthews's eventual successor. Similarly, in "The Associate Director and the Controllers," the stakes of the game are higher for James Joel, the ambulatory care manager, and for Percy Oram, its controller, than for Milton Schlitz, the medical center director of finance, and for Miller Harrang, the chief executive officer of the ambulatory care program.

Why must Joel decide to do anything at all? In "A New Faculty Practice Administrator," Francis must choose a new faculty practice administrator. But in "The Associate Director and the Controllers," Joel cannot get involved and allows Harrang and Schlitz to deal with the consequences of Oram's ineffectiveness. How much should it matter to Joel whether Oram remains on the job or not, so long as Joel can protect his own job? On the other hand, Joel is paid to manage, not to observe or protect himself.

Good management generally makes a difference to the patient, as well as to the organization's ruling coalition. How much of a difference is open to question. But who will look after the manager's interest if she doesn't look after it herself? This is the first rule of managerial survival. Looking after one's own interest does not mean that the manager should close her office door, read reports, and tell subordinates what to do. Instead, there are opportunities to strategically plan one's professional development, as considered in the case "Now What?"

Healthcare managers often face tremendous pressures from government to move in certain directions, and resistance from physicians who do not wish to move one step further than that required by law. How much value do managers add to performance? Not much, according to Pfeffer and Salancik (1978), who argue that the contribution of managers accounts for only around 10 percent of the variance in organizational performance, and who agree with the sportscaster cliché that "managers are hired to be fired." An increasing amount of evidence, however, indicates that managers *do* make a difference in organizational performance, if only because they play a key role in obtaining the resources necessary for organizational survival and growth.

If the healthcare manager can never meet all the expectations of key organizational stakeholders, she can at least be seen as taking stakeholder interests into account in policy formulation and implementation. This requires regular communication, which takes valuable time. What makes for an effective healthcare manager? This depends on perceptions of various stakeholders as well as performance or motivation. Sometimes—as in the short case "The Nowhere Job"—the right move for a manager *is* to resign. Clearly, managers must acquire information, learn skills, and have values consistent with an organizational context and its ruling coalition. Deciding what actions to take after receiving disquieting information is not always easy, as in the short case of "Managing Morale at Uptown Hospital." Similarly, the realities faced by new managers in "A Sure Thing," "The First Day," "Conflict in the Office," and "Annual Performance Evaluation" all create challenges in managing expectations as well as in job performance.

Evaluating managerial effectiveness or contribution carries a cost. All pertinent information may not be available at a reasonable cost. Reliance on measurement may divert attention inappropriately away from what is easily measured. Evaluating managers, like management itself, involves judgment, which in Ray Brown's (1969) phrase, is "knowledge ripened by experience."

For management students, case discussions are an excellent way of obtaining safe experience in forming managerial judgments.

References

Brown, R. 1969. *Judgment in Administration*. New York: McGraw-Hill.
Pfeffer, J., and G. R. Salancik. 1978. *The External Control of Organizations*. New York: Harper & Row.

Case A
A New Faculty Practice Administrator for the Department of Surgery

David M. Kaplan and Anthony R. Kovner

Donald Matthews recently announced he was leaving his role as the administrator for the department of surgery at Wise Medical Center to move to a chief operating officer position at another local medical center. Dr. Francis, who is the chair of surgery, asked Matthews to assist in the selection of his successor prior to leaving for his new position.

The faculty practice in the department of surgery has been in place since 2006, when Dr. Francis took over as chair and Matthews joined him as the administrator.

Wise Medical Center is regarded as one of the largest and best-managed hospitals in Eastern City. The CEO, Dr. Dante, was appointed in 2001. He has elevated the medical center from the depths of financial despair to one of the most successful in the country. His philosophy has been one of growth and investment in new faculty, clinical programs, research, and teaching programs. Dr. Dante also worked to replace nearly all the department chairs. The department of surgery is one of the medical center's largest departments. Dr. Francis is a vascular surgeon, world-renowned for his ability to treat aortic aneurysms, but also is regarded as a savvy businessman.

Over the past five years, Dr. Francis and Matthews have developed a tremendous partnership as they have significantly grown the department of surgery. Specifically, they have recruited more than 30 faculty and increased total faculty practice revenue by more than 150 percent. In 2010, the department earned more than $40 million in physician receipts for the first

EXHIBIT I.5 FPG Surgery Practice Suites Billing and Collections

Month	Billings	Collections	Contractual Allowances	Gross Collection Rate	Net Collection Rate
September	$8,241,151	$3,899,226	$4,532,633	47%	105%
October	$8,213,040	$3,749,477	$4,517,172	46%	101%
November	$10,864,25	$3,459,275	$5,975,338	32%	71%
December	$9,203,564	$3,513,639	$5,061,960	38%	85%
January	$8,514,687	$2,927,637	$4,683,078	34%	76%
February	$7,847,159	$3,852,977	$4,315,937	49%	109%
March	$8,268,573	$3,430,401	$4,547,715	41%	92%
April	$9,358,751	$3,212,200	$5,147,313	34%	76%
May	$7,046,892	$3,136,728	$3,875,791	45%	99%
June	$6,781,441	$2,968,865	$3,729,793	44%	97%
July	$7,813,332	$3,553,466	$4,297,333	45%	101%
August	$9,215,116	$3,263,895	$5,068,314	35%	79%
Total	**$101,367,957**	**$40,967,788**	**$55,752,376**	**40%**	**90%**

time in its history (see Exhibit I.5). Dr. Francis is praised for his leadership skills, his business intelligence, and his loyalty to his faculty and staff. This loyalty sometimes inhibits his ability to make tough decisions regarding his less-productive faculty, such as reducing their salaries or moving them out of the institution. Both the department and the medical center face increasing financial pressures as the state and federal government look to reduce funding for Medicare, Medicaid, and other related programs. As such, Dr. Dante and others are trying to determine the most effective response to these increased financial pressures.

Simultaneously, the faculty practice group (FPG) for Wise Medical Center is also grappling with significant space constraints due to the rapid expansion of all departments, consistent with Dr. Dante's growth strategy. The FPG has more than 800 faculty across 26 different clinical departments. The FPG generates nearly $450 million in patient revenue and schedules more than 530,000 outpatient visits per year.

The FPG building has 15 specialty floors, and each department is responsible for providing the staff for its clinical practice. The department of surgery has two clinical floors, with a total of five specialty-specific suites. Each suite is staffed with a front desk receptionist, two medical assistants, and two medical billers. The suites are roughly 5,000 square feet apiece, and each has four exam rooms and two consult rooms. The suites were designed to accommodate two physicians for each session (defined as a four-hour time block).

EXHIBIT I.6 FPG Surgery Practice Utilization Statistics, September 2009–August 2010

Division/Suite	Percent Utilization 2009	Percent Utilization 2010	Total Exam Rooms	Total Available Sessions 2009	Total Available Sessions 2010	Total Actual Sessions 2009	Total Actual Sessions 2010
General surgery	92	94	4	104	156	96	147
Vascular surgery	94	94	4	208	208	196	196
Plastic surgery	100	100	4	156	208	156	208
Surgical oncology	75	77	4	104	104	78	80
Colon and rectal surgery	87	87	4	104	104	90	90
Bariatric surgery	63	67	4	104	104	66	70
Transplant surgery	65	62	4	104	156	68	96
Pediatric surgery	65	62	4	104	156	68	96
Total	83	82	4	988	1,196	818	983

Note: Utilization defined as Total Actual Sessions/Total Available Sessions.

Dr. Francis has asked Matthews to compile the utilization statistics for the surgery practice for an upcoming meeting with Dr. Dante. Matthews has assessed that the visits over the past year have increased from 25,000 to 32,450, representing 30 percent growth. Overall the department has a utilization rate of 90 percent for its practice suites (see Exhibit I.6), above the benchmark for acceptable utilization across the FPG, which was set at 85 percent. But numbers only tell one side of the story. Two of the suites—plastic surgery and colon and rectal surgery—are particularly busy, leaving many of the surgeons to complain they cannot get adequate time to see their patients.

At present, the surgery suites are open from 9:00 a.m. to 5:00 p.m. Monday through Friday, and Matthews has estimated that if the office hours were to be expanded to include nights and weekends, these suites could increase their volume by 10 to 15 percent. Matthews also estimated that this increase in volume could increase practice receipts by about $15,000 per month, or $180,000 per year. Altering these hours would, of course, require additional staff costs, and possible overtime costs, plus additional space charges for off-hour access.

Dr. Dante has also asked all chairs to prepare a plan to address possible reductions in clinical revenue caused by budget reductions for their departments. These plans should include possible reductions in expenditures as well as projections for growth and investments in key strategic programs that expect large returns within a short period of time.

In the midst of these competing demands, Dr. Francis and Matthews were getting ready to embark on the interview process for Matthews' replacement. Their discussion went as follows:

Dr. Francis: Donald, you have been an incredible partner during our five years together. While I am excited about your new opportunity, I have great trepidation about your departure. Given the new financial landscape that is evolving, I need a candidate who is financially savvy and not afraid to take risks. I also need someone who is operationally adept and can relate well to both the faculty and the staff. What do you think?

Matthews: Well, Dr. Francis, as you know, I have truly enjoyed working with you and members of the department, and I will be sorry to leave. But I am also looking forward to my new challenges. I agree with your general assessment of the type of person you need. In addition, I would suggest you seek someone who can "put out fires" as well as being resourceful. Given that people are going to be asked to do more with less, having someone who can keep the place running with limited resources is going to be essential.

Dr. Francis: I agree with you. As you perform your initial interviews of these candidates, I want you to look for all these qualities, but recognize that we also need someone who is personable and energetic, who isn't afraid to work, and perhaps someone who is considered a rising star in the industry.

Matthews: No problem. I have started the recruitment process and will send you all the good candidates. I have spoken to several directors of healthcare administration programs and to the hospital human resources department. I have also been in touch with many of my personal contacts to identify any additional candidates. I will let you know how I am progressing.

Dr. Francis: Good. I know you will do an excellent job of identifying someone. I have to run to the operating room, so I will catch up with you tomorrow to discuss this further. Try to pull together the rest of the materials for my meeting with Dr. Dante as well. I would like to be able to give Dr. Dante an update on our search when I meet with him later this week.

Matthews: OK, talk to you later. I will work with Cindy, your assistant, to schedule interviews for you with any good candidates.

Fortunately, Matthews was able to quickly identify several candidates whom he was able to schedule for interviews for this position over the next few days. In total, Matthews was able to interview eight people for this role. With the permission of these candidates, he recorded all the initial interviews to assist him with the selection process going forward.

Matthews was able to quickly eliminate two of these candidates because of their lack of experience or irrelevant experience for this position. He was also able to remove another set of two internal candidates who worked in the finance department and did not seem to have the people-management skills required to manage one of the largest departments in the medical center. Matthews was able to identify four potential candidates whom he felt might be appropriate for the position, but he was having a tough time choosing one of them.

Matthews' first viable candidate was David O'Brien, currently assistant director for the medical center finance department at the medical center. The second was Sal Sorrentino, currently the divisional administrator for cardiology at Westside Hospital. The third was Marcia Rabin, the director of ambulatory services for the Partner's Health Group, also in Eastern City. Finally, there was Bonnie Goldsmith, currently the vice president of surgical services at Rochester Medical Center. Matthews decided to review the initial interview recordings with the vice chair for the department of surgery, Dr. Harris, who also practices in the FPG surgery suites, before scheduling follow-up interviews for the possible candidates with Dr. Francis.

David O'Brien

Matthews (to Dr. Harris): The first candidate is David O'Brien, age 28. He wears conservative glasses and dresses conservatively. When I spoke to Michael Scanlon, Wise Medical Center chief financial officer, he said that David is energetic and conscientious, and that he was able to get things done. He recommended David for this position. If there is any weakness, Michael said that David is a bit intense, and sometimes intimidates and antagonizes others. He continued to say that David has no problems, it seems, in getting along with his superiors, but has limited experience working with physicians. (Matthews plays the interview recording for Dr. Harris.)

Matthews: David, thank you for coming in today for this meeting. Can you please tell me a little bit about your background and why you feel it might be a good fit for this position?

O'Brien: Sure, Mr. Matthews. I went to Upstate College where I was a business major. Then I started working here in the finance department for Mr. Scanlon as a reimbursement analyst. After a couple of years, I was appointed as the assistant director for the finance department, where I oversee all budget and reimbursement activities for the medical center. Given my understanding of the medical center's finances, I am now looking for operational experience, which I feel this role will provide.

Matthews: I see that you are currently enrolled in school. What are you studying, and why?

O'Brien: I am currently working on getting my master's in public administration from the City University. I am enrolled in their part-time program.

I feel that this will be important for my future career prospects. I am scheduled to finish this May, so I'm almost done.

Matthews: What would you say are your biggest accomplishments in your role in the finance department?

O'Brien: I would say that my biggest accomplishment is the recent simplification and redesign of the budget process. There were a lot of complaints about how complicated this process had become, and people were begging for an upgrade to the system. Based on this feedback, we were able to automate and simplify the system, and many folks are now singing praises for the newly designed system—wouldn't you agree?

Matthews: Fair point. I think the system is much improved, but far from perfect. We certainly recognize your contributions to the new system. If you were in this position, what would you consider to be your greatest asset?

O'Brien: I would say it's my ability to get a job done. There are too many people in this industry who are just willing to live with the status quo until there is a "fire" that requires them to take action. By that point, it is often too late. I prefer to be proactive in my approach to fix things.

Matthews: What would you say is your greatest liability?

O'Brien: Well, you know, in every organization some people are against change, either because it affects their own interests or because they just are averse to change. After all, every change in somebody's department has to affect everyone involved in a relative if not in an absolute way. As one of my professors once said, "You don't make an omelet without breaking a few eggs." And I guess I must rub some people the wrong way who are against me as a change agent.

Matthews: What aspect of this new position do you believe is the most important?

O'Brien: I think it will be improving the overall revenue of the department. I've spoken to Mr. Scanlon, and he preaches this to all of us in the finance department. While I think that you and Dr. Francis have done a tremendous job over the past several years, I think by looking at the revenue cycle operation, and exploring the day-to-day expenses, we could possibly identify further opportunities that will help us achieve this goal.

Matthews: Before you go, is there anything you would like to ask me about the job?

O'Brien: As a matter of fact there is. We've talked about the salary and benefits, but if I perform as expected, what is the likelihood of an annual bonus and/or increase after the first year? You know I have a wife and two young children.

Matthews: Well, I'd say the chances are pretty good. Dr. Francis is fair and I think he would be generous if the practice results improved significantly. (Matthews turns off the recorder.)

Harris: He seems like a fine candidate.

Salvatore Sorrentino

Matthews (to Harris): Sal Sorrentino is the next candidate. Sal is 27. He is presentable, although he dresses a bit on the flashy side—fast-talking and enthusiastic. Sal is currently the divisional administrator for cardiology at Westside Hospital. When I spoke to his reference, Dr. Plotkin, he recommended Sal highly for the position. He said that Sal is idealistic, energetic, and pleasant. If there is any weakness, Dr. Plotkin thought that Sal has a tendency to initiate or implement new initiatives without understanding the possible implications. I asked him to clarify, or to provide an example, and he said Sal had decided to change the way patients were scheduled without getting sufficient input from the physicians, nurses, or secretarial staff. The result was that patients were being triple-booked and, in some cases, having to wait for more than two hours for their appointments. The issue was quickly resolved, and Dr. Plotkin believed that Sal had learned his lesson. Dr. Plotkin did reiterate that he highly recommends Sal for this position. (Matthews plays the recording of the interview.)

Matthews: Sal, can you tell me, in a few words, something about your background and experience?

Sorrentino: Yes. I have been in healthcare for about six years. I started my career as a physician biller, where I learned about revenue cycle. I then quickly moved into the role of division administrator for cardiology. Dr. Plotkin and I have really formed a solid partnership and have accomplished many things together. However, he has decided to take another position in California, and I am unable to relocate. That's why I am searching for a new position, because I am sure the new chief will want his or her own administrator.

Matthews: And what would you say, Sal, was your greatest accomplishment while working as the administrator of cardiology?

Sorrentino: Well, one of the things I am proudest of is the development of a new marketing program to promote our cardiologists. This took a tremendous amount of time and effort, but the rollout was successful and has made our division incredibly successful.

Matthews: Can you tell me more about this marketing program?

Sorrentino: I independently crafted a number of marketing brochures and letters for our faculty and developed the mailing lists from our billing system. We opted to distribute these via e-mail as well as using traditional mailings to effectively canvass the area. Some of the physicians didn't particularly love their brochures, but overall I think the benefits far outweighed any negative feedback.

Matthews: I see. In the position you are applying for, what do you think would be your greatest asset?

Sorrentino: Well, it seems like your biggest concern is increasing sales and profitability. This is clearly something that I have some experience with as a divisional administrator. I believe that my analytical ability, along with my experience, would be my greatest asset to this position.

Matthews: Another question, Sal. What do you think would be your greatest liability, if any, if you were chosen for this position?

Sorrentino: I don't know. I want to get things accomplished, so perhaps I move a little too fast. Sometimes I act without thinking of the consequences as I try to enact change. I also believe in delegating to empower your staff, and sometimes I assume things get done once assigned to people. I could do a better job at verifying that tasks get completed.

Matthews: Ensuring people are accountable for their responsibilities is certainly important. What do you think is the most important aspect of the job you're applying for in terms of the work that needs to be done?

Sorrentino: I guess first you have to get all your systems working properly, such as billing and reporting. I think the next most important thing is to increase your revenues. Based on your description, it sounds like Dr. Francis's plan for the department is for the faculty practice to generate enough revenue to help support faculty member salaries.

Matthews: You're right there. Is there anything now you want to ask me about the job?

Sorrentino: Two things, really. First, what kind of person is Dr. Francis to work for? And, second, what are your best ideas, Donald, about how to increase departmental revenue?

Matthews: In answer to your first question, I think Dr. Francis is an excellent person to work for, as long as you produce for him. He's loyal, and gives you enough autonomy to do your job. Perhaps my only complaint is that it is sometimes difficult to see him because he is so busy. I often don't want to bother him with trivial issues. I have recommended to him that he appoint another physician within the department as head of the faculty practice, a plan that I know Dr. Francis is considering. As to your second question, I would probably say that the largest opportunity to enhance departmental revenues is to open a satellite surgical center. I feel ambulatory surgery is the future for surgical departments to successfully grow their business. (Matthews turns off the recorder).

Harris: Well these first two candidates have quite contrasting backgrounds, yet it seems clear to me that either of them might do a perfectly respectable job. Nonetheless, the outcomes resulting from their work might be quite different.

Marcia Rabin

Matthews (to Harris): Yes, that's so. The third candidate is Marcia Rabin. Marcia is 26 years old and energetic. Les Carson, the CEO of Partner's Health Group, highly recommended her for the position. Ms. Rabin is the director of ambulatory services for the group, which consists of 50 physicians and 20 support staff. Carson said she is hardworking and gets along well with both professional and nonprofessional staff. If there is any fault to find with her, Carson said that Rabin takes her work too seriously, drives herself too hard, and, as a result, has taken her full quota of sick days. But Carson stressed that Rabin has performed very well on all the big jobs that he has given her to do, and that she has been both reliable and competent. He continued to say that she has demonstrated the ability to positively relate to the staff and faculty to drive change. (Matthews plays the recording of the interview.)

Matthews: Ms. Rabin, can you tell me, in a few words, something about your background and experience?

Rabin: Certainly. I guess you don't want me to go back to high school, but I was president of my student government at Suburban High. In college I majored in psychology, and for a while I thought I would like to be a psychologist. But my father works in a hospital—he is director of housekeeping at Sisters' Hospital—and he encouraged me to go into healthcare management. After attending the City University master's program, I was hired as the director of ambulatory services at Partner's. Previously they didn't have this position, but when the group bought two additional practices and expanded from 20 to 50 physicians, the position was established. While at Partner's, I worked under the tutelage of Mr. Les Carson, the CEO.

Matthews: What would you say your greatest accomplishment was in this position?

Rabin: I think my greatest accomplishment in this position has been working to maximize the patient volume in the practice. We had to work on mapping out patient flow, revising physician schedules, and evaluating the hours of the practice. Our efforts helped the practice to realize a roughly 50 percent growth in practice volume within a six-month period.

Matthews: That sounds interesting. In terms of the present position with Dr. Francis, what would you say would be your greatest asset?

Rabin: I don't know exactly how to answer that question. My first response would be to say I like and am good at doing systems work—creating order out of chaos and working effectively with people so that they feel it is their system, not something that I pushed on them. I feel that I am particularly skilled at building consensus around new initiatives. I relate well to people, and this helps to get things accomplished.

Matthews: And what, if you'll pardon my asking, would you say is your greatest liability?

Rabin: Well, if you must know, Mr. Matthews, I'm not aggressive enough. Sometimes I think my efforts aren't properly appreciated, and I don't push myself to the front the way some people do. I work hard and I work well and it annoys me—sometimes more than it should—that others who don't work as hard and don't do as well still push themselves forward and move ahead faster.

Matthews: What aspect of the job, as I have tried to outline it to you, would you say is the most important at this time in the history of the faculty practice?

Rabin: I think you have to set up more clearly defined ways of doing things—systems, if you prefer the word. I noted in the materials that you shared with me that your collection rate isn't what it should be, and that your utilization of examining rooms in certain areas can be improved. I don't think that this kind of systems work is that different from my work at Partner's.

Matthews: Are there any questions that you would like to ask me?

Rabin: Well, one question is how the physicians might relate to having a woman in this position. Second, when can you let me know if you are offering me the job? I have been offered a job as assistant director of human resources at King Hospital, and although they aren't pressing me that hard, I would like to be able to tell them something soon.

Matthews: With regard to the first question, I do not think this will be an issue. Our physicians are amazing to deal with, and as long as you are logical, honest, and transparent with them, they will align with whomever is in this position. To answer your second question, I think it will take about a month for Dr. Francis to decide on a candidate. I can't tell you what you should say to the King people. You are one of the four candidates whom I am sending on to see Dr. Francis. (Matthews turns off the recorder.)

Bonnie Goldsmith

Matthews (to Harris): Permit me to introduce our last candidate, Bonnie Goldsmith. She dresses conservatively and gives the impression of a modest, unassuming, kind young woman of 27. Bonnie is currently the vice president of surgical services at Rochester Medical. Her boss, Mr. Robert Muldoon, who recently left Rochester Medical as their chief operating officer, recommended Bonnie as hardworking, modest, and reliable. He said Bonnie gets along with people, but she tends to lack drive and needs to be motivated occasionally. However, Mr. Muldoon says that once a task is clearly outlined, Bonnie is thorough, dedicated, and relentless. As an example, he praised Bonnie's work on a recent report related to improving operating room utilization. (Matthews plays the recording of the interview.)

Matthews: Bonnie, can you tell me a few words about your background and experience?

Goldsmith: Yes. I was a zoology major at City University. Originally, I wanted to be a physician. In fact, I attended medical school for one year, and then I decided it just wasn't for me. I didn't know what I wanted to do. I don't know why, but I thought that working in a hospital admitting department might be interesting, and I did that for a while. My father is a psychiatrist. The administrator is a good friend of my father's, and he talked to me and convinced me to apply to City University's graduate program in health policy and management. Back in school, I really enjoyed the coursework related to quality improvement, information systems, and statistical analysis. A whole new world opened up to me, although I must confess I had a bit of difficulty with some of the heavy reading and writing courses. After graduation, I was fortunate to get a position at Rochester Medical in the surgical services department as an analyst. Once again, my father's connections helped to open some doors for me. After being there for a few years, I was promoted to department head for surgical services, and for the past two years, I have been fortunate to serve as the vice president for surgical services. Of course, Rochester is a small institution, but I am ready to consider working for a larger academic center. Also, the role on the hospital side is a bit limited compared with what I would expect for a department administrator role.

Matthews: What would you say has been your greatest accomplishment at Rochester?

Goldsmith: I would say my greatest accomplishment has been working to maximize the utilization of our operating rooms. One of the biggest challenges that any medical center has is ensuring the ORs are utilized to make sure the case volume and associated revenue are also realized. We worked with the faculty closely to revamp the entire OR schedule.

Matthews: What kind of solutions did you come up with?

Goldsmith: Well, we first looked at which surgeons were not using their assigned times on a regular basis; these folks were then bumped. We then reviewed the volume of cases per surgeon, and the lower-volume surgeons were bumped from having assigned block time. Lastly, we took the existing faculty members and lined them up on the schedule. We now have roughly a 95 percent utilization rate overall, which is tremendous.

Matthews: I see. What do you think would be your greatest asset in the open position here within the department of surgery?

Goldsmith: Perhaps it's my ability to get along with and to understand the needs and problems of the surgical profession. I don't have a big ego. I like analytical work, solving operations problems, and I think I'm pretty persistent in trying to solve them. I also think my surgical management experience could be an asset.

Matthews: And your greatest liability?

Goldsmith: Well, some people think I'm not driven to succeed at work, and that I don't sufficiently express my opinions. Others may think that I don't work that hard, but I don't want work to be an obsession, as it is for my father. I mean I'm married, with a nice husband and a young son, and I want to enjoy my work and perform well, but I also want to enjoy my family. From my perspective, this also helps me remain calm and even-tempered when managing staff and faculty, especially surgeons.

Matthews: If you do the job well, what you say makes sense. What aspects of the job strike you as most important?

Goldsmith: Well, I don't know. Certainly, we have to improve surgeon and patient satisfaction, and of course increase overall revenues. I'd like to assess each of these elements to determine where the opportunities for improvements exist. This might require a number of meetings, and I don't know how feasible such meetings would be because of people's time requirements. There are a few questions I would like to ask you.

Matthews: Please go ahead.

Goldsmith: My first question is, do you think the surgical practice is going to grow? The second is incidental, but I would like to know more about the benefits, such as tuition remission, as I was thinking about furthering my education at City, perhaps taking some more courses in statistical analysis.

Matthews: I think the surgical practice will continue to grow. Space is our key constraint now, and the medical center will have to figure out how we are going to better deal with managed care and possible reductions in reimbursement given the economic climate. With respect to your second question, yes, I believe tuition remission for such purposes is available, although I don't see where you will have the time to fit everything in with the demands of this job—which are quite considerable—along with your commitment to your family. (Matthews turns off the recorder.)

The Recommendation

Harris: Well, Donald, now all you have to do is tell Dr. Francis whom you recommend for the job.

Matthews: I need to sleep on it. This selection process is much more difficult than I had envisioned, but that's also what makes it so much fun.

Harris: I agree with you there. Sorry, but I've got to leave now. I will also mull this over and I'll give you my opinion tomorrow.

Case Questions

1. What criteria would you use in evaluating the four candidates?
2. What are the strengths and weaknesses of each candidate?
3. What were Matthews's criteria for evaluating the four candidates?
4. Whom would you recommend to Dr. Francis as your selection for the position?
5. What is the evidence that you used in making this recommendation?

Case B
The Associate Director and the Controllers

Anthony R. Kovner

Fortunately for Jim Joel, he didn't lose his temper often. Otherwise, he might not have been able to function as associate director of the Morris Healthcare Program of the Nathan D. Wise Medical Center (NWMC) (see Exhibit I.7). But now, he had become so enraged at the Morris program controller, Percy Oram, that he had to concentrate hard to keep from yelling. Joel had just been informed by Felix Schwartzberg, an assistant director, that the accounting department was not collecting cash from the billing assistants in the family health units as previously agreed. Unfortunately, Oram did not usually keep Joel informed of his actions. But in any case, Joel knew his own reaction was excessive—an aspiring health services executive did not throw a tantrum, which is what he now felt like doing.

EXHIBIT I.7
Organization
Chart:
Nathan D. Wise
Medical Center

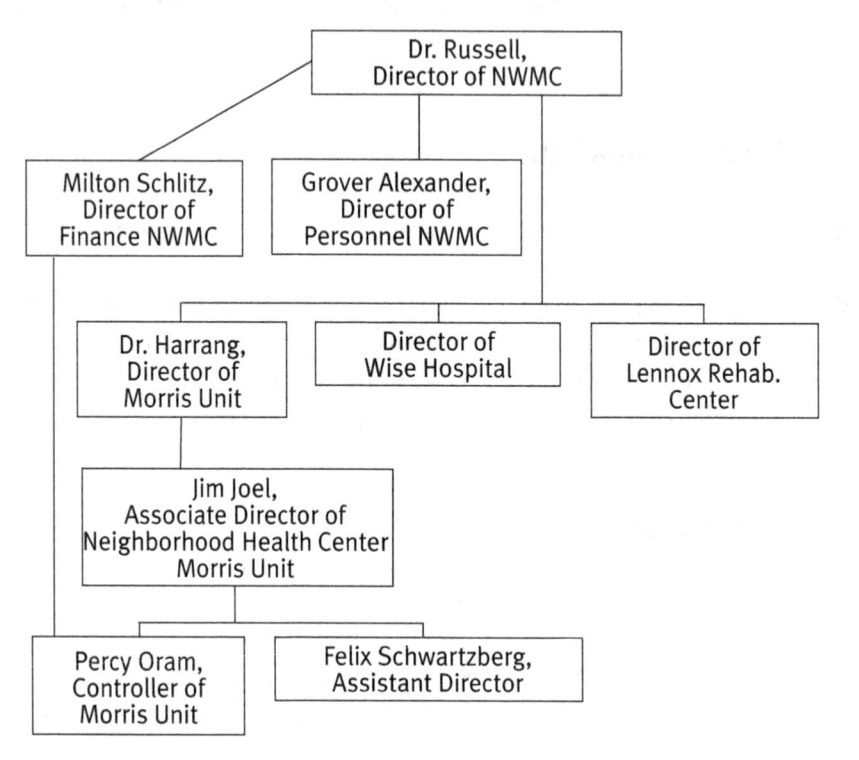

Joel was 30 years old, ambitious, and a recent graduate from Ivy University's master of healthcare administration program. Before returning to school, he had worked as a registered representative on Wall Street, where he had found the work remunerative but uninteresting. The director of the Ivy program, Dr. Leon Russell, assumed the post of director of the Nathan D. Wise Medical Center three years ago. Joel, one of his best students, asked to join Russell toward the end of that year, and he was hired shortly thereafter as an assistant hospital administrator. The Nathan D. Wise Medical Center is located in New York City and comprises three large programs: the Nathan D. Wise Hospital, the Lennox Rehabilitation Center, and the Morris Healthcare Program. The hospital and the rehabilitation center are owned by the Wise Medical Center, but the Morris Healthcare Program is operated by the Wise Medical Center under contract with the City of New York and is located in a city-owned facility.

Russell had been impressed with his former student's drive and promise and had originally created a job for Joel—half-time as a staff assistant at Wise Hospital and half-time as an evaluator at the Morris unit, where new methods of delivering ambulatory medical care were being developed and demonstrated. Eventually Russell offered Joel the position of associate director of the Morris unit. The director of the Morris unit was Dr. Miller Harrang, a 45-year-old physician.

Joel felt ambivalent about Russell's offer. He knew he would take the position, even before requesting a night to think it over, but at the same time he had certain reservations. Joel enjoyed his work at the hospital. He had submitted an in-depth plan for increasing efficiency of the operating room, which had been enthusiastically accepted by the medical staff executive committee, and he was just starting an evaluation of patient transport in the hospital. His key interest was implementation of findings from his master's thesis on nurse staffing. Joel believed that by assigning rooms to patients on the basis of their nursing needs, one-third fewer registered nurses would be required. Joel wished to be director of a large general hospital within ten years. He wasn't sure how working at the Morris unit would advance him toward that goal, nor how comfortable he would feel working in a facility serving the poor in a low-income section of the city.

However, after taking the job, Joel found before long that he liked working at the Morris unit immensely. Morris was rapidly expanding—in the past year, the number of physician visits had increased 25 percent to 215,000. Through a generous grant from the Office of Economic Opportunity (OEO), the budget had increased from $15 million to $25 million. Joel worked 65 to 70 hours a week. There was so much to do. He liked Harrang and the others who worked at Morris. The atmosphere was busy and informal, a nice change of pace from Wise Hospital, where things happened more slowly. Dramatic change was the norm at Morris, whether this was conversion of the medical and pediatric clinics to family health units, or confrontations with a community health council resulting in increased participation in policymaking by the poor.

There was no formal division of responsibility between Harrang and Joel. Harrang spent most of his time in community relations (time-consuming and frustrating), in individual conversations with members of the medical staff at Morris, and in working out problems with Wise Hospital. Harrang also took responsibility for certain medical units such as the emergency room, obstetrics-gynecology (ob-gyn), and psychiatry. Joel's primary responsibility lay in the area of staff activities such as finance, personnel, and purchasing. He also supervised several departments or units, including laboratory, X-ray, pharmacy, dental, housekeeping, and maintenance. Responsibility for the family health units was shared by the two top administrators.

Before Harrang became director, the Morris unit had been run as a unit independent of Wise Hospital. The unit was decentralized, with departments such as laboratory and internal medicine handling their own personnel and often their own purchasing. It was Russell's wish to create a more integrated medical center, and Joel saw an important part of his job as creating staff departments (such as personnel and purchasing) and upgrading these functions with the help of medical center experts.

When Joel arrived, the controller's department consisted of four individuals: Bill Connor, the controller, who promptly resigned (Joel never met this individual, whom he was told had personal problems of an unspecified nature); Peter Stavrogin, an industrious bookkeeper, who was a 55-year-old Eastern European refugee with a limited knowledge of English; a payroll clerk; and a secretary. This was the staff for an organization of more than 400 employees that was funded by five different agencies under five different contracts. The accounting department had heavy personnel responsibilities as well, at least so far as payroll was concerned, because no personnel department as such existed. One of the first things Joel did was hire Connor's replacement. In doing so—and to conform with Russell's policy of an integrated medical center—Joel enlisted the help of the medical center staff: Milton Schlitz, the director of financial affairs, and Grover Alexander, the director of personnel. Alexander volunteered to place the ads and check the references of applicants for the controller position, and Schlitz suggested that he screen the applicants. The best three or four would then be reviewed by Joel and Harrang who, between them, would select the new controller. Joel was pleased with this arrangement, although he thought the recommended salary for the position was too low. He agreed to go along, however, based on the recommendations of Alexander and Schlitz, who had considerably more experience in these matters.

However, because of what Schlitz and Alexander believed to be a shortage of qualified accountants, and the undesirable location of Morris, they found only two prospective applicants. Albert Fodor, a 55-year-old certified public accountant (CPA) with no hospital experience but good references, was the obvious first choice to be Morris's new controller. Fodor was pleasant and industrious. It took him six months to learn the job. Fodor then resigned, claiming that the tremendous pressure and workload were too great for a man of his years. The payroll clerk also resigned at this time for a higher paying job at another hospital.

During the next three months, Joel employed three new billing clerks as well as a personnel assistant and a purchasing agent. Most of the accounting department's work, which would have been done by the controller, was performed by Joel, who handled the budgetary aspects, while Stavrogin covered the accounting aspects. This system was unsatisfactory, however, because both felt Joel should spend less time troubleshooting financial problems and more time on the programmatic aspects of the job. Also, Joel wanted to conduct and supervise a variety of special studies for contract purposes and cost comparisons, an undertaking hardly feasible under the present setup.

So Joel went back to Schlitz and Alexander, insisting that the salary for the controller job be raised $3,000 per year because of the complexity of the job and the distance from Schlitz's direct supervision. Schlitz agreed reluctantly; he knew this meant he would have to raise salaries or face morale problems in the accounting department at Wise Hospital.

After advertising the job extensively, Schlitz screened eight to ten candidates and sent three candidates to Joel and Harrang, of whom Percy Oram seemed the best. Oram was 40 years old; though not a CPA, he had solid accounting experience in a medium-sized business firm. Oram had no hospital or healthcare experience. Schlitz and Joel did not feel that such experience was necessary for the job, although, of course, they would have preferred it. Oram was physically attractive, well dressed, and married with no children. He said he was interested in advancing himself in the expanding hospital field. Joel went over the Fodor experience with Oram, stressing the work pressures. Oram responded that he was looking for a job where he would have more autonomy, where he was in charge and responsible, and where he knew he would be rewarded (or blamed) based on his performance. Of course, he would like to spend a lot of time at first learning the ropes with Schlitz. Joel told Oram he would let him know later that week if the job was his. Afterward, Joel and Harrang agreed that Oram was the best of the three candidates. However, Harrang had a vague feeling of unease—Oram seemed too good, too qualified for the job. Independently, Schlitz also agreed that Oram was the best of the three candidates. Alexander checked Oram's references, who confirmed the high opinion of Schlitz and Joel. Oram was then offered the job as controller of the Morris unit, which he accepted.

From Joel's point of view, things went fairly well at first, perhaps because Joel was busy with other matters and Oram was spending a lot of time at Wise Hospital with Schlitz. The first sign of trouble was the lateness of the monthly statement that Joel had instituted and required. The statement included detailed categories of departmental costs, comparing costs (Joel hoped eventually to compare costs with performance as well) for this month, last month, and this month last year, as well as cumulative totals for this year. Joel had reviewed with Oram how he wanted the statement done (in what categories), with a cover sheet that would suggest the reasons for any large variances. Oram agreed to furnish such a report, but one month later, Joel still hadn't received it. When asked about the report, Oram said that he was too busy, and that he was working on it. When the statement finally did arrive on Joel's desk, there was no cover letter about variances, and there were large variances caused by sloppy accounting (items in one category last year, for instance, that were in another this year, causing large discrepancies). Even some of the amounts were incorrect, such as salaries of certain individuals that had not been counted in the proper categories. Joel, patiently but with irritation, explained that this was not what he wanted. He told Oram why he wanted what he wanted, and when he wanted the report—15 days after the end of the month. Timeliness, he emphasized, was especially important because, although the city contract remained at the same sum every year, changes in the OEO budget had to be individually approved by Washington, and OEO funds had to be spent by the year's end. This meant that a lot of shuffling had to be done (e.g., transfer of city positions because of increased salary costs to the OEO budget) based on correct information. Oram apologized and agreed to improve his performance.

At the same time, Joel had begun to hear complaints about Oram from other staff members. Linda Lee, the personnel assistant, and Felix Schwartz-berg, the assistant director, complained about his rudeness, arrogance, and insensitivity to the poor—such as his repeated statements about "welfare chiselers." Such terminology was at odds with the philosophy of the unit. When changes in employee paychecks had to be made because of supervisory mistakes or because of inadequate notice concerning an employee's vacation, Oram reluctantly did the extra work. He warned those involved, without clearing it with Joel, that eventually checks would not be issued on this basis.

Joel had been approached by Oram two weeks previously about a personal matter. Oram explained that he had to come to work an hour and a half late twice a week because of an appointment with his psychiatrist. The psychiatrist couldn't see him before or after work, and Oram hoped Joel would be sympathetic. Oram was willing to stay late to make up the time. Joel said he wanted to think it over before responding, and then discussed Oram's situation with Schlitz and Harrang. They all agreed that they would have liked to have known this before Oram was hired, but that if the work was done and he made up the time, it would be permitted. It was agreed that Joel would check occasionally in the account-ing office, which was located in a separate building a block away from the health services facility, to see if Oram was indeed putting in the extra time.

For about the next six months, Oram's performance remained essen-tially the same. The cover letter was superficial and the statements were late and often contained mistakes. (The statements did, however, eventually arrive and were eventually corrected.) The special studies requested of Oram were done late and Joel often had to redo them. In checking on Oram, Joel never found him in the office after 5:00 p.m., but he did not check every day. The routine work of the accounting department was being done effectively, but this had been the case before the current situation with Oram, when no con-troller had been present. Oram had added another clerk, and Joel suspected that Stavrogin was still performing much of the supervisory work as he had been prior to Oram's arrival. Joel was not happy. He discussed the situa-tion with Harrang, who agreed that the statements were less than acceptable. Harrang told Joel to do as he liked but to clear it first with Schlitz.

Soon after, Joel went to Wise Hospital to discuss Oram with Schlitz. Schlitz, a CPA, had been controller of Wise Hospital, now Wise Medical Center, for 27 years. Schlitz was talkative but often vague, hardworking, basically conservative, and oriented primarily to the needs of Wise Hospital (at least in Joel's opinion) rather than to the medical center at large. This was reflected in the allocation of overhead in the Morris contracts (administrative time allocated was greater than that actually provided) and in the high price of direct services, such as laboratory, performed for Morris by the hospital. More important, Schlitz saw his job almost exclusively as worrying about "the bottom line"—whether the hospital or the Morris Unit ran a deficit or broke even—rather than in terms of performance relative to costs. Nevertheless, Joel thought he had established a cordial relationship with Schlitz, and their discussion about Oram was indeed cordial for the most part. Schlitz agreed that Oram's performance left something to be desired. He was particularly unhappy about the time Oram put in. On the other hand, Schlitz felt that the Morris unit was in good financial shape and that there was nothing to worry about. In view of the experience with the previous controller, Fodor, Schlitz wondered if indeed they could find a better man for the salary. Schlitz urged that they talk to Oram together but said that he would go along with whatever Joel wanted to do.

Acting on Schlitz's recommendation, Joel set up a meeting with Schlitz, Oram, and Harrang to discuss his dissatisfactions. During the course of the meeting Joel admitted that the monthly statements were improving, but only after extensive prodding. Oram remarked that the reason for this meeting surprised him; he had thought, on the basis of previous meetings with Joel and Schlitz, that they were pleased with his work. He then asked to be included in more top-level policy meetings, as he felt that controllers should be part of the top management group. Oram said he felt isolated, in part because the accounting department was located in a separate building. Joel responded that he would welcome Oram's participation in policy meetings after the work of the accounting department had been sufficiently upgraded, and that Oram would be kept informed of and invited to all meetings that concerned his department.

Returning to the Morris facility, Joel discussed his perplexity with Harrang. Actually, he asserted, he did not understand what was going on. Oram never gave him what he wanted. He had no way of knowing how busy Oram actually was. Lately, Oram had said that he couldn't produce certain studies by the stipulated dates because he was busy doing work for Schlitz or attending meetings at the hospital with Schlitz and the controllers of the other units of the medical center.

Harrang replied that he believed that Schlitz was indeed responsible in part for Oram's lack of responsiveness. Schlitz had probably told Oram not to listen to Joel but to do what he, Schlitz, recommended, because Oram's salary and benefits were largely determined by Schlitz rather than by Joel. Schlitz didn't want the accounting department at Morris to use more sophisticated techniques than the hospital because this would reflect badly on Schlitz. Moreover, Schlitz wanted his "own man" at the Morris unit so that the hospital benefited in all transactions with Morris (e.g., there should be enough slack in the city budget to meet any contingency, with as many staff as possible switched to the OEO budget).

Joel had to agree with Harrang's observation. On the other hand, Harrang had become increasingly bitter toward Russell over the last six months. This concerned a variety of matters, most specifically Harrang's salary. Harrang was working much harder than he had bargained for at Morris, and he didn't feel he was getting the money or the credit he deserved. Nevertheless, Joel did think that Schlitz might be part of the problem; he had never been particularly impressed with Schlitz.

Several weeks later, a new state regulation was passed stating that for city agencies to collect under Medicaid, all efforts must be made to collect from those who, by state edict, could afford to pay. This was in conflict with Morris's philosophy of providing free service to all who said they couldn't pay, and there was much opposition to implementation of the policy by the professionals at Morris. The professional staff felt that no special effort should be made to collect from those who had formerly received free services. Oram disagreed with this philosophy and said that Morris should make every effort to collect.

When it came to implementing collections, Oram requested that the registration staff who were to collect the money be made part of his department, or that a separate cashier's office be set up on the first floor of the health facility. Otherwise his department didn't wish to be involved. Schwartzberg, the assistant director in charge of registration, argued that the registration staff should continue as part of the family health units because of other duties, that no space was available on the first floor for a cashier's office, and that it was not fair to patients to make them stand in two lines, as they would have to under Oram's arrangement, before seeing a health professional. Joel and Harrang sided with Schwartzberg and discussed with Oram a plan under which he would be responsible for the cash collection aspects of the registrar's work. It was agreed that Oram would devise, within a week, a plan for implementation. After two weeks, Schwartzberg reported to Joel that Oram had not devised a plan and was unwilling to cooperate with the plan Schwartzberg and the chief registrar had devised.

Joel pounded his desk. What concerned him was not so much this specific matter, which he knew he would resolve, but what to do in general with Oram. Joel was working Saturday mornings with a militant community group over next year's OEO budget and was still working 60 to 65 hours per week. He didn't think Oram's performance would improve unless Schlitz agreed with Joel's priorities and, even in that event, sufficient improvement was unlikely. On the other hand, Joel did not look forward to hiring a fourth controller in the two years he had worked at Morris. Moreover, the routine work of the accounting department was being performed to Schlitz's satisfaction. Joel decided to go for a walk by the river and make his decision.

Case Questions

1. What is the problem from Joel's point of view? From Oram's point of view? From Schlitz's point of view? From Harrang's?
2. In what ways should Oram be accountable to Joel and Schlitz?
3. Given that Oram's performance is not acceptable to Joel, what options does Joel have to affect Oram's performance?
4. What do you recommend that Joel do now? Why?
5. What is the evidence that you used in making the above recommendation?

Case C
Now What?

Ann Scheck McAlearney

Kelly Connor had been working at West Liberty Health System for four years, and she was starting to wonder about what was next for her career. She remembered her graduate school experience in health administration fondly, especially now that she had been in the same position for three full years since her first promotion. The excitement of learning new things—and the terror of exams and presentations—were seemingly distant memories. Instead, she felt stuck in her present job as manager of operations for the division of cardiology.

While West Liberty was a multihospital health system, Connor's expectation that she could grow and learn within the health system was not becoming a reality. She found that the real day-to-day existence of this operations management position was about as unglamorous as she could imagine, and she was unable to envision a promotion in her near future. Connor had tried to continue to read and learn on the job, but there just wasn't enough time in the day. The firefighting of operations and real-time crises were always priorities, and she was afraid that she would soon be unable to remember how to analyze the business case for a new venture or how to think strategically about anything.

As Connor returned home at the end of the week, she decided things had to change. Even though West Liberty seemed like a good and caring employer when she had interviewed all those years ago, they now seemed much better at talking about caring for employees than actually doing something about it. When Connor looked back on the past three years, she realized that she had yet to successfully participate in any seminar or educational class offered by the health system because she could never seem to get away from her job. Yet she also realized that she was not alone. Her friends in other departments had similar complaints, and it seemed that the only way they were able to take a break was to leave the country—but nobody had enough time or money to do that very often.

Feeling burned out and disappointed, Connor knew she needed to do something different, but she didn't know what. She wanted to take the educational programs West Liberty offered, but she needed to find some protected time, and she needed to figure out how to better navigate the politics and chaos of West Liberty.

Connor set up a meeting with her boss, Patricia Miller, director of cardiology, to voice her concerns. While she told Miller that the reason for the meeting was "professional development," she wasn't sure that Miller understood what Connor meant by that term, and she wasn't confident that Miller would be able to provide the guidance Connor sought. Connor, though, knew that she had to get Miller's support before she could reallocate her time to focus on her own professional development. And since Miller was only swayed by evidence and data, Connor knew she had to do her homework before the meeting.

Considering Her Options

Connor's first step was to investigate the professional development opportunities provided through West Liberty Health System. Looking at the online course catalog, she was amazed at the long list of courses. As she started to look at the individual course titles, though, she found that most of the courses seemed focused on the needs of frontline staff and new managers. Courses with titles such as "Avoiding Needle Stick Injuries" and "Compliance Education" weren't really appropriate for her role, and the management classes such as "Skills for New Managers" and "How to Motivate Your Nursing Staff" seemed too basic. She was encouraged when she found a list of course offerings "under development" in the areas of quality management and performance improvement, but she didn't know when the courses would be available or whether they would be appropriate for her when they were rolled out. For now, Connor felt she needed to find courses geared toward mid-level managers, especially those focused on people management skills, but these didn't appear on the West Liberty list.

Expanding her search outside the health system, Connor pulled up websites from organizations such as the American College of Healthcare Executives (ACHE) and the American Management Association to see if their offerings were any more appropriate. She was delighted to find titles such as "Managing Conflict" and "Improving Your Negotiation Skills" that were offered through some of the professional conferences and meetings. Given her latest performance evaluations, she knew that Miller felt she had opportunities to improve in these areas in particular, and the course descriptions sounded fantastic. However, finding the courses themselves was only the first step. To take these courses, she had to gain support from Miller in the form of both financial resources and free time.

Strategically Planning Her Professional Development

Connor knew that the best approach to obtaining Miller's endorsement for her professional development was to develop a plan. By creating a formal plan, Connor would be able to outline her professional development goals and build a case for why achievement of her goals would be important. Further, development of a formal plan would force her to build the evidence case for her professional development, drawing from the available research literature she knew Miller respected.

Determining the Perspective

Connor's project management skills came in particularly handy as she began to sketch out a plan for her professional development. As she remembered from her strategic management course in graduate school, she knew that one of the first decisions she needed to make was about the time horizon of the plan. While she was certainly concerned with both long-term and short-term goals, she decided to focus on two specific time frames for this plan: a two-year horizon for the short term and a five-year horizon for the mid-range term. Another immediate decision she needed to make concerned the perspective of the plan. Despite seeming a bit unorthodox, she decided that she would frame this strategic planning process with herself as the "entity" to be planned, and use her own perspective to base considerations about other stakeholders and so forth.

An Environmental Analysis

Immersing herself in the planning process, Connor began to consider how an environmental analysis would look from the perspective of an individual. She decided that a good next step would be to perform a stakeholder analysis for her professional development. Sketching on a piece of paper, she put herself in the center box, and began to consider other stakeholders in her development. Clearly, West Liberty Health System as an employer could be listed as an important stakeholder, as well as her own division and her professional colleagues. She also considered the perspectives of stakeholders outside the health system —such as members of the community, members of her professional community, and so forth—but decided it would be better to focus on the West Liberty environment as a start. Exhibit I.8 shows the results of her preliminary analysis.

Internal Analysis

Satisfied that this stakeholder analysis would help make her case for how her own professional development could impact others within the health system, she then turned to an internal analysis, using her own ideas and hopes to guide her planning process. She was aware of research in management and leadership development, and selected a framework from McCall, Lombardo, and Morrison (1988) that recommended three particular action steps: (1)

EXHIBIT I.8
Stakeholder
Map for
Connor's
Professional
Development

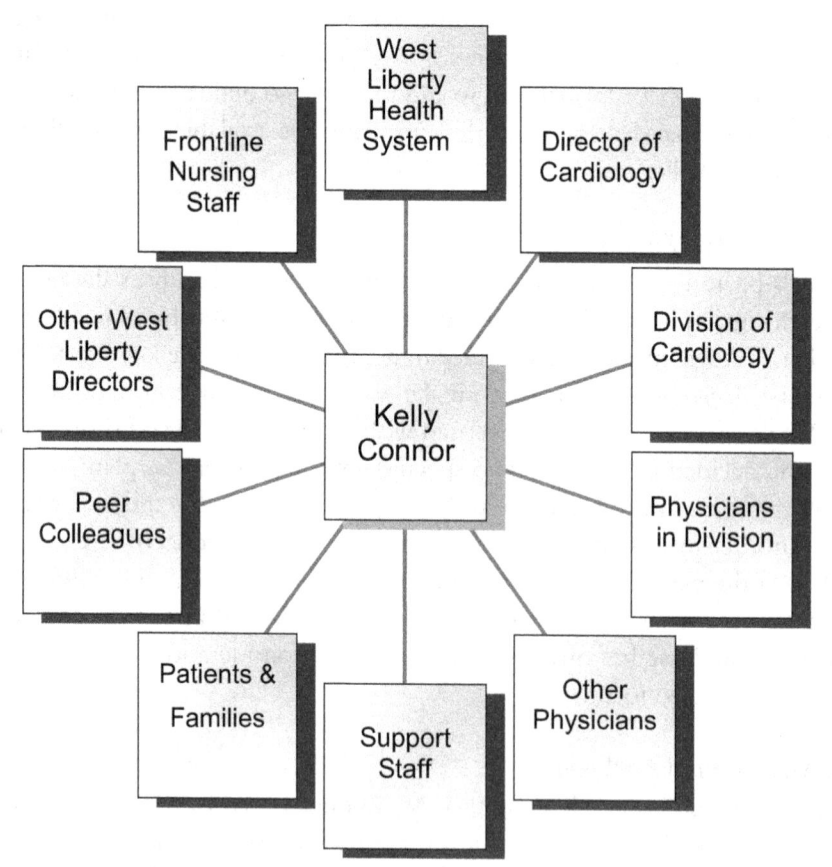

learn about personal shortcomings; (2) accept responsibility for shortcomings that result from a lack of knowledge, skills, or experience, or because of personality, limited ability, or situational misfit; and (3) decide what to do about shortcomings. While none of these three steps was easy, she knew there were several available sources of information to help in her personal analysis.

Connor first reviewed the feedback she had received in her performance evaluations, highlighting patterns that showed opportunities for development. She remembered the uncomfortable moments of each past review when she and the director had come to the sections of "Managing Conflict" and "Building Professional Teams." She had never been comfortable with conflict and was acutely aware of taking the "easy way" out of most conflicts by capitulating to the other person or referring the issue to her director. Not surprisingly, this tendency was reflected fairly clearly in her last two evaluations. However, she also noted a disturbing pattern in her annual reviews with respect to her ability to work with established nurses in cardiology. With this group, in particular, she never felt comfortable asserting authority, and, as a result, typically let them walk all over her, often bullying her to get their way. This trend had resulted in several difficult situations over the past year when this group of long-term nurses presented strong resistance to the introduction of a new electronic health record system with electronic medication administration records embedded in the system. Reflecting on a number of examples, Connor realized that this was certainly an area in which she could improve.

Connor also took some time to do a more formal evaluation of her strengths and weaknesses with respect to professional development, and used a competency assessment tool she found available on the web to assess her capabilities for leadership in health administration (Robbins, Bradley, and Spicer 2001). This tool had been developed, tested, and published in the peer-reviewed *Journal of Healthcare Management*, thus offering the kind of credibility Miller appreciated. The tool assessed 52 competencies that were categorized into four different domains: (1) technical skills, (2) industry knowledge, (3) analytic and conceptual reasoning, and (4) interpersonal and emotional intelligence. Completing the assessment, Connor found that she seemed to have an appropriate level of competency in the technical skills areas of operations, finance, and information resources, but had technical skills gaps in the areas of human resources and external affairs. Further, she noted several areas in the domain of interpersonal intelligence where her competence level could be improved.

This competency assessment tool was even more helpful than Connor had anticipated, though, because it provided suggestions about how she could develop different competencies through either on-the-job experience or formal graduate training. For example, in the area of human resources technical skills, one competency area she lacked was the ability to "demonstrate understanding of the governance function including structure and fiduciary responsibility and impact on management decisions (for both for-profit and not-for-profit organizations)" (Robbins, Bradley, and Spicer 2001). To address this deficiency, the assessment tool suggested the straightforward work-based experience of "attend board and board committee meetings" (Robbins, Bradley, and Spicer 2001). Connor knew that while access to board meetings at West Liberty might not be easy to obtain, evidence about the effectiveness of the work-based experience would help convince Miller and others that this type of experience might be worth arranging to support Connor's professional development.

Goal Planning

Armed with the results of her first personal internal analysis, Connor decided a good next step would be to develop a personal mission statement and several goals for her professional development in the coming years. While this process was also difficult, it helped her to focus her own goals so that she could be clear and compelling when she presented her case to Miller. By focusing on the two- and five-year time horizons she had established, she was able to keep herself from feeling completely overwhelmed. Knowing that the best goals were those that were measurable, Connor outlined her professional development goals and their associated metrics as a start for her discussion with Miller. This preliminary outline is presented in Exhibit I.9.

EXHIBIT I.9
Professional
Development
Goals

Two-Year Goals
- Improvement in conflict management skills, reflected in improvement in Annual Performance Evaluation section of "Managing Conflict"
- Improvement in team-building skills, reflected in improvement in Annual Performance Evaluation section of "Building Professional Teams"
- Successful completion of cross-system project, involving collaboration outside Division of Cardiology
- Expanded professional network to include at least two West Liberty executives
- Higher personal job satisfaction (personal perspective)
- Promotion of at least one direct report to manager at West Liberty

Five-Year Goals
- Promotion to director at West Liberty
- By year three, Annual Performance Evaluation strong in all areas
- High job satisfaction of direct reports, reflected in Annual Employee Work-Life Survey
- Promotion of at least two direct reports to manager at West Liberty in years 3–5

Strategic Options

Once Connor had outlined her goals, she saw that the next step in her strategic professional development planning process was to highlight specific areas of development necessary to achieve her goals. Several areas needing focus jumped out at her in particular: (1) conflict management, (2) building professional teams, (3) internal networking, (4) cross-system collaboration, (5) leadership development, and (6) employee development.

Considering each of these areas, she was aware that they could be addressed by a variety of approaches, so she built a list of alternative tactics by which she could develop skills and competencies in each area. Connor's preliminary list for the first three focus areas is shown in Exhibit I.10.

A Scenario Analysis

Finally, Connor recognized that Miller, similar to many others, was a visual thinker. One tool she knew of that might help both her and Miller envision alternative professional development options for Connor was a scenario analysis exercise that described what success might look like if things did or did not go as planned. Connor got herself a glass of iced tea and imagined how things might happen for good or bad, considering whether she was able to enlist the support and make the personal and behavioral changes she believed were necessary. Exhibit I.11 shows how she envisioned these three scenarios for the two-year time horizon.

EXHIBIT I.10
Alternative Professional Development Approaches

Focus Area	Approach
Conflict Management	• External course offering (e.g., ACHE) • Internal course offering (when developed) • Reading and discussion • Structured assignment and feedback • Coaching
Building Professional Teams	• External course offering (e.g., ACHE) • Internal course offering (when developed) • Reading and discussion • Action learning project requiring team development • Structured assignment and feedback • Coaching
Internal Networking	• Attendance at systemwide meetings • Assignment to systemwide task force or project • Lunch invitation to interested directors, other executives, to help mentor informally

Scenario 1: Stormy Weather

Unable to enlist sufficient support for her own professional development, Connor was forced to continue the development process on her own. She signed up for multiple class offerings through West Liberty's education division, but was limited by both the course catalog and her own schedule. While she successfully completed several online courses that introduced her to focused topics, she was unable to complete any courses that required in-class sessions due to her inability to get away from her job. The director of cardiology was supportive of Connor's efforts, but unable to provide additional resources to enable her to travel to off-site conferences or participate in courses that required time away from operations. Connor's performance evaluations continued to be positive, but the director's comments consistently indicated room for improvement in her people skills. The director was particularly concerned about Connor's ability to work with established nurses and her inability to create and sustain productive teams that involved clinicians. On Connor's part, she remained frustrated about her lack of free time, and about a seemingly endless career as a manager who would never be promoted. She started to look outside West Liberty for new positions, but realized her lack of professional development had limited her job possibilities to lateral moves.

Scenario 2: The Long and Winding Road

While initially frustrated by her job's incessant demands that she be continually available, Connor began to see windows of opportunity for her development. With her director's support, she was able to sign up for a new mentoring program at West Liberty, and developed an interesting professional connection with the director of food services in the health system. This director had been at West Liberty for her entire career, and was able to provide advice about important topics such as negotiating the politics of the health system and using the performance evaluation process as an opportunity for shameless self-promotion. As she pointed out to Connor, West Liberty did not like to lose good people, so building one's professional image as one of the "stars" of the system was an excellent first step toward getting promoted. In addition, through her mentor, Connor was able to find a similarly minded manager of operations in food services who was interested in learning more about West Liberty. With the help of both directors, Connor and her colleague negotiated a job switching arrangement whereby the managers would spend two hours each day in the other's role for a three-month period. During these three months, the managers also agreed to have lunch together at least twice per week to ensure that they had direct opportunities to coordinate with each other so that their job rotation hours would not result in lost productivity for either department. While the job rotation itself did not directly lead to a promotion, this creative arrangement helped reduce Connor's frustration with West Liberty and enabled her to see opportunities throughout the system for the coming years.

Scenario 3: Sunny Side of the Street

Connor's meeting with the director went better than she could have hoped. The director was in complete agreement about the need for Connor to focus on her professional development, and she offered to provide whatever resources she could to help Connor succeed. After reviewing Connor's professional development plan, the two agreed on a plan of attack for the coming year and were able to identify two specific off-site conferences that were well aligned with Connor's need to develop her conflict management and negotiation skills. In the meantime, the director suggested that Connor read several books related to these topics, and offered to serve as a sounding board to discuss the books at a series of monthly lunches they would schedule. The director also offered to recommend that Connor be placed in the new program that was being developed at West Liberty for "high potentials," ensuring that she would receive executive-level attention to her leadership development in the coming two years. At the end of the meeting, the director handed Connor a copy of one of her recommended books, *Crucial Conversations*, and they agreed on a date for the first book lunch meeting in the coming month. Nine months flew by, and at Connor's annual performance evaluation meeting, she had her next formal opportunity to discuss professional development with the director. They agreed that the book discussion lunches were both productive and fun, and they listed the next three books they would plan to read and discuss. However, their frank discussion about Connor's ability to apply what she had learned from the external courses she had taken at a recent professional meeting highlighted several opportunities for Connor to further develop her leadership skills and practice new behaviors over the coming months. While the new West Liberty Leadership Development program was yet to begin, the director suggested that Connor

(continued)

seek other leadership development opportunities within and outside the health system, to continue making progress toward her own professional development goals. In particular, the director recommended that Connor enroll in a course through the Center for Creative Leadership focused specifically on leadership development for women, and promised to provide Connor with her full support to attend. Together, they laid out a plan for the next year and highlighted a possible promotion for Connor within the coming year as a goal toward which to strive.

Preparing for the Meeting

In getting everything together for her meeting with Miller, Connor considered what she should forward to Miller ahead of time and what she should leave for the actual meeting. Knowing Miller hated to be surprised or caught off guard, Connor decided to compile all of her preliminary planning ideas in a "for your eyes only" document that she could send Miller a week in advance of the meeting. This document contained the results of all her analyses, as well as brief paragraphs introducing the various sections and analytic approaches. She knew Miller's time was limited, but she wanted to make sure Miller understood how important this was to her future at West Liberty. Connor was dependent on Miller's buy-in to help her achieve her professional development goals, and felt that her personal strategic plan would provide a solid framework with which she could guide the discussion.

Case Questions

1. What constraints does Connor face within her position? What options does she have to overcome those constraints?
2. What can Connor do within her present job to learn on the job?
3. How has Connor's strategic planning exercise built or weakened her case for spending time away from operations to develop her professional skills?
4. How much of professional development is one's personal responsibility, and how much is the responsibility of the employer?

References

McCall, M. W., M. M. Lombardo, and A. M. Morrison. 1988. *The Lessons of Experience: How Successful Executives Develop on the Job.* Lexington MA: Lexington Books.

Robbins, C. J., E. H. Bradley, and M. Spicer. 2001. "Developing Leadership in Healthcare Administration: A Competency Assessment Tool." *Journal of Healthcare Management* 46 (3): 188–202.

Short Case 1
Nowhere Job

David Melman

Jack Ernest works for a young and growing healthcare company. The company has successfully developed a market niche by contracting with colleges and universities to manage and operate their campus health centers. Ernest has been hired to develop the operational structure for a new product that will link students' managed care health insurance coverage to services provided by their campus health centers. This new product will result in cost savings as well as improved service delivery. It is a new concept in the industry and while Ernest does not have significant healthcare experience, he does have a great deal of energy and enthusiasm, and he is expected to learn on the job.

Ernest has not been given a formal job description. He was originally given a list of performance objectives verbally, but these objectives have been subsequently changed without his input, and there have been no new objectives put in place. Ernest's work environment is unusual in that he mostly works out of a home office, with occasional trips to the corporate office 70 miles away. Ernest reports directly to the corporate medical director of the company, but this director is located in Miami, 1,200 miles away. Communication with his boss occurs almost exclusively by e-mail, telephone, or fax.

Ernest has made progress toward achieving organizational objectives, but he is now facing obstacles that are largely caused by his isolation from others in the company. He is not informed when changes are made to project objectives, nor are the underlying reasons for these changes ever explained to him. Ernest finds that his isolation limits his ability to grow professionally, and he has trouble contributing to the work of the company because he is unable to describe his company's needs accurately to outside vendors without being properly informed himself.

Ernest has asked to have a formal job description and stated performance objectives based on the format suggested by a human resources consultant hired by the company, but he has received no response. Meanwhile, Ernest has been asked to complete the contracts he has negotiated with several outside vendors, and he is told he now reports to an outside consultant who has been hired to help coordinate technical operations, including information systems. This outside consultant tells Ernest not to proceed with these contracts the very day after the CEO tells him to complete them.

Ernest attempts to contribute to the sales and marketing efforts of his company by proposing that the company sponsor an institute at a prestigious university, and he wants to contribute his time and energy to make this project a success. He is told it is a good idea, but the vice president of sales and marketing does not keep his commitment to respond to Ernest's proposal. Ernest sends reminders and continues to develop the idea with the university. He is trying to expand his job responsibilities to include business development, but he knows he needs the support of others in his organization to make a meaningful contribution.

Case Questions

1. What should Ernest do?
2. What are the risks to Ernest?
3. How could Ernest have anticipated these problems before accepting his current position?
4. What should Ernest's priorities be in evaluating an alternative career opportunity? Why?

Short Case 2
Manager Morale at Uptown Hospital

Sofia V. Agoritsas

John Robbins, MD, the savvy and scholarly chief executive officer of Uptown Hospital, minimized the window on his computer just before his monthly department chiefs meeting was about to start. He was concerned about the results of the latest employee satisfaction survey that the vice president of human resources had e-mailed him. The survey results were going to be an important part of the report on "Manager Development at Uptown Hospital" that was being produced by the newly hired consulting group, Coaches Like Us, in response to the board chair's special request.

Robbins stared intently at the light fixture in his office and wondered what would happen when the chairman of the board saw the report that included these survey results. Robbins knew the chairman was eager to see the consultants' report, especially since a close colleague of the chairman owned the consulting group.

Uptown Hospital

Uptown Hospital, a 500-bed community teaching hospital, is one of two tertiary-care centers in the area; its main competitor is University Hospital, which focuses more on its medical school and research. Robbins recently became chief executive officer, having been promoted from his previous position as chief medical officer. He had been asked to fill the CEO role last year on an interim basis after the former CEO left for a new position in a major health system. After a year-long executive search failed to produce any viable external candidates, Robbins was offered the permanent position. For the most part, Uptown Hospital has been a financially sound organization, largely because of its location. People in the area are not interested in driving far to get to the next closest health system, and they seem to be satisfied with the care provided at Uptown Hospital. Cost management has not been a major focus of the organization, but this has recently become an area of increased attention as costs for labor and supplies seem to be escalating uncontrollably.

If one were asked to describe the organizational culture at Uptown, that individual would likely say the place is both comfortable and familial. This is partially attributable to the fact that turnover among Uptown employees has historically been low. On average, about 15 percent of employees leave Uptown annually, compared with a national average of 23 percent. Internal movement within the organization is typically slow, but given the relative stability of the workforce, most of Uptown's managers and even many of the physicians seem to have "grown up" at Uptown. Over the past year, though, multiple department and nurse managers have resigned, and this has been noticed.

Community voluntary physicians have a strong influence on the care provided at Uptown Hospital. They are the core referral source for the organization, and these physicians play an integral role in the patient care process. The nursing staff know the voluntary physicians personally, as the patient care areas are open units and the physicians round regularly on their patients.

Recently, many of the major physician practices in the area have become affiliated faculty practices within Uptown Hospital. Now, though, physician faculty members seem to be increasingly at odds with hospital residents and administrative managers because of the different practice patterns and care practices used by the voluntary physicians. This has led to a number of complaints filed by the department chiefs, since this lack of standardization results in considerable variation in care. Staff loyalty has also seemed to sway because of constant confusion about care practices. Further, many of the administrative managers and hospital employees have become frustrated by the seemingly noncooperative and noncollaborative environment. The staff's willingness to take on new responsibilities usually depends on how the attending physicians are acting, but not everyone is on good behavior anymore. As a result, the managers are often unable to hold their staff accountable for various job responsibilities.

The Survey Results Are In

Robbins was struck by the survey results on several dimensions. First, he wondered how the people in his organization could not know about the key strategic initiatives of Uptown Hospital. It was not as if the executive team was hiding its activities, and the modernization of the patient care building had been an area of focus day in and day out for the past year. However, he was more surprised that on average the managers stated they were unhappy in the organization.

According to the survey results, the managers' chief complaints included the following:

1. The goals of the organization are not well defined.
2. Staff are reluctant to take on new responsibilities.
3. There is limited use of a team approach to patient care.
4. The overwhelming number of noncooperative employees makes it difficult to hold the staff accountable.
5. Managers feel the majority of their staff perform at an average to below-average level.

Robbins thought about how these results reflected the perspectives of the different managers throughout the hospital. He could name them all. Most had been at Uptown for more than 15 years. He reflected on the brief instances he had run across these individuals and knew that he usually got to see them all at his quarterly management meetings. In contrast, he was able to foster a more personal relationship with each of Uptown's department chiefs.

Robbins swiveled around in his black leather executive chair and realized he needed to take responsibility for this situation at the hospital. He plastered a welcoming smile on his face as the department chiefs entered his office. He knew he needed to become the hero who would save the day, but he wasn't sure how to begin.

Case Questions

1. What should the CEO do with these survey results?
2. How could morale have declined so quickly at Uptown?
3. What constraints would you face in implementing your recommendations to the CEO?
4. What are ways to overcome these constraints?

Short Case 3
A Sure Thing

David A. Kaplan and Anthony R. Kovner

Doug Williams received his master's degree in health management from Kings University in 1997. Since then he has enjoyed a successful healthcare career, having worked at some of the city's most prestigious academic medical centers. Williams even spent some time as a healthcare consultant, traveling across the country performing financial turnarounds at multiple medical centers. Williams was always considered to be somewhat of a risk-taker and was willing to give up stability if it meant moving to the next level in his career. The following case study is based on a real-life situation that happened to Williams.

****

Williams had left consulting and had landed a position as divisional administrator of cardiology at St. Lucy's University Hospital. The division was the largest within the department of medicine, and University Hospital was working to make cardiovascular medicine its leading service line. Williams reported to the division chief, Dr. Fishman, as well as to the department of medicine administrator, Linda Carter.

Williams worked tirelessly helping Fishman, a relatively inexperienced division chief, to develop a strategic framework for building the division. This included increasing the number of faculty, increasing the clinical practice volume and associated revenues, building a robust research arm, and improving the reputation of the training program.

After nearly two years of achieving tangible results across all of these areas, Williams felt it was reasonable to request a salary increase and/or promotion within the organization. Williams first approached Fishman and had the following conversation:

Williams: Dr. Fishman, I have really enjoyed working with you over the past couple of years and I feel that together we have accomplished a great deal, wouldn't you agree?

Fishman: I absolutely agree, and I can't thank you enough for all your efforts in helping me to achieve my vision of making this one of the top programs in the nation.

Williams: Well, after all my efforts, I was hoping that you might be able to help me. I really would like to be considered for a salary increase. I feel that I have earned this and, in all honesty, with everything going on at home, I really could use it.

Fishman: Have you talked to Linda about this?

Williams: I have, but she sent me to discuss this with you.

Fishman: Okay. I agree that you deserve an increase, especially given all your hard work. Let me look into this and get back to you shortly.

Williams: Thanks so much. I really appreciate your help.

* * * * * * *

Nearly two months went by without any mention by either Carter or Dr. Fishman of an increase. In the meantime, Williams, who lived outside the city, was approached about becoming vice president of hospital operations at State Hospital. State Hospital was a government-sponsored academic hospital within minutes of his house. However, the state institution was known to be a political land mine, and many people who worked there spoke about their negative experiences. In addition, several people who had worked there had had their careers shattered by controversy.

These legendary stories did not deter Williams from exploring the new opportunity. In fact, with every interview Williams became more and more enthralled with the notion of working at State Hospital. To think that at the age of 30 he could be a vice president of hospital operations overseeing ten hospital departments. What a dream come true! On top of it all they were offering a salary 30 percent higher than his current salary and the place was located within minutes of his house. His father always told him that any job had three components—money, location, and the role itself. He would say that if you found a job that had two of these aspects, it would be a wonderful opportunity; amazingly, this job had all three.

A couple of days after his final interview, Williams received a call from the chief operating officer (COO) of State Hospital, Alex Roberts, who offered him the position. Without blinking, Williams accepted the position, and was set to start his new job in two weeks.

Williams was so excited that he even called his professor from his health management program to tell him the good news. His professor, who was also aware of State Hospital's reputation, warned Williams to reconsider his decision, but it was too late. Williams had already accepted.

* * * * * * *

Later that week, Williams went to talk with Fishman about his decision:

Williams: Dr. Fishman, I again want to thank you for the opportunity to help you rebuild this division. I have had the time of my life working with you and the members of this team. That being said, I have decided to accept an offer to become a vice president at State Hospital starting in a couple of weeks.

Fishman: Wow. I wasn't expecting this, but I suppose that a person with your skills is bound to move up the ranks quickly. Congratulations. I don't suppose there is any way to convince you to stay?

Williams: No. This new job just has too much going for it. I would be hard-pressed not to take on the new and challenging role.

Fishman: Well, I want to wish you the best of luck. Please keep me informed about your future success.

* * * * * * *

A few weeks later, Williams started in his new role at State Hospital. The first year for Williams read like a textbook. He connected with all of his managers, evaluated the operations of his services, and worked hands-on with his managers to make operational improvements. In addition, he worked closely with his boss, COO Alex Roberts, and the CEO, Bob Swanson, to further grow and build his service lines. Williams didn't understand what all the fuss was about working at this organization. As far as he could tell, this new life was perfect. That was until he received the news.

* * * * * * *

Williams was in his regular 8:00 a.m. meeting with the other vice presidents reviewing the weekly agenda items. Roberts strolled into the meeting and made the announcement that he had decided to take a new position as COO at UCLA Medical Center in California. Williams felt his heart fall into the pit of his stomach. Williams knew that Roberts had been the individual primarily responsible for recruiting him, and, in fact, had made the decision that he would pull several service lines away from one of the other long-standing vice presidents for Williams to manage. The transition of Roberts away from State Hospital could have major implications for Williams.

To make the matter even worse, within a week of the COO's announcement, the CEO, Swanson, decided that he, too, would be leaving to become the CEO at Boulder University Hospital in Colorado. If anyone could have helped Williams without Roberts to intercede, it was sure to be Swanson. Swanson's announcement was disastrous, as Williams would surely be exposed now.

* * * * * *

Williams was in a quandary with both of his supporters and mentors gone. It soon became evident that the long-standing vice president was going to get her services back at any cost. She tormented Williams by sabotaging his programs, and even recruited some of his managers to aid her in her efforts. Williams, who was inexperienced with these types of politics, was no match for this vice president and she eventually won her services back. Williams saw his dream job start to unravel and quickly realized that he made a mistake in coming to work at State Hospital. Williams ultimately resigned his position, knowing he could not win at this game.

******

You will be happy to know that following this experience, Williams eventually found a successful position as a department administrator for another academic medical center in the city. He is happy in his position and has learned that while the grass always appears greener on the other side, it isn't. As for Williams's father's saying that a job has three components—money, location, and the role itself—if you find a job that has all three, it is probably too good to be true. In Williams's case, it certainly was.

Case Questions

1. Should Williams have pushed harder to get an increase and/or promotion at St. Lucy's University Hospital?
2. Should Williams have done anything differently before accepting the position at State Hospital?
3. What could Williams have done differently once faced with the change in leadership at State Hospital?
4. Once faced with adversity, what should Williams have done to possibly preserve his position at State Hospital?
5. Do you think Williams made the right decision in accepting the new position at State Hospital? In leaving his position at State Hospital?

Short Case 4
The First Day

Ann Scheck McAlearney

Susan was both thrilled and terrified. Tomorrow was her first day as a manager. Having recently completed her master of health administration degree at a prestigious local university, a thorough job search had resulted in her being hired as the new manager of patient accounts at University Health System. She had had numerous interviews with various directors and other managers in the health system, as well as a lunch interview/meeting with six people who would report to her, but those interviews seemed very far away. Susan wanted to make a good impression and get off to a positive start, yet she wasn't sure what to do first. She had learned the importance of listening in management, but she also knew she was the boss. Further, her own boss, the director of patient care services, had emphasized the importance of getting her employees to improve productivity at any cost. Susan had heard that while her new direct reports were nice to one's face, they had a tendency to complain and scapegoat, and this had led to the sudden departure of the previous manager of patient accounts. She was particularly nervous about being younger than all of her new employees. To quell her fears, Susan decided to list what she wanted to accomplish in her first days and weeks on the job.

Case Questions

1. As a friend of Susan's considering a similar position, what would you recommend that she put on the list?
2. How would you suggest that she prioritize her goals?

Short Case 5
Conflict in the Office

Ramya Rao and Ann Scheck McAlearney

Trisha Olsen has been an assistant director at Liberty Research Hospital for the past seven years. She currently manages eight people in the protocol department, which is responsible for ensuring that all research studies are compliant with research regulations and institutional review board requirements. Unfortunately, the protocol department has a reputation for having high turnover rates, and many workers are rumored to leave because of how they have been treated by their boss. However, two of the protocol specialists have been with the department for more than ten years, and these two specialists have been promoted to team leaders in the past year.

Recently, the department changed its approach to quality control, requiring more involvement and oversight of work by different employees.

Workers must now circulate their work and have it reviewed by all coworkers, including team leaders, instead of the former process that required circulation only among the protocol specialists. This new approach has introduced some tension within the department and raised issues about work quality that had not been concerns in the past. Team leaders had become particularly critical of others' work, but they were also unhappy when their own work was returned to them with others' criticisms that had to be addressed.

Yesterday, tension within the department was particularly high. Olsen was out of the office at the time, but apparently Stephanie, a protocol specialist, and Bella, a team leader, were overheard arguing about whether a comment should be made in a database about a minor change in the research protocol. The argument was heated enough so that coworkers started to pay attention to the altercation, and Olsen heard rumors about the incident after she returned from her meeting. To make matters worse, both Stephanie and Bella then e-mailed Olsen to describe the situation and give their points of view about the disagreement.

Olsen wasn't sure how to handle the situation. She knew that Bella had a history of getting into arguments with coworkers and could hold a grudge for months. The department would certainly suffer if the tension remained, and Olsen could not handle further turnover among protocol specialists.

Case Questions

1. What should Olsen consider prior to addressing the conflict?
2. How can she help to resolve the conflict?

Short Case 6
Annual Performance Evaluation: Can You Coach Kindness?

Ann Scheck McAlearney

Bob Carter, RN, has been working at New Hope Hospital for six years, ever since he finished nursing school. He has always planned to become a manager at some time in his career, and it seems that the opportunity might soon be available. As a floor nurse, Carter has earned the respect of his peers, never taking no for an answer and, in many cases, saving patients' lives because of solid clinical instincts. At this point Carter has been working for two years as a case manager in the clinical case management department, participating in case management and discharge planning within the hospital. Carter is considering applying for a promotion to manager of discharge planning to fill a newly vacated position in the clinical case management department, and he is looking forward to his upcoming performance review with the director of clinical case management as an opportunity to discuss this possible promotion.

Sally Valen is the vice president of clinical operations, and the clinical case management department is one of her areas of responsibility. She is particularly concerned about the role of this department in ensuring appropriate discharge planning for all patients, especially in light of the new attention focused on discharge planning through the Centers for Medicare & Medicaid Services (CMS) Core Measures Program.

You are the director of clinical case management, and eager to fill the vacant manager of discharge planning position. You know that any manager in the department will require a strong clinical background, but you are also aware that this individual must have the ability to work well with others in process improvement activities needed to strengthen discharge planning and clinical case management services throughout the hospital.

In reviewing Carter's file before his performance evaluation, you are reminded of several issues that might affect your decision about his promotion. First, you are aware that Carter's attitude toward social workers within the department has been less than collegial. Your observations of his work style would indicate that he feels superior to the social workers, but you have not discussed this directly with him. Second, you are somewhat concerned about Carter's potential management style. While he has yet to be tested as a manager, you have seen him verbally reprimand other nurses in front of other employees, and this has frustrated some of his coworkers. On the positive side, though, you know that Carter has excellent clinical instincts. Further, while he may seem to have a superior attitude in interactions with some of his coworkers, his interactions with patients have been consistently outstanding. His ability to help patients manage challenging health issues and take responsibility for their care postdischarge has been noted several times in his file.

Your reflections about Carter's possible promotion have left you confused. You have several considerations.

Case Questions

1. What is the relative importance of clinical competence and patient focus over one's ability to work as a member of a clinical team in this department?

2. Do you want Carter to be a manager in your department?

3. What should you tell Carter to help him improve and develop his managerial skills regardless of your recommendation for him to apply for the manager position?

4. Based on your recommendation about Carter's possible promotion, what do you do now to help him succeed in a managerial role, or how do you encourage his professional development within New Hope so that he does not leave for a different job?

II

CONTROL

You may regard as a Utopian dream my hope to see all our hospitals devoting a reasonable portion of their funds to tracing the results of the treatment of their patients and analyzing these results with a view to improving them. You may prefer to ponder over the voluminous discussions now appearing in our journals and in the lay press about the pros and cons for state medicine and who is to pay the cost of medical care. I read these discussions, but they seem to be futile, until our hospitals begin to trace their results.
—*E. A. Codman (1935)*

I envision a system in which we promise those who depend on us total access to the help they need, in the form they need, when they need it. Our system will promise freedom from the tyranny of individual visits with overburdened professionals as the only way to find a healing relationship; will promise excellence as the standard, valuing such excellence over ill-considered autonomy; will promise safety; and will be capable of nourishing interactions in which information is central, quality is individually defined, control resides with patients, and trust blooms in an open environment.
—*Donald Berwick (2002)*

COMMENTARY

Hospital cafeteria manager to counter staff before the start of the workday: Give our customers what they want from our daily menu and kitchen selections.

First customer to counter staff: I want a hot dog with mustard and relish. (Counter staff hands out a hot dog with mustard.)

Customer: There is no relish on my hot dog.

Staff: Sorry. (Takes back the hot dog and adds relish.)

Customer: Thanks. (Proceeds down the cafeteria line to the cashier at the end.)

This simple example raises a lot of the concepts related to control in healthcare or in any other organization. Let us set this example into the context of a hospital's mission, vision, and values.

The *mission* of the hospital in this case is to provide the finest care by skilled and pleasant staff. The *vision* is that care will always meet best-practice standards and be timely, error-free, appropriate, and provided at a reasonable cost. The key *values* are that patients come first and employee satisfaction is valued.

The cafeteria fits into these goals by providing hospital workers a meal they want at a reasonable price. The hospital leadership is pleased that staff brag about working at the hospital, including the good food in the cafeteria. The cafeteria manager sets rules for appropriate work for the counter staff, leaving it up to them to match food to customer requests. There are clear limits to what the staff can do. The price of one hot dog does not buy two. Chocolate sauce is not offered for your hot dog. These rules are not burdensome because the customers are socialized to know the first rule and don't ever ask for chocolate sauce on their hot dogs.

From an organizational point of view, this example is similar to the nursing supervisor saying to the staff nurse: "These are your patients. With your good skills and education I am confident you can care for them. Call me if you need help."

Management in healthcare means creating the space and support systems that allow skilled people to meet the needs of the people they serve. If the relish jar is empty, the best counter staff cannot meet their customers' wishes. If the procedure kit is not in the examining room ready to use, the patient may not get a Pap smear test.

In our cafeteria example, an *error* was made and because of the customer's rapid *feedback*, it was corrected. If the quality is measured as the end result of this transaction (a hot dog with mustard and relish), the quality score was perfect, the transaction succeeded, and the customer was satisfied. The error was recognized—"Sorry"—and corrected: "Thanks."

Using a more accurate measure of quality, this transaction did not get a perfect score. Ideally, the error should not have occurred. There is a *cost of poor quality* here in the fraction of a minute used by staff, this customer, and other customers backed up in line, while the error was corrected.

This quality problem was observed in time and corrected by the customer. Patients are usually unable to provide such corrective feedback to caregivers. Professional caregivers—not the patients—are expected to define appropriate care. Therefore, caregivers carry a greater burden and responsibility for avoiding errors.

Human beings are bound to make mistakes, and errors will occur. The goal of error reduction is to create systems that stop errors. For example, a self-serve condiment station can be placed beyond the cashier so customers can help themselves. This requires a system for regularly replenishing the supply. This kind of system redesign is sometimes called *reengineering* the process.

Did this employee make a mistake due to lack of *motivation?* The vast majority of workers want to do a good job and not make mistakes. In this example, most likely the employee simply forgot. It may do more harm to criticize this employee for negligence and more good to create a system that makes it easier to avoid errors.

The genius of the McDonald's franchise is that it is a system designed to produce an identical package of French fries in thousands of locations using relatively unskilled employees. Such a system works with farmers to produce the right kind of potato, creates a standardized package, and uses a special metal scoop for filling the package. By such attention to the details of its system design, McDonald's can convince millions of people that they make the best French fries, which gives them a great market advantage. Healthcare has a long way to go to create such systems to reduce error.

Standardization and Variation

A hundred years ago, the hot dog might have been handmade, and no two were exactly alike. Shopping then was a more complicated process: "I want the fifth hot dog from the left; it looks bigger." Now that hot dogs are standardized and identical, there should be no reason to choose one over another. Although variation is still possible—how well cooked, how hot, how much relish, what kind of mustard—we do not expect this kind of customer-driven variation in a hospital cafeteria line. Hospital care is a combination of standardized activities (hernia surgery) with variation (left or right side). Best-practice standards combined with appropriate variation are required for good quality of care.

Standardization Can Be Cheaper and Variation Expensive

Back to our cafeteria: What about the attractiveness of the plate and napkin? What about the interpersonal relationship between the server and the customer? Does the server smile? Here, quality is in the mind of the customer.

Quality in healthcare is not defined by the customer alone. The hospital nutritionist might say the hot dogs have too much cholesterol and it would be healthier to replace them with meatless "veggie" dogs, and that the employees should set an example of healthy eating. This changes the definition of quality from customer preference to expert knowledge about nutrition and health. A distinctive feature of healthcare is that professional quality criteria are used. Healthcare organizations (HCOs) must sometimes balance patient satisfaction and adherence to expert definitions of quality.

A System of Control

Healthcare delivery where professional judgment, cost, and the patient's perceptions all matter have led to the concepts of the "value compass" and "balanced scorecard." Outcomes are measured in terms of patient satisfaction, cost of care, physical functioning (e.g., less pain, the ability to climb stairs), and physiological measures such as blood pressure and cholesterol levels (issues the patient may be unaware of, but that are key indicators for a future healthy life).

A system of control comprises five elements:

1. *Goals and objectives* (in our example, meeting customer needs)
2. *Information* used to measure performance
3. *Evaluation of performance in relation to goals and objectives.* Did the customer get what she wanted?
4. *Expectations.* Two levels of expectation were described in our cafeteria example. Did the customer eventually get what she wanted? Is this good enough? Or do we have a higher expectation of getting it right the first time? If this is the case, this transaction fell short.
5. *Incentives.* These can be based on an internalized desire to do a good job, or on external rewards. The desire to make the customer happy and

the desire to please the supervisor in hopes of a merit raise ideally go together without a conflict. The manager is delighted when good care is given. Problems start where there is a disconnect between satisfying the customer and satisfying the manager.

Goals and Objectives

Mission, vision, values, goals, and objectives are widely used concepts (see Exhibit II.1). Our mission is to meet the needs of our customers; our vision is to be the best; the values we live by are our religious beliefs; our goal is to survive this year; and our objective is to break even.

A goal is a broadly stated intention or direction—to improve the quality, for example, by lowering the infection rate. Organizational goals are determined by the preferences of individuals with power. Organizations are collectives of people and things brought together to achieve a common purpose. Individuals with similar goals create the organization. Goals are important because they provide organizational focus. They provide a long-term framework for dealing with conflict, and they encourage commitment from those who work in the organization. Goals are implemented by individuals working together on budgets, involve the allocation of functions, and may be influenced by the authority structure.

The individual wants housing and food and health and entertainment. This person decides he can do his best by working for pay as a nurse in a clinic. Nursing can be both a means (paycheck) and an end in itself (the satisfaction

EXHIBIT II.1
Organizational
Directions

Concept	Definition	Example	Requirement
Mission	Reason for existing	To meet the primary healthcare needs in our town	System maintenance
Vision	What we hope to do	People will move to our town because our care is so good.	Adaptive capability
Values	The philosophy that guides behavior	Mutual respect for both caregivers and care receivers	Values integration
Goal	An intention or direction	To open a new clinic this year	Goal attainment
Objective	A measurable intention	The new clinic will see 200 patients a week by the end of the year.	

of helping people in a friendly work environment). The clinic's goal of good quality and reasonable cost assumes that this nurse continues to have an enjoyable job and a paycheck. It is the role of the manager to make this happen.

Organizations may have objectives to measure production, sales, profit, and quality. Unit or organizational objectives can be determined by reading formal official goal statements or by observing what is happening in an organization. These observations may reveal shifts in resources or decision-making power among units or individuals, what types of individuals are leaving or being recruited to the organization, and what the organization is not doing and which population it is not serving. Many large corporations expend a lot of effort in goal specification.

What happens if HCOs do not specify objectives? Organizations may lack focus in their programs and may be less likely to abandon products and services that are neither effective nor efficient. The powerful and their short-term interests will tend to be favored over the weak and the long term; there will be less adaptation to the environment; and there will be a greater tendency to retain the status quo.

Healthcare managers should determine their organization's operative objectives. Official goals may not always provide reliable guidelines for managerial behavior. When those in power go against what a manager sees as the long-range interests of an organization, the manager should be careful, speaking out only if he or she is willing to pay the price and is certain about the facts.

Information

Healthcare managers must obtain information for key product lines about volume of services, the quality of care, service and production efficiency, market share, system maintenance, and the health status of the population served. They may use the following measures to assess performance: cost per case, cost per visit, cost per day, profit, fixed and variable costs, market share, capital expenditures as a percentage of sales, days of receivables and payables, top admitting physicians and their characteristics, staff turnover and overtime, sick time, and disability and fringe benefits costs. In addition, healthcare information systems are being expanded to include revenue by service line, budgeting and variance reporting, and clinical performance review. Computerized medical records are linked to cost and revenue data, concurrent review for quality of care, and final-product cost accounting for groups of similar patients at alternative levels of demand. Risk management relies on incident reports of untoward events, which are then aggregated and analyzed.

With the continuing investment in electronic medical records, required performance reporting, and standardized patient satisfaction surveys, healthcare is entering an era of information overload. Instead of the previous lack of quality of care data, now management has more information than it can cope with. What measures should take priority? What are the key quality characteristics?

Performance Evaluation

One of the problems with control systems is that they may measure the wrong thing. They may also measure the right thing inaccurately. These issues are particularly relevant for outcomes-of-care measurement. The easiest response to information we do not like is to say the data are wrong. No information is accurate enough to be accepted in a hostile, fearful environment. One of the important aspects of quality improvement (QI) is to create a climate "free from fear," where data can be accepted for what they are despite their inaccuracies and still be used to make improvements.

Increasingly, healthcare managers have access to performance data comparing their organizations to other similar ones. In the past, a nursing home board of directors may have simply believed without question that its care was outstanding, but now comparative data allow the board to see how the nursing home stacks up. The first step is to measure its care; for example, the frequency of bed sores or the percentage of patients under physical restraint. The next step is to compare measures. Why are 15 percent of our patients under restraint while the statewide average is 8 percent? The third step is to make this information public on accessible websites. This step is being done by third-party payers such as by Medicaid for nursing homes and by Medicare for hospitals (www.hospitalcompare.hhs.gov). Concurrent with these steps is a change from denial (our patients are sicker) and fear to a desire to improve. Managers can visit another similar nursing home with a very low restraint rate to learn how to improve their own situation. This requires collecting performance data over time to track improvements. This process of systematic comparison to best-practice organizations is called *benchmarking*.

Expectations

It is well documented that medication errors occur frequently in hospitals. The wrong medicine, the wrong dose, and the wrong time are all parts of this problem. Although no clinic wants medication errors, there are different ways to respond to this problem. What is the level of expectation for good performance? It could be "zero tolerance for error." It could be that "we will make yearly improvements to continuously reduce our error rate." It could be "everyone has this problem and we are no different" or "we have the best nurses and physicians, so I am sure our error rates are lower than anyone else's." One's performance expectations make a difference. Six Sigma is one method for reducing unwanted events.

Incentive Systems

How does the manager transform the individual worker's desire for a paycheck into a pursuit of organizational goals so that both are achieved exactly together? Incentives are stimuli to affect performance. Adoption of incentives is usually based on the answers to the following questions: Does the incentive contribute to the desired results? Is the incentive acceptable to those workers whose behavior managers wish to affect? Could implementation of the incentives produce other dysfunctional consequences (e.g., rewards for cutting costs might lead inadvertently to reduced quality of care)?

Organizations use both positive and negative incentives. Incentives can be monetary or not. One of the underlying ideas of QI is that monetary incentives are often disruptive. The assumption is that people want to do a good job and that faulty systems, not the intentions or abilities of the employees, prevent that from happening. How can the admissions clerk rapidly process an admission when the computer has crashed? How can the dietary department provide hot food at the bedside when the patient is waiting in the X-ray department? QI calls for management to lead the effort in improving these systems, whereas rewarding individuals monetarily may create rivalry rather than teamwork.

Improving care requires "just in time" data about key quality characteristics and an observer who has the expertise to understand this information, whose job it is to improve care, and who is given the power to do so. For example, say the goal is to reduce the burden of asthma for kids. This is measured by the number of school days missed in a particular area due to asthma. A just-in-time information system would show how many children missed school yesterday (not last year or even last month). An asthma expert has the assignment to reduce this rate and is given the power to do something about it. This would likely be an effective system, but there are too few examples of such management approaches in healthcare.

References

Berwick, D. 2002. *Escape Fire: Lessons for the Future of Healthcare.* New York: The Commonwealth Fund.

THE READINGS

How do hospitals and health systems continually improve? HCOs have many stakeholders, including patients and future patients, family, government, payers, insurers, employers, labor unions, professionals, and accreditation agencies, and they all have an interest in the quality and safety of the care given and its cost. The challenge for management is to improve performance while meeting the needs of these multiple stakeholders.

The Malcolm Baldrige National Quality Award recognizes performance excellence by HCOs based on seven areas of focus: leadership; strategic planning; customer focus; measurement, analysis, and knowledge management; workforce focus; operations focus; and results. "Finding the Frontier of Hospital Management" describes how hospitals that have achieved Baldrige recognition have excelled by emphasizing certain areas: communicating the mission, promoting a learning culture, focusing on measurement and benchmarking, and instituting systematic approaches to process improvement. These areas of emphasis have set them above other hospitals and HCOs and have led them to be recognized as among the best.

Finding the Frontier of Hospital Management

John R. Griffith
From *Journal of Healthcare Management* 54 (1): 57–73

Summary

The frontier of demonstrated high-performance community hospital management is a valuable guide to the potential of this important healthcare sector. The best documented frontier cases are recipients of the Malcolm Baldrige National Quality Award, a varied set of 34 US community hospitals in nine states. As validated by trained independent examiners, recipient data suggest that performance at or near the best decile of current distributions can be sustained simultaneously across several critical dimensions. However, these hospitals operate substantially differently from tradition, emphasizing a broadly communicated mission, a supportive learning culture, universal measurement and benchmarking, and systematic process improvement.

A few community hospitals and their associated medical staffs are known to deliver high quality, delight their patients and caregivers, and keep their costs low enough to thrive financially on standard Medicare and insurance payments. Their success has been consistent and stable. They operate across a broad spectrum of metropolitan and rural America (Griffith and White 2005). The best documented and audited members of this set are the recipients of the Malcolm Baldrige National Quality Award (MBNQA): SSM Health Care (based in St. Louis, Missouri) in 2002; Baptist Hospital, Inc., (Pensacola, Florida) in 2003; Saint Luke's Hospital (Kansas City, Missouri) in 2003; Robert Wood Johnson University Hospital (Hamilton, New Jersey) in 2004; Bronson Methodist Hospital (Kalamazoo, Michigan) in 2005; North Mississippi Medical Center (Tupelo, Mississippi) in 2006; Sharp HealthCare (San Diego, California) in 2007; and Mercy Health System (Janesville, Wisconsin) in 2007.

Other than SSM Health Care (SSMHC), Sharp, and Mercy, the recipients are relatively large community hospitals. SSMHC is a system of 20 acute care hospitals (17 at the time of application) and other healthcare enterprises in four states. Sharp is a multihospital integrated health system providing comprehensive services, including health insurance, to a large metropolitan area. Mercy is also an integrated health system that serves a largely rural area around Janesville, a city of 60,000, in southern Wisconsin and northern Illinois. In all, recipients operate in nine states and a range of communities from very rural (Mercy and SSMHC) to large and urban (Sharp). While academic medical centers and impacted urban areas are underrepresented, the set reflects a broad spectrum of American healthcare. The organizations and their settings are described in Exhibit II.2.

Application for the MBNQA requires a 50-page document that responds to its Criteria for Performance Excellence, which cover seven major elements of the organization: (1) leadership; (2) strategic planning; (3) focus on patients, other customers, and markets; (4) measurement analysis and knowledge management; (5) workforce focus; (6) process management; and (7) results. Scoring is based on evidence of *approach*—appropriateness, effectiveness, replicability, and knowledge foundation of work methods; *deployment*—consistency and universality within the organization; *learning*—refinement through cycles of evaluation and encouragement of breakthrough change; and *integration*—alignment with organizational needs across processes and work units and across measurement, information, and improvement systems (Baldrige National Quality Program 2007a, 53).

All Baldrige applications are reviewed and scored by consensus of several individual examiners trained in using the criteria. Forty-five percent of the score is based on measured results in the six process elements

EXHIBIT II.2 Descriptive Characteristics of Malcolm Baldrige National Quality Award Recipients, 2002–2007

Award Year	Organization	Activity Measures	Location	Services
2002	SSM Health Care	151,000 admissions, 22,000 employees	Missouri, Oklahoma, Illinois, Wisconsin	17 hospitals, physician practices, extended care
2003	Baptist Hospital, Inc.	18,000 admissions, 2,270 employees	Pensacola, FL (metropolitan area 500,000)	Comprehensive acute general hospital
2003	Saint Luke's Hospital	3,200 employees, $350 million net revenue	Kansas City, MO (metropolitan area 2,000,000)	Comprehensive acute general hospital affiliated with University of Missouri–Kansas City School of Medicine
2004	Robert Wood Johnson University Hospital	14,000 admissions, 1,650 employees, $160 million net revenue	Hamilton, NJ (suburban community of 100,000 near Trenton)	Comprehensive acute general hospital, affiliated with the Robert Wood Johnson Health System and Network
2005	Bronson Methodist Hospital	22,000 admissions, 3,200 employees, $683 million operating revenue	Kalamazoo, MI (metropolitan area of 300,000)	Comprehensive acute general hospital
2006	North Mississippi Medical Center	142,000 admissions, 56,000 emergency, 249,000 outpatient, 3,900 employees	Tupelo, MS (metropolitan area of 130,000); 72% market share in 7 counties with a total population of 235,000	Comprehensive acute general hospital
2007	Sharp HealthCare	$1.8 billion net revenue	San Diego, CA	Integrated health system, 350,000 insured lives
2007	Mercy Health System	3,700 employees, $500 million net revenue	Janesville, WI	Integrated health system

Note: Data are as of time of application. The Baldrige Criteria allow the applicant to choose measures of performance; the applicants did not report uniformly.

Source: MBNQA Application Summaries, available at www.quality.nist.gov/Contacts_Profiles.htm.

(Health Care, Patient and Other Customer Focused, Financial and Market, Workforce Focused, Process Effectiveness, and Leadership). A few potential recipients are selected from consensus review and site visited by teams of seven or eight examiners who undertake a rigorous 300-hour audit to "verify" the application statements and to "help ensure that the applicant can provide role model practices to the public" (Baldrige National Quality Program 2008a, 2). By Baldrige rules, the recipients must make their applications public, although they are allowed to suppress competitive proprietary details.

Although exact counts are not available, several hundred community hospitals are believed to be making "the journey" to the Baldrige, generally a multiyear series of local (and later national) submissions. Only the national award recipients are obligated to release their applications; the submissions and names of others are deliberately kept confidential.

This article analyzes the published applications to summarize results and identify the most recent developments in the processes recipients use to achieve and sustain excellence.

Findings

Achievements of Baldrige Recipients

In the Results section, applicants are expected to provide data on actual performance in six categories of outcomes—Health Care, Patient and Other Customer Focused, Financial and Market, Workforce Focused, Process Effectiveness, and Leadership—reflecting the applicant's core business requirements and strategy, with benchmarks and evidence of improved results over time. "The use of this composite of measures is intended to ensure that strategies are balanced—that they do not inappropriately trade off among important stakeholders, objectives, or short- and longer-term goals" (Baldrige National Quality Program 2007a, 7).

Exhibit II.3 shows the achievements of the first eight healthcare recipients. Recent (2006–2007) recipients have averaged 150 different measures, about two-thirds higher than the initial (2002–2003) recipients. The greatest growth has been in the two categories of Health Care and Patient and Other Customer Focused. Financial and Market measures remained stable, and Leadership grew only slightly. The percentage of measures subject to external comparison (i.e., excluding the "no benchmark" measures) has increased, as has the number actually achieving best quartile or better comparative performance. Mercy's 89 percent of reported comparable measures actually in the best quartile, and more than half in the best decile, have become the new standard of excellence.

EXHIBIT II.3 Results Data Reported by Baldrige Recipients, 2002–2006

Outcomes	Healthcare	Patient and Other Customer Focused	Financial and Market	Workforce Focused	Process Effectiveness	Leadership	All Measures
SSM Health Care	—[a]	16	9	15	22	—[a]	62
Best quartile[b]		0	2	1	3		6
Best decile[b]		8	0	1	0		9
No benchmark[c]		3	5	3	11		22
Best quartile attainment		62%	50%	17%	27%		38%
Baptist Hospital, Inc.	17	13	13	13	15	5	76
Best quartile	0	3	0	5	2	0	15
Best decile	4	5	0	0	1	0	5
No benchmark	2	2	9	5	3	5	26
Best quartile attainment	27%	73%	0%	63%	25%	0%	40%
Saint Luke's Hospital	16	13	11	13	14	6	73
Best quartile	0	0	2	0	3	0	5
Best decile	5	8	2	2	1	0	18
No benchmark	0	0	6	3	1	4	14
Best quartile attainment	31%	62%	80%	20%	31%	0%	39%

Outcomes	Health Care	Patient and Other Customer Focused	Financial and Market	Workforce Focused	Process Effectiveness	Leadership	All Measures
Robert Wood Johnson University Hospital	26	20	17	25	17	14	119
Best quartile	2	1	3	0	1	1	8
Best decile	14	15	0	12	10	8	59
No benchmark	1	4	10	1	1	0	17
Best quartile attainment	64%	100%	43%	50%	69%	64%	66%
Bronson Methodist Hospital	25	30	30	25	23	31	164
Best quartile	1	2	15	0	0	0	18
Best decile	15	17	1	13	5	0	51
No benchmark	0	0	6	0	0		6
Best quartile attainment	64%	63%	67%	52%	22%	0%	44%
North Mississippi Medical Center	69	22	8	31	33	11	174
Best quartile	10	1	4	0	0	0	15
Best decile	23	13	0	14	9	0	59
No benchmark	0	2	3	11	1	3	20
Best quartile attainment	48%	70%	80%	70%	28%	0%	48%
Mercy Health System	36	38	18	29	21	10	135
Best quartile	11	14	8	3	1	0	37
Best decile	27	0	0	20	3	5	55
No benchmark	0	4	10	5	9	4	32
Best quartile attainment	100%	78%	100%	96%	33%	83%	89%
Sharp HealthCare	33	27	13	25	25	11	134
Best quartile	4	17	2	3	3	0	29
Best decile	12	2	1	14	11	2	42
No benchmark	4	5	6	3	1	7	26
Best quartile attainment	55%	86%	43%	77%	58%	50%	66%

[a]The MBNQA Criteria established different categories for results reporting in 2003. SSM Health Care reported several measures appropriate to the missing categories in other categories.

[b]Application summaries indicate comparative performance, usually as "averages," "best quartiles," "best deciles," or "benchmarks." The Baldrige Criteria defined *benchmarks* as follows (Baldrige National Quality Program 2007a, 67):

The term "benchmarks" refers to processes and results that represent best practices and performance for similar activities, inside or outside an organization's industry. Organizations engage in benchmarking to understand the current dimensions of world-class performance and to achieve discontinuous (nonincremental) or "breakthrough" improvement.

In this table, any entry in "best decile" exceeds the 90th percentile, or is a perfect score, or exceeds a "benchmark" identified by the applicant.

[c]Two kinds of measures cannot reasonably be benchmarked: (1) embedded in local situation, such as volume or market share, and (2) uniquely defined by applicant, such as "ethical behaviors" or "governance principles." Category 1 is several times more common than category 2.

Applicants are free to choose their own measures, and they obviously select their best examples. Examiners will expect documentation of all critical operations and important business units. The Baldrige recipients documented balanced excellence across the following areas:

1. *Process and outcomes measures of quality of care.* The measures selected varied widely in early years. Recent recipients have reported selectively from the

Centers for Medicare & Medicaid Services' (CMS) Hospital Compare measures, often showing benchmark performance. Overall, on the subset of ten measures selected by the Dartmouth Institute for Health Policy and Clinical Practice (2008), MBNQA recipients exceeded means for their referral regions in 14 of 19 hospitals with sufficient data.

2. *Patient and customer satisfaction.* Six of the recipients achieved best decile performance on overall patient satisfaction measures. All eight were above the third-quartile level. Baptist (2003, 36) noted that it had "consistently ranked among the top percentile for the inpatient database over five years."

3. *Financial stability.* All recipients documented substantial financial performance, reflected in earnings, funds available for expansion and community service, and bond ratings.

4. *Worker satisfaction and retention.* The last six recipients documented best decile performance in both satisfaction and retention. Most had turnover rates less than 10 percent per year in nursing and in all personnel.

5. *Physician satisfaction.* Measures of physician satisfaction were not reported until 2006. The last four recipients showed that their physicians were satisfied and loyal to the organization.

6. *Efficiency and cost control.* Recipients routinely documented below-average length of stay and cost per case. They did not report more global, population-based costs. Mercy and Sharp operate health insurance companies, but these were not the focus of their applications. The Dartmouth Institute for Health Policy and Clinical Practice (2008) has developed per capita measures for the last two years of life. The recipient hospitals tended to be higher than their referral region and slightly higher than national averages on both total Medicare expenditures and intensive care unit days. (The regional comparison may reflect selection mechanisms within the region.)

Processes Supporting Recipient Achievement

Across all industrial sectors, the Baldrige Criteria expect rigorous implementation of "management by fact," "focus on results and creating value," and "systems perspective" (Baldrige National Quality Program 2007a, 1). They expect strategic management based on extensive, ongoing environmental surveillance; an explicit process for setting quantitative goals at all levels of the organization; and intensive continuous monitoring. They expect systematic, ongoing analysis and improvement of work processes and a growing battery of measures, trends, and goals. In working toward these goals, the health-care recipients also emphasized increased understanding of workers' needs for training, support, and incentives. The recipients also deliberately changed supervisor roles and behavior, pursuing a "service excellence" concept, whereby meeting worker needs assists and motivates them to seek and meet customer needs (Heskett, Sasser, and Schlesinger 1997). While these basic concepts are now the recommended standard of hospital operation (Griffith and White 2007), it is not clear how widely they are practiced outside the Baldrige group.

The model that emerged from all eight healthcare recipient applications incorporates the following elements:

a. *Emphasis upon mission, vision, and values.* Mission, vision, and values (MVV) statements become a point of consensus for all stakeholders and a touchstone for resolving priorities in a continuous improvement environment. All eight recipients referenced "best," "excellent," or "exceptional" care (see Exhibit II.4). Many organizations use these terms in MVV statements but do not use the MVV in daily operations. The Baldrige alignment, deployment, and integration criteria demand that the MVV are frequently referenced, used as a basis for organizational decisions, and used explicitly to shape the culture. Recipients drew on the MVV constantly to identify areas for improvement where measured performance falls short of those goals.

The words "profit," "earnings," or "financial" do not appear in any of the MVV in Exhibit II.4. The recipients' statements expanded on and redirect "no margin, no mission," saying instead, "the right mission is the path to satisfactory margins." They recognized the more fundamental importance of satisfying patients, employees, and physicians. One way or another, all recipients noted that they must maintain financial stability under pricing and competitive pressures. They noted the threats of personnel shortages, declining payment, competition with physicians, and rising stakeholder expectations. The path they chose to meet these challenges was "excellence in patient care."

b. *Responsive leadership and worker empowerment.* All recipients made extensive, structured efforts to listen to and communicate with their stakeholders, particularly their patients, employees, and physicians. Much management time was consumed in listening, communicating, and negotiating. Several hours per week of "rounding"—face-to-face contact with frontline personnel—were mandatory for all higher management levels. Sharp claimed that its "leaders regularly walk around in their functional area to visit and communicate with employees/customers/ partners, including suppliers/partners, to connect on a personal level, validate values/direction, solicit upward communication, identify needs for tools and equipment, provide recognition, and ensure satisfaction." Logs or diaries of rounds were analyzed for improvement opportunities (Sharp HealthCare 2007, 9). At North Mississippi Medical Center

(NMMC) and Baptist, "servant leadership" was expected (Calhoun, Griffith, and Sinioris 2007). The concept here is that managers are obligated to respond to worker and other stakeholder needs. This empowers the workers, allowing them to remove handicaps to performance. Recipients used a wide variety of communications devices in addition to rounding.

EXHIBIT II.4 Mission, Vision, and Values of Baldrige Recipients

Organization	Mission	Vision	Values
SSM Health Care	Through our exceptional health care services, we reveal the healing presence of God.	Communities, especially those that are . . . marginalized, will experience improved health in mind, body, spirit and environment.	Compassion, respect, excellence, stewardship, community
Baptist Hospital, Inc.	To provide superior service based on Christian values to improve the quality of life for people and communities served.	To become the best health system in America.	Integrity, vision, innovation, superior service, stewardship, teamwork
Saint Luke's Hospital	Highest levels of excellence in . . . health services to all patients in a caring environment.	Best place to get care, best place to give care.	Quality excellence, customer focus, resource management, teamwork
Robert Wood Johnson University Hospital	Excellence through service. We exist to promote, preserve and restore the health of our community.	To passionately pursue the health and well-being of our patients, employees and the community.	Quality, understanding, excellence, service, teamwork
Bronson Methodist Hospital	Provide excellent healthcare services.	National leader in healthcare quality.	Care and respect, teamwork, stewardship, commitment to community, pursuit of excellence
North Mississippi Medical Center	To continuously improve the health of the people of our region.	To be the provider of the best patient-centered care and health services in America . . .	Compassion, accountability, respect, excellence, smile
Mercy Health System	The Mission of Mercy Health System is to provide exceptional healthcare services resulting in healing in the broadest sense.	Quality—Excellence in patient care Service—Exceptional patient and customer service Partnering—Best place to work Cost—Long-term financial success	Healing in its broadest sense, patients come first, treat each other like family, strive for excellence
Sharp HealthCare	To improve the health of those we serve with a commitment to excellence in all that we do. Sharp's goal is to offer quality care and services that set community standards, exceed patients' expectations, and are provided in a caring, convenient, cost-effective, and accessible manner.	Sharp will redefine the health care experience through a culture of caring, quality, service, innovation, and excellence. Sharp will be recognized by employees, physicians, patients, volunteers, and the community as the best place to work, the best place to practice medicine, and the best place to receive care.	Integrity, caring, innovation, excellence

Source: MBNQA Application Summaries, available at www.quality.nist.gov/Contacts_Profiles.htm.

The emphasis on listening and responding creates a culture in which the contract between the individual and the organization is negotiated, rather than imposed. Agreement is reached, rather than orders being given. Subordinates are encouraged to ask questions and can expect to have those questions answered. This characteristic is critical to building worker satisfaction and loyalty, and it is a relatively recent development in organizations in general. It is reinforced by frequent rewards for desired behavior and formal incentive payments.

Baldrige Criteria expect all organizations to "exceed requirements and excel in areas of legal and ethical behavior" and to partner with other organizations for the benefit of their communities. All the healthcare recipients pursued the highest standards in governance. They specified and achieved goals for community benefit, collaborated extensively with physician organizations and also with competing hospitals and community agencies, and voluntarily accepted relevant Sarbanes-Oxley Act provisions.

c. *Strategic planning.* The recipients followed a rigorous yearly planning cycle of environmental analysis; opportunity identification; and a cascading system of goal setting, process improvement teams, and results deployment. Saint Luke's graphic model is simpler than reality, but it illustrates the process (see Exhibit II.5).

d. *Patient, customer, and healthcare market knowledge.* All the recipients pursued a deliberate strategy of market growth through excellent patient service. Baptist claimed to have a "culture obsessed with patient care and

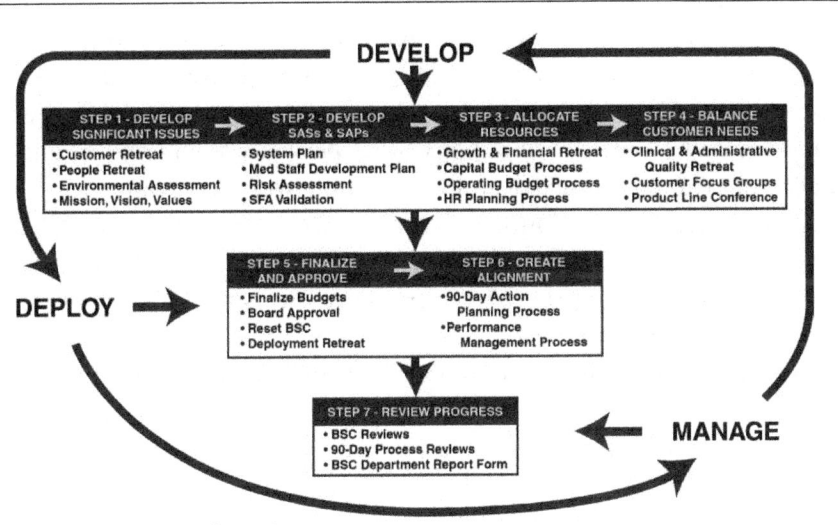

EXHIBIT II.5
Saint Luke's Hospital Strategic Planning Process

Source: Saint Luke's Hospital of Kansas City.

customer satisfaction." Each patient was encouraged to call the clinical unit leader's cell phone or the hospital president's home phone at "any time of the day or night, if they have an issue." In the event of an adverse customer event, any employee could call a special hotline to log the event, get financial assistance for service recovery, and document action. A team of two employees made approximately 120 calls per month to referring physicians, systematically inquiring about service needs and service experiences of their patients (Baptist Hospital, Inc. 2003, 10, 14, 20).

What distinguishes Baptist is the extent of deployment. The core—contacts, service recovery, event analysis, and risk reduction—is universal for Baldrige recipients. The result is a steadily declining rate of unfortunate incidents of all kinds.

e. Measurement, analysis, and improvement of performance. Every work team in these organizations had benchmarks and short-term goals for multiple measures of performance. All the recipients had careful procedures to define, capture, validate, and audit the measures. Managers received extensive training and direct support to use measures effectively. Formal systems of process analysis and improvement, such as Lean and Six Sigma, were often used, but their use was as a supplement to a general program of continuous improvement. The result is an environment where objective measures and data drive performance, rather than history, tradition, or professional domains of authority. The recipients all had concrete plans to expand electronic medical records, but they made measurement and process improvement the foundation of their information strategy.

f. Workforce focus. All the Baldrige recipients' workforce management strategies emphasized creating a stable, enthusiastic workforce that was responsive to training and made training cost effective. Beginning with careful selection and orientation, recipients provided 80 or more hours of training per worker per year, flexible hours and benefits, assurance of a safe and comfortable work environment, competitive compensation, and bonuses. They carefully trained first-line supervisors in responsive behavior. They implemented their value of respect with programs to promote diversity and cultural competency and with personal development plans. Bronson listed 33 communication and training mechanisms, including instant messaging, daily huddles, employee neighborhood meetings, computer-based learning, self-study modules, skill fairs, and learning labs. Each employee developed three work-related personal goals (Bronson Methodist Hospital 2005, 19–20).

Discussion

The reported results show that Baldrige recipients frequently achieved best decile responses that simultaneously met a broad spectrum of stakeholder needs. Many of the measures presented show high performance sustained over several years prior to receiving the award. The Baldrige approach is shown to benefit all constituents in a variety of operating situations and over several years, strongly suggesting that it is both stable and replicable. In 2007 interviews, the CEOs of the first six recipients indicated that their organizations were working to reapply. That is, the Baldrige approach not only moved their organization to excellence, but they viewed it as an effective way to sustain excellence (Calhoun, Griffith, and Sinioris 2007, 18).

Studies of the validity of the Baldrige approach are supportive of that conclusion. Baldrige recipients in other industries outperform similar organizations (Prybutok and Cutshall 2004). A study of public corporations generally supports the approach taken in the Baldrige Criteria, finding that the linkage of the strategic quality planning process with performance measures and analysis is associated with improved performance (Ghosh et al. 2003). A survey of healthcare organizations identified significant positive relationships between hospitals' adherence to the Baldrige Criteria (independent of actual Baldrige applications) and their results in patient and customer satisfaction, staff and work systems, and organization-specific results (Goldstein and Schweikhart 2002).

The processes documented in the applications describe an approach to management that is a radical departure from hospital traditions, which have tended to emphasize static domains of authority rather than formally measured performance, goal setting, and continuous improvement. The underlying mechanisms that support the results can be grouped into three interacting dynamics:

1. Empowerment and the emphasis on learning generate strong worker loyalty and improved capability. These workers provide better patient care and customer satisfaction.
2. Steadily improved work processes create an efficient organization that is easily capable of success within prevailing market prices.
3. Strategies are carefully developed, and trustees are attentive to identifying and responding to market trends.

As these dynamics evolve and interact, better work processes reduce worker frustration and injuries, supporting loyalty. They also reduce costs, improving financial performance. Better patient and physician satisfaction increase patient volumes, further improving finances. The funds are used in part to reward the workforce. Strategic monitoring keeps the organization responsive to all stakeholder needs, supporting long-term success.

The sample is small and incomplete, but not atypical. There is no obvious reason that the recipients' model cannot be replicated; the critical resources are mastery of the concepts and commitment rather than capital, a preferred location, or a specific scarce resource. Several hundred hospitals seem to be doing so.[1]

The model provides a powerful vehicle to focus hospital operations, improving quality, pleasing patients, eliminating waste, and improving work attractiveness. Hospitals like NMMC that are intent on change report substantial improvements in two or three years (Griffith and White 2003). Overall, the recipients started their programs incrementally and received returns incrementally. Implementing the model does not require a large reserve of surplus capital.

Several important issues deserve consideration.

1. *The cultural transition is a dual change,* from a static relationship featuring domains of authority to a dynamic one featuring measured performance, and from one that emphasizes rank and power to one that emphasizes objective evidence and egalitarian relationships. From a public policy perspective, the transition looks extremely attractive. From the perspective of those currently holding power, it is disruptive and potentially threatening. Managing the transition requires a substantial grasp of detail, probably best acquired by practice in a successful site. It also requires a firm resolve and, for many individuals, a change in professional behavior.

2. *Incentives to encourage hospitals to make the transition are limited.* The recipient organizations made extensive use of rewards, including incentive pay, to encourage and sustain the necessary behavior changes. Important potential gains were visible for patients, doctors, nurses, and other hospital workers. Evidence of actual gain in cost per capita, important to health insurers, is lacking. In the not-for-profit structure of American community hospitals, the only corporate incentive to make the transition is the commitment to service. Improved safety and efficiency resulting from process improvement offer the promise—sustained by the record of the recipients—of improved financial performance. As governing boards contemplate the transition, these potential rewards may not be sufficient to overcome the magnitude and uncertainty surrounding the change.

3. *There are clear potential dangers to using the model in socially dysfunctional ways.* The Baldrige recipients and others pursuing this and similar paths clearly believe the missions and visions solidly within a tradition of Samaritanism and communitarianism. One can easily envision using the model as a powerful marketing tool to sell services with high financial return and low contribution to health. Similarly, a highly effective healthcare organization could deliberately target paying patients to the exclusion of those less well financed.

4. *Standardized national measures can improve both the rate of transition and the likelihood of socially useful results.* Common measures establish a de facto control on the direction of improvement. Benchmarking requires careful standardization of data and audited results. As consensus emerges on measures, the existence of valid comparisons becomes a strong incentive. CMS's Hospital Compare measures and generally accepted accounting measures such as net income and EBITDA (earnings before income, taxes, depreciation, and amortization) are good examples. Additional measures that are standardized and reliably calculated will be accepted and will shape the definition of high performance. Developing measures for community benefit, cost per capita, and health effectiveness will shape the direction of growth.

5. *Public reporting and incorporation into payment could stimulate transitions.* Current trends in payment plans and public release of data have increased attention to quality and safety. Payment plans and public release of comparative data tracking the outcomes measure established in the Baldrige Criteria are likely to be a powerful stimulus. Most important, they would allow governing board members a substantially clearer picture of corporate performance.

As the criteria argue, balance is important. Ideally, payment plans should reward excellence on all the Baldrige Results dimensions. Omissions of measures or careless implementation of rewards could create serious imbalances. For example, the Leadership outcome should include measures to promote community health and to provide for uninsured patients. Publicizing or compensating these measures will predictably raise attention; ignoring them will increase per capita cost. Public reporting of composite measures of cost per capita or insurance benefit costs per member could have several beneficial effects. It would increase focus on a core issue—financing our national healthcare. It might encourage health insurers to pursue Baldrige concepts. (There are no insurance companies among the 75 MBNQA recipients.) Increased attention to end-of-life care measures, such as those developed by the Dartmouth Institute, would encourage consensus on this complex question.

In the markets where Baldrige recipients compete, these organizations are generally capturing market share. Their competitors are losing share. The CEOs of these organizations noted continued progress and universally expected to file additional Baldrige applications (Calhoun, Griffith, and Sinioris 2007). If the approach these hospitals have developed becomes more widespread, hospitals that do not follow the trend will ultimately face two basic solutions—recover, probably by adopting the model that has proven successful, or merge with other organizations. Both solutions have substantial merit in an environment where success reflects superior ability to meet stakeholder needs.

Note

1. The Baldrige National Quality Program (2008b) reported 43 healthcare applicants out of a total of 85 for 2008. Most applicants begin at the state level; 43 states have programs. In 2006, the states had a total of 426 applications, but sector-specific counts are not available (Baldrige National Quality Program 2007b). The ratio of 43/85 suggests that at least 200 hospitals are in some stage of the journey.

References

Baldrige National Quality Program. 2008a. *Site Visit Manual*. Accessed July 6, 2012. www. quality.nist.gov/Word_files/2007_Site_ Visit_Manual.doc.

———. 2008b. "Baldrige Process News." Accessed July 6, 2012. www.quality.nist .gov/Baldrige_Process_ news.htm.

———. 2007a. "Criteria for Performance Excellence." Accessed July 6, 2012. www .quality.nist.gov/Criteria.htm.

———. 2007b. *Malcolm Baldrige National Quality Award: Program Impacts*. Accessed July 6, 2012. www.quality.nist.gov/Ambassador/Slides/2007_ Program_Impacts.ppt.

Baptist Hospital, Inc. 2003. "Baldrige National Quality Award Application Summary." *Baldrige Performance Excellence Program*. Accessed July 9, 2012. www .quality.nist.gov/PDF_files/Baptist_Hospital_Application_Summary.pdf.

Bronson Methodist Hospital. 2005. "Baldrige National Quality Award Application Summary." *Baldrige Performance Excellence Program*. Accessed July 9, 2012. www.quality.nist.gov/PDF_files/Bronson_Methodist_Hospital_Application_ Summary.pdf.

Calhoun, J., J. Griffith, and M. Sinioris. 2007. "New Insights in Leadership Strategies: Achieving Organizational Excellence Using the Baldrige Framework."

National Center for Healthcare Leadership Supplement. *Modern Healthcare* December 13, 9–19.

Dartmouth Institute for Health Policy and Clinical Practice. 2008. *Dartmouth Atlas of Health Care*. Accessed July 9, 2012. www.dartmouthatlas.org.

Ghosh, S., R. B. Handfield, V. R. Kannan, and K. C. Tan. 2003. "A Structural Model Analysis of the Malcolm Baldrige National Quality Award Framework." *International Journal of Management & Decision Making* 4 (4): 289.

Goldstein, S. M., and S. B. Schweikhart. 2002. "Empirical Support for the Baldrige Award Framework in U.S. Hospitals." *Healthcare Management Review* 27 (1): 62–75.

Griffith, J. R., and K. R. White. 2007. *The Well-Managed Healthcare Organization*, 6th ed. Chicago: Health Administration Press.

———. 2005. "The Revolution in Hospital Management." *Journal of Healthcare Management* 50 (3): 170–200.

———. 2003. *Thinking Forward: Six Strategies for Highly Successful Organizations*. Chicago: Health Administration Press.

Heskett, J. L., W. E. Sasser Jr., and L. A. Schlesinger. 1997. *The Service Profit Chain: How Leading Companies Link Profit and Growth to Loyalty, Satisfaction, and Value*. New York: Free Press.

Mercy Health System. 2007. "Baldrige National Quality Award Application Summary." *Baldrige Performance Excellence Program*. Accessed July 9, 2012. www.quality.nist.gov/PDF_files/2007_Mercy_Application_Summary.pdf.

Prybutok, V., and R. Cutshall. 2004. "Malcolm Baldrige National Quality Award Leadership Model." *Industrial Management & Data Systems* 104 (7): 558–66.

Sharp HealthCare. 2007. "Baldrige National Quality Award Application Summary." *Baldrige Performance Excellence Program*. Accessed July 9, 2012. www.quality.nist.gov/PDF_files/2007_Sharp_Application_Summary.pdf.

Discussion Questions

1. How would you advise the CEO of a 75-bed hospital who is interested in becoming a Baldrige winner? Where should she start?

2. How can the Baldrige Criteria be used to improve care in all hospitals?

3. As CEO, how would you react if the competing hospital in your market won the Baldrige Award? What would you focus on in your institution?

4. Suppose your neigbor came to you and said, "I have just been diagnosed with X condition (for example, diabetes, multiple sclerosis, or the need for heart surgery). Can you help me find a high-quality provider for my condition?" Pick a condition and see what you can find on the Internet about good care.

Required Supplementary Readings

Berwick, D. M. 2005. "My Right Knee." *Annals of Internal Medicine* 142 (2): 121–25.

Bradley, E. H., E. S. Holmoe, J. A. Mattera, S. A. Roumanis, M. J. Radford, and H. M. Krumholz. 2003. "The Roles of Senior Management in Quality Improvement Efforts: What Are the Key Components?" *Journal of Healthcare Management* 48 (1): 15–28.

Curry, L. A., E. Spatz, E. Cherlin, J. W. Thompson, D. Berg, H. H. Ting, C. Decker, H. M. Krumholz, and E. H. Bradley. 2011. "What Distinguishes Top-Performing Hospitals in Acute Myocardial Infarction Mortality Rates? A Qualitative Study." *Annals of Internal Medicine* 154: 384–90.

James, B., and L. Savitz. 2011. "How Intermountain Trimmed Health Care Costs Through Robust Quality Improvement Efforts." *Health Affairs* 30 (6): 1185–91.

Jha, A. K., J. B. Perlin, K. W. Kizer, and R. A. Dudley. 2003. "Effect of the Transformation of the Veterans Affairs Healthcare System on the Quality of Care." *New England Journal of Medicine* 348 (22): 2218–27.

Discussion Questions for the Required Supplementary Readings

1. For any specific HCO, what are the most important things for the information system to measure?
2. Errors are frequent in healthcare. They often have serious consequences. What would you recommend to reduce medical errors?
3. What is the role of senior management in promoting quality improvement?
4. What are the barriers to cost containment in HCOs, and how can these be overcome?

Recommended Supplementary Readings

Batalden, P., and P. Stoltz. 1993. "Performance Improvement in Healthcare Organizations: A Framework for the Continued Improvement of Health Care." *The Joint Commission Journal of Quality Improvement* 19 (10): 424–52.

Berwick, D. M. 1995. "The Toxicity of Pay for Performance." *Quality Management in Health Care* 9 (1): 27–33.

Black, J. 2008. *The Toyota Way to Healthcare Excellence*. Chicago: Health Administration Press.

Eisenberg, J. M. 1996. *Doctors' Decisions and the Cost of Medical Care*. Chicago: Health Administration Press.

Gawande, A. 2004. "The Bell Curve." *The New Yorker*, December 6, 82–91.

Glandon, G. L., D. Smaltz, and D. J. Slovensky. 2008. *Austin and Boxerman's Information Systems for Healthcare Management*, 7th ed. Chicago: Health Administration Press.

Griffith, J. R., and K. R. White. 2010. "Creating Excellent Governance." In *Reaching Excellence in Healthcare Management,* 61–79. Chicago: Health Administration Press.

———. 2007. *The Well-Managed Healthcare Organization*, 6th ed. Chicago: Health Administration Press.

Hebert, C., and D. Neuhauser. 2004. "Improving Hypertension Care with Patient Generated Run Charts: Physician, Patient and Management Perspectives." *Quality Management in Health Care* 13 (3): 174–77.

Institute of Medicine. 2001. *Crossing the Quality Chasm*. Washington, DC: National Academies Press.

Lewis, L. E. 1996. "Improving Productivity: The Ongoing Experience of an Academic Department of Medicine." *Academic Medicine* 71 (4): 317–28.

Longo, D. R., J. A. Hewett, B. Ge, and S. Schubert. 2007. "Hospital Patient Safety: Characteristics of Best-Performing Hospitals." *Journal of Healthcare Management* 52 (3): 188–204.

McDonagh, K. J. 2006. "Hospital Governing Boards: A Study of Their Effectiveness in Relation to Organizational Performance." *Journal of Healthcare Management* 51 (6): 377–89.

McGlynn, E. A., S. M. Asch, J. Adams, J. Keesey, J. Hicks, A. DeCristofaro, and E. Kerr. 2003. "The Quality of Health Care Delivered to Adults in the United States." *New England Journal of Medicine* 348 (26): 2635–45.

McLaughlin, D., and J. Hays. 2008. *Healthcare Operations Management*. Chicago: Health Administration Press.

Pointer, D. D., and J. E. Orlikoff. 2002. *Getting to Great: Principles of Health Care Organization Governance*. San Francisco: Jossey-Bass.

Rindler, M. E. 2007. "Extraordinary Success at Northeast Georgia Medical Center." In *Strategic Cost Reduction,* 33–44. Chicago: Health Administration Press.

Rundall, T. G., P. F. Martelli, L. Arroyo, R. McCurdy, I. Graetz, E. B. Neuwirth, P. Curtis, J. Schmittdiel, M. Gibson, and J. Hsu. 2007. "The Informed Decisions Tool-Box: Tools for Knowledge Transfer and Performance Improvement." *Journal of Healthcare Management* 52 (5): 325–41.

Umbdenstock, R. J., and W. M. Hageman. 1990. "The Five Critical Areas for Effective Governance of Non-profit Hospitals." *Hospital and Health Services Administration* 35 (4): 481–92.

Watts, B., R. Lawrence, D. Litaker, D. C. Aron, and D. Neuhauser. 2008. "Quality of Care by a Hypertension Expert: A Cautionary Tale for Pay-for-Performance Approaches." *Quality Management in Health Care* 17 (1): 35–46.

Yap, C., E. Siu, G. R. Baker, and A. D. Brown. 2005. "A Comparison of Systemwide and Hospital-Specific Performance Tools." *Journal of Healthcare Management* 50 (4): 251–62.

Zelman, W. N., D. Blazer, J. M. Gower, P. O. Bumgarner, and L. M. Cancilla. 1999. "Issues for Academic Health Centers to Consider Before Implementing a Balanced Scorecard Effort." *Academic Medicine* 74 (12): 1269–77.

* * * * * *

In addition to the readings, these three journals about quality and safety are worth following:

The Joint Commission Journal on Quality and Patient Safety, www.jcrinc .com/Periodicals/. (At this site, also check out the Codman Award videos for interesting examples of excellence in care improvements.)

BMJ Quality and Safety, qualitysafety.bmj.com.

Quality Management in Health Care, www.qmhcjournal.com.

THE CASES

Peter Drucker (1973) commented, "The basic problem of service institutions is not high cost, but lack of effectiveness." In those days, all hospitals believed they provided the best care with the best nurses and doctors, and patients believed these claims in the absence of any information to the contrary. However, three recent trends with glacier-like power have changed this perception. First is the development and acceptance of evidence-based medicine. How do we know the care we give is beneficial? The Cochrane Collaboration (www.cochrane.org) has now published more than 5,000 reviews (Cochrane Reviews) summarizing the results of thousands of randomized clinical trials that demonstrate treatment effectiveness or the lack of it. Now that much more evidence-based agreement exists about what works, creating clinical guidelines for best-practice care and asking that they be followed are easy.

The quality and safety movement is the second major force for change. The quality improvement movement encourages the use of best practices for all patients, and disparity research focuses on who and what groups do not get such good care.

The third and most important force in the long run is the steady, relentless growth of computer capacity combined with the declining cost of computing power. While the first health management applications were for insurance billing and finance, the new wave emerging is related to clinical information.

The three case studies that follow reflect the process of control in different healthcare organizations. Case D by D'Aquila, Follows, Zaccagnino, and Kovner describes the implementation and results of a program designed to improve patient flow in a hospital. Case E by McAlearney shows the importance of focusing on people and high-performance work practices to improve patient safety and quality of care, specifically in the area of reducing healthcare-associated infections. Case F by Victory examines the process and impact of efforts to introduce rigorous performance management expectations in the Visiting Nurse Service of America. These cases all show that we are moving from Drucker's absence of data to information overload.

The six short cases consider parallel issues. These include the introduction of performance measurement concepts for a hospital board (Short Case 7), the introduction of a new piece of equipment designed to reduce staff injuries at a hospital (Short Case 8), analysis of existing budget information (Short Case 9), examination of the issue of handoffs from a hospital emergency department (Short Case 10), and the introduction of an electronic medical record system (Short Case 11).

Reference

Drucker, P. 1973. "Managing the Public Service Institution." *The Public Interest* 33: 43–60.

Case D
Moving the Needle: Managing Safe Patient Flow at Yale–New Haven Hospital

Richard D'Aquila, Peter Follows, Michael Zaccagnino, and Anthony R. Kovner

Executive Summary

The purpose of this qualitative case study is to help decision makers learn how to better manage safe patient flow from the experience of Yale–New Haven Hospital (YNHH), a large academic medical center in New Haven, Connecticut. This process had important quality and financial consequences for a hospital constrained by limited capacity. Hospitals have to make tremendous changes to cope with circumstances under healthcare reform that include lower payments relative to higher costs of providing services.

What follows is a description of how YNHH's Safe Patient Flow (SPF) Project achieved significant decreases in average lengths of stay and in waiting times for beds in the emergency department (ED) and in the post anesthesia care unit (PACU) during a period of considerable growth in hospital admissions. These improvements were accomplished in part by changes such as discharging patients earlier in the day, decreasing bed turnaround times, and improving patient job transportation turnaround times. YNHH improved safety, quality, patient and staff satisfaction, and efficiency—all while achieving significant positive financial results.

For more information about this case study, please contact Professor Kovner at anthony.kovner@nyu.edu.

The Challenge: Implementing Significant Change Without a Crisis

How can a hospital ensure safe patient flow while improving safety, quality, patient and staff satisfaction, and financial health? How can a large academic medical center accommodate incremental admissions volume without adding positions?

This case study suggests that positive results can be achieved through more effective management.

The results achieved during a two-year period starting July 2008 are impressive indeed:

- Average length of stay (ALOS) decreased from an average 5.23 to 5.02 days year to date through June 2009.
- LOS in the ED for patients being admitted was decreased by 25 minutes, despite significant increases in ED volume.
- Percentage of discharges by 11:00 a.m. increased 50 percent, from 12 to 18 percent on average.
- Median time of discharge decreased by 45 minutes.
- PACU length of stay decreased by approximately 25 minutes, and the percentage of "red phones" (an indication of a transfer delay out of the PACU) was further decreased by 8 percent in the past nine months.
- Bed turnaround time decreased by 35 minutes, on average, for priority 1 bed assignments (those bed assignments that are higher priority because a patient is awaiting a bed).
- Patient transport time (i.e., transport turnaround time) remained within 30 minutes, despite the addition of a new Cancer Hospital Pavilion. (Transport turnaround time has two components: (1) how long it takes to assign the transport job after it has been requested, and (2) how long it takes to complete the transport from when it is assigned to when it ends.)

An example of improved outcomes involves the times when patients were actually discharged. The hospital uses green, yellow, and red indicators to predict likely readiness for discharge the next day. Green indicates very likely to be discharged the next day; yellow indicates clinically ready for discharge the next day but recognizes that this readiness will be contingent on certain things (e.g., pending laboratory results or the ability to tolerate a diet); and red indicates not likely to be clinically ready for discharge the next day or an appropriate disposition is not available. The disposition requires that the interdisciplinary team be in close communication with one another regarding both clinical status and appropriate disposition resources. Opposition by some physicians had to be overcome as they said they needed to see their sickest patients first (rather than those most ready for discharge).

Implementing this process change at YNHH had six phases: (1) creating the urgency for change, (2) framing the process properly, (3) ensuring proper staff support and systems, (4) engaging physicians, (5) building accountability and transparency, and (6) ensuring sustainability of change. We discuss these phases and conclude with lessons learned from the initiative.

1. Creating the Urgency for Change

YNHH had a backlog of patients, resulting in part from physician recruitment and program development that had temporarily outpaced facilities development (i.e., the opening of a new cancer center). Rick D'Aquila, the YNHH chief operating officer (COO), actively participated in and sponsored the SPF initiative, which included creating "a burning platform" for planning and implementing the change.

> *Associate chief of staff and vice president of performance management:* "In 2008, The Joint Commission said YNHH lacked an organized way of responding to capacity problems. I was the first director of bed management before I moved into my present job. The initiative was not so much about discharging patients faster as it was about getting the right patient into the right bed at the right time. The sickest patients were in the ED, and the critical staff to take care of them were waiting for them on the patient floors. The question was which patients should these physicians be seeing."

2. Framing the Process Properly

A steering committee was appointed as the ultimate authority for decision making. Carpedia International was hired as a consulting firm. Nursing leadership conducted weekly meetings prior to steering committee meetings. Safety was the first priority. The second priority was actively managing organizational resources. Frontline leaders and employees met daily to review schedules (i.e., in "huddles") and provide daily operating reports. Accountability was data driven relative to targets and time frames.

Prior to their engagement, Carpedia carried out an "opportunity analysis" to identify areas of particular gain, in terms of quantifiable financial results. This analysis took five consultants nearly three weeks to complete. Carpedia began by identifying and quantifying specifically what processes needed improvement. It next identified functional areas and support departments that would need to be involved. Support departments included transport, environmental services, admissions, and bed management. Outcomes were set for each area: for example, room turnover time (for environmental services) and turnover time (for patient transportation). Carpedia identified the main database indicator as reduction of ALOS from 5.23 to 5.02 days—primarily for adult medical and surgical patients.

Nurse directors quantified reasons for variances. Unit huddles were conducted three times a day for ten minutes each to review which patients were going home and which patients could go home if barriers were overcome (e.g., nursing home transfer or organizing rides home).

3. Ensuring Proper Staff Support and Systems

To assess YNHH's readiness to carry out the project, Carpedia's opportunity analysis set up targets and time frames relating to performance gaps in current processes. The seven-person operations support (OS) department provided consulting, behavior audit, support, and coaching. Execution controls were established to allow managers to monitor and prioritize assignments for both clinical and nonclinical managers. Daily operational supports gave a balanced set of key performance indicators, comparing actual to planned performance.

OS partnered with Carpedia, and four internal YNHH staff members were pulled out of their jobs to work with the six Carpedia consultants. Carpedia used the client's own performance data to describe current and desired states rather than relying solely on industry benchmarks:

> *Carpedia consultant:* "Carpedia spends 50 to 60 percent of its time in the pre-proposal phase, observing processes. This allows us to quantify "lost time." We can then play it back to the client so they can see what their employees are going through to get certain processes completed. We also observed the patient's experience through her eyes. We followed through an entire process for 20 patients and for 30 eight-hour employee shifts, observing managers, nurses, and physicians."

4. Engaging Physicians

YNHH augmented the Carpedia team (which lacked physicians and nurses) with a team of two physicians, one nurse, one pharmacist, and one financial analyst. Different service lines wanted to "own" their own beds. Centralized bed placement proved more effective in reducing wait for the PACU and for the ED.

For the first year, the associate chief of staff was chair of the steering committee. He explained to physicians that the basic premise of the initiative was to reduce crowding of the PACU and the ED by discharging patients earlier in the day. When patients were admitted later in the day, house staff could not treat these patients promptly. These delays caused a poor match of resources, as house staff were needed for discharge summaries, prescription orders, and counsel on postdischarge care. The early discharge initiative was also in conflict with the scheduled teaching program because the house staff had educational responsibilities that might not be well timed with the need for early discharges. Under the SPF initiative, the discharge process begins the evening before the scheduled discharge. Residents huddle together and identify patients likely to leave and then work to facilitate earlier discharge by completing tasks such as notifying the family. Success in reducing waiting times generated a cascade of support for the SPF initiative.

Associate chief of staff and medical director of hospitalist service: "When physicians in the ED saw improvements in waiting times for beds, this was a motivator.... Now there was less delay in moving patients from interventional radiology, no cancelling of elective surgery cases, and more patients moving quickly through the system. ORs had been on hold because patients were sitting in the PACU. We now track all the waits. And we discharge every surgery patient to their floor of preference, such as oncological surgery, for more specialized care, post-op."

5. Building Accountability and Transparency

Carpedia met with the YNHH leadership team on a weekly basis. The steering committee navigated much of the work. Carpedia presented the work that had been done last week and what was going to be done in the next two weeks. Teams used dashboard and targets and reviewed variances for identified performance measures. (See Exhibit II.6 for excerpts from the YNHH executive throughput scorecard, which tracks throughput for the week ending November 6, 2010.)

Units and departments reported to the steering committee, followed templates, and established desired outcomes. For example, 11:00 a.m. was set as the target discharge time because this was a time when the OR, the PACU, and the ED got congested and when patients were waiting for treatment on the floors. The number of patients discharged by 3:00 p.m. was also measured. The goal was to increase the percentage of patients being discharged earlier rather than changing the hour of discharge for all patients. The median patient discharge time was moved from 3:00 p.m. to 1:30 p.m. Discharge is one of the hospital measures for the performance incentive program, common for all employees and managers and representing 80 percent of the annual performance bonus.

The COO, the steering committee, Carpedia, and OS pushed active management.

Associate director of nursing: "This was not just managing to meet targets, but holding the huddles three times daily, looking at the facility boards...so more patients were ready for earlier discharge. This meant actively managing physicians who were resistant, and managing communications with families so they were better about rides. The tools we used included daily operating reports, variance reports, audit reports on methods changes, and weekly committee meetings."

6. Ensuring Sustainability of Change

The YNHH senior leadership management team has institutionalized regularly scheduled meetings with accountability for results going forward as the

EXHIBIT II.6 Executive Throughput Scorecard, Week Ending November 6, 2010

Area	Metric	Threshold (R1)	Target (R2)	Max (Stretch)	Last Week (Actual)	Direction (Last week compared to YTD performance)	YTD Performance	YTD Performance Compared to Target
Patient Services	Surgery–11:00 a.m. discharges	13.0%	15.0%	17.0%	20.0%	Better	17.0%	Above Max
	Surgery–Median discharge time (hour)	13:57	13:42	13:27	13:55	Better	14:03	Below Threshold
	Medicine–11:00 a.m. discharges	19.0%	19.5%	20.0%	22.0%	Same	22.0%	Above Max
	Medicine–Median discharge time (hour)	14:11	13:56	13:41	14:18	Better	14:30	Below Threshold
	Oncology–11:00 a.m. discharges	18.9%	20.0%	20.0%	24.0%	Better	13.0%	Below Threshold
	Oncology–Median discharge time (hour)	13:50	13:40	13:30	13:52	Better	14:07	Below Threshold
	Children's–11:00 a.m. discharges	19.0%	20.0%	21.0%	14.0%	Worse	21.0%	Above Max
	Children's–Median discharge time (hour)	13:53	13:43	13:33	14:31	Worse	13:38	≥ Target, Below Max
	OB–11:00 a.m. discharges	13.4%	15.0%	17.0%	8.0%	Worse	11.0%	Below Threshold
	OB–Median discharge time (hour)	12:23	12:08	11:53	12:33	Worse	12:24	Below Threshold
	Psych–11:00 a.m. discharges	31.0%	35.0%	37.0%	37.0%	Better	34.0%	≥ Threshold, < Target
	Heart & Vascular– 11:00 a.m. discharges	24.0%	24.5%	25.5%	22.0%	Worse	26.0%	Above Max
	Heart & Vascular–Median discharge time (hour)	13:41	13:26	13:11	13:17	Better	13:21	≥ Target, Below Max
	Hospitalwide–11:00 a.m. discharges	19.0%	20.1%	21.1%	19.0%	Same	19.0%	≥ Threshold, < Target
	Hospitalwide–Median discharge time (hour)	13:41	13:27	13:17	13:31	Better	13:34	≥ Threshold, < Target

organization tackles additional areas for improvement. One such area is a transforming patient care initiative. YNHH nurses are familiar now with the safe patient flow methodology and trust that this initiative will not primarily be a cost-cutting initiative ending with layoffs of nurses and nurse practice associates.

Associate director of nursing: "The new transforming patient care initiative is about regulatory readiness, to take off the nurse's plate all the non-value-added tasks that nurses do so that nurses can focus on compliance, for example with more and better patient education…. We want 60 minutes of nurse time per shift for every patient. Nurses are on this new and separate steering committee. The work is data-driven, focusing on patient satisfaction; the support staff will support patient care, not nursing, but allow nurses to do effective nursing."

Lesson Learned

YNHH has achieved significant results in increasing throughput without adding positions. Patients benefit by being in the right bed at the right time. Management initiatives are often resisted by clinicians who have observed past manager rhetoric as facades for one-time efforts to cut costs, including not filling vacant positions. YNHH senior leadership was constantly engaged in articulating and rearticulating purpose. Data were generated to show that patients were waiting less for needed treatments on the floors as a result of new schedules and targeting. Success in reducing wait times built support for changes in physician schedules. Transparency and accountability were accomplished largely through formation of a steering committee with ultimate decision-making authority for the initiative. The steering committee was chaired by a respected physician, and half of the members of the committee were physicians. Extra resources—obtained both externally from Carpedia and internally by temporarily reassigning key staff—were essential in implementing new methods that spanned many departments and involved major changes in schedules and work flow. Sustainability was assured before the external and internal consulting services were withdrawn (although they are still available as needed). The purpose of the project was to provide safer care for the patients.

Acknowledgments

The authors would like to acknowledge the contribution of Sandra Bacon, director, operations support, Yale–New Haven Hospital, for her contributions to the content of this case. Ms. Bacon, of course, had a great deal to do with the success of the actual project as well.

Anthony R. Kovner wrote a first draft of this article as a consultant for Carpedia.

Part II: Moving the Needle, at Our Place?

Your administrative fellow, Timmy Fields, has just brought to your attention the case study, "Moving the Needle: Managing Safe Patient Flow at YNHH." You are Joe Miller, CEO at Jones Memorial Hospital, a 450-bed community hospital in Eastern City. Your first response is to think of all the reasons you shouldn't do it. "Moving the Needle" is a big initiative. This means it will cost a lot and certainly be met with resistance. And where's the gain in it?

Besides, this is a community hospital, not an academic medical center. You don't need to build a new wing. Jones Memorial is making money. You like the idea of shortening length of stay, but you think you are going to pass at this time. Maybe you will forward the case study to your chief medical officer, Dan Farber, and see what he thinks about it.

Case Questions

1. What would it take to change Joe Miller's response?
2. What adaptations to the initiative would have to be made at Jones Memorial Hospital to make it work?
3. What response would you make to this situation at Medicare's Center for Innovation (i.e., would staff at Medicare's Center for Innovation think it would be a good idea to replicate and expand what YNHH is doing)?

Case E
Reducing Healthcare-Associated Infections at Academic Medical Center: The Role of High-Performance Work Practices

Julie Robbins and Ann Scheck McAlearney

Late one Tuesday afternoon, Don Patterson, the CEO of Academic Medical Center (AMC), sat in his office putting the final touches on a board presentation. The presentation highlighted AMC's latest quality scores—and the scores were the best they had ever been at AMC. Patterson was particularly proud of these results because he had made a conscious effort over the past two years to make quality and patient safety top priorities for the organization.

Just as Patterson was about to leave for the day, his assistant stuck her head into his office. "I'm sorry to interrupt what you're doing," she began, "but I have the governor on the line. She wants to talk to you about AMC's infection rates."

As his assistant left, Patterson picked up the phone with confidence and asked, "Governor, what can I do for you?"

"Patterson," the governor answered, "I know you and your team at AMC are doing great work. You are an incredible resource for this state and the region. However, I am very concerned about central line–associated bloodstream infection [CLABSI] rates in your hospital."

As the governor continued, Patterson's confidence began to wane. She explained, "I just spoke to my health commissioner, Sally Slater. She had been at a national meeting where she learned that our state has the highest CLABSI rates in the country. Slater was surprised by this information, so she and her team further reviewed the data. They found that because AMC is the largest hospital in the state, AMC's CLABSI rates are a major contributor to our state's high CLABSI rates. That means that AMC's high infection rates have pulled our state's rankings to the bottom. This is absolutely unacceptable!"

Stunned but attempting to recover, Patterson interjected, "Governor, you must be mistaken. Our rates may be higher than those of other hospitals in the state, but that's because the patients we treat are much more complex and therefore much more prone to bloodstream infections. When we compare ourselves to our academic medical center peer institutions, we do as well or better than they do with respect to CLABSI rates."

The governor sighed and stated, "Look, Patterson, that may be true. But I don't care about other academic medical centers. I care about my state, and I know you do, too. Also, my health commissioner tells me that there are some states—states that also have large medical centers—that have not had *any* CLABSI infections in the last year. So don't tell me that it can't be done. You need to fix this. We have enough problems in this state without becoming known for giving people infections when they come to our hospitals!"

After the call ended, Patterson knew he needed to do something, but he was still in shock about the governor's revelation. Given the lateness of the hour, he packed his briefcase, turned off his office lights, and walked toward the stairs to head home. He needed some time to think about how best to address the governor's concerns.

AMC's Commitment to Quality

When Patterson had been hired as AMC's CEO, he came into an already-strong organization that was widely recognized for clinical excellence and that was routinely recognized as one of the country's best medical centers. Locally, AMC served as a hub for specialty and subspecialty services within the state and surrounding region, particularly trauma, cardiac, neonatal, and other complex services. AMC had been a leader in quality, comparing favorably to its academic medical center peers across the country on key quality indicators.

Of course Patterson recognized that there was always room for improvement, and he tried to do everything possible to ensure that patients at AMC got the best possible care, had good outcomes, and, most important, were not made worse during their stays. Like most healthcare leaders, Patterson was appalled by the national statistics showing that more than 98,000 people die every year from preventable medical errors in hospitals, and this motivated him to set the ambitious organizational goal to make AMC the safest medical center in the country.

As part of this commitment to safety, Patterson hired an executive-level chief quality officer, Kristin Dempsey, MD, to lead the organization's ambitious quality and safety efforts. During her two-year tenure with AMC, Dempsey had helped the organization make significant progress toward improving safety, and had developed a quality report card to track progress. In addition to sharing the quality report card with the board of directors, Patterson reviewed these quality data at his monthly leadership meetings. He encouraged managers and staff to make changes necessary to make AMC the safest medical center in the country, and then he held them accountable for results, celebrating successes along the way.

Given his personal commitment to quality and safety, Patterson was unsettled by the governor's phone call about AMC's CLABSI rates. When Patterson got to work the next day, he met with his executive team, told them about the call with the governor, and let them know, in no uncertain terms, that he expected them to improve AMC's CLABSI rates. Specifically, he charged Dempsey with developing an aggressive CLABSI prevention plan within the week and told her that he intended to review CLABSI rates and improvement progress at their biweekly updates.

Could AMC Improve Its CLABSI Rates?

Like Patterson, Dempsey was upset by the governor's call and its implications. When she got back to her office, she asked her assistant to set up a meeting with the intensive care unit (ICU) leadership team. The ICU leadership team included Brigid King and Mary Hughes, the respective directors of the medical and surgical ICUs, and Dr. Brian Robinson, the medical director for both ICUs.

Although CLABSI rates had not been included on AMC's organizational-level quality report card, they had been tracked as unit-level indicators for the ICUs. Dempsey knew that AMC's CLABSI rates met the organization's standard of being within the top tenth percentile when compared with its academic medical center peers. Dempsey shared the view of others in the organization that some CLABSIs were virtually unavoidable, seeing some infections as part of the cost of doing business, for AMC's complex patient population.

At the unit level, ICU leaders had long recognized the importance of trying to minimize CLABSI rates and therefore had been tracking CLABSI rates as an important quality metric. In fact, several years earlier, the ICUs' rates had been out of line compared with the rates of ICUs in AMC's benchmark peer institutions, but the ICU team had implemented a coordinated effort to reduce CLABSI rates. This effort had been successful, and AMC's rates had dropped to an acceptable level and remained steady since then. In practice, the ICU team believed that as long as CLABSI rates remained low and hit the benchmark targets there was very little need to discuss CLABSIs at all.

When Dempsey met with the ICU leaders, she conveyed the concerns of both the governor and Patterson. She acknowledged that perhaps she and others in the room had gotten too complacent about CLABSIs and suggested that their collective belief that some level of infection was inevitable might have been shortsighted.

Since her talk with Patterson earlier in the day, Dempsey had done some research on CLABSI prevention and had found that the clinical team at the Johns Hopkins Medical Center had virtually eliminated CLABSIs. Dempsey told the team about Johns Hopkins' success and said, "I know we have complex patients with many problems and I certainly know that preventing infections may be difficult. Nonetheless, if Johns Hopkins, one of the nation's top medical centers, can do it, so can we!"

Even more compelling were data from the state of Michigan that indicated that Michigan hospitals had gone for more than a year without a CLABSI after they launched a collaborative to implement the Johns Hopkins approach in hospitals across the state. After presenting these data to her team, Dempsey continued: "The Michigan experience demonstrates that it is possible to get to zero CLABSIs. I think that we here at AMC need to change our thinking. Rather than accept that infections are a cost of doing business and comparing ourselves to peers who may be stuck in the same way of thinking as we are, we need to aim higher and decide that we can get to zero CLABSIs too!"

Despite Dempsey's pep talk, not all members of the ICU team agreed. As Dr. Robinson started to explain why getting to zero would be impossible at AMC, Dempsey stopped him midsentence: "Look, I know it will be hard, and we can sit around and argue and grumble all day. However, I have a clear directive from Don Patterson. He has made a commitment to the governor and has charged me with turning this around. Based on the evidence I've just shared with you from other states and academic medical centers, I am convinced we can improve our CLABSI rates. Further, based on what I know about the quality of the leadership in this room and the level of commitment we have from the physicians and nurses in our ICUs, I don't see any reason why we can't eliminate CLABSIs from our hospital altogether. I have to give Patterson a plan by the end of the week explaining how we aim to address this issue, and I need your help to do it. I know that you all have already put a lot of effort into reducing CLABSI rates, so now I want you to build on those efforts to take our initiatives to the next level."

Brigid King, RN, was the first to respond and said, "I think we all know that even though we have a good plan in place and have made some progress on the units, we could be more consistent and vigilant in our processes. We definitely have areas in which we could improve. None of us likes it when something we do or did gives our patient an infection. If we can change our practices to make sure that never happens, then we need to do it."

After some reflection, Dr. Robinson also appeared to come around commenting, "I guess it's hard to argue. If Johns Hopkins can do it, why can't we?"

Dempsey, pleased with the responses of her team, then forged ahead. "Great! I appreciate your support and commitment. Now, why don't the three of you work off-line to put together a plan for eliminating CLABSIs from our ICUs and we can meet again next week?"

Leaving the meeting, Dempsey called Patterson to let him know that she had met with the ICU leaders and, as a result, could assure him that they were collectively committed to eliminating CLABSIs at AMC.

Reinvigorating CLABSI-Prevention Efforts Through Management and Accountability

Setting and Attaining CLABSI Prevention Goals

After meeting with the ICU leaders, Dempsey turned her attention to the CLABSI data. She knew that one of the keys to getting to zero would be to make sure that the ICU clinicians and staff were aware of their own unit's CLABSI rates and their ability to improve those rates. In the past, some ICU clinicians had grumbled about how CLABSI rates were reported and tracked. She was concerned that her improvement initiative might get derailed if staff argued about the data.

For several years, AMC had used the state's CLABSI definition to calculate a rate that was expressed as the number of infections per 1,000 line days in the ICU. A few vocal physicians believed that this definition inflated the ICU CLABSI rates. Mostly they were concerned the ICU had infections counted against them if a patient received a central line in another department (e.g., the emergency department or surgery) and then developed a CLABSI shortly after arrival in the ICU. Not only did these physicians believe that this counting method overstated the ICU CLABSI rates, they also believed it assigned responsibility for infections that were not really the ICU's fault because the central line insertions had not been under the control of the ICU. Dempsey knew that the state's definition wasn't perfect, but she also knew that every definition had its own problems.

Dempsey pulled together a small group that included the most vocal ICU physicians, the ICU directors, and members of her own quality improvement department to develop an internal CLABSI report card that would include unit-level data. At the first meeting of this group she opened the meeting by saying, "I know that the state's CLABSI definition is not perfect, but it is the best we've got. Since we have to use this definition to collect and report our data externally, I suggest that we use the same definition and data collection methods as the basis for our internal reporting and quality improvement efforts."

As expected, several of the physicians challenged the definition. Yet when they failed to provide a more suitable alternative, Dempsey redirected the conversation. She explained, "We need to focus all of our attention on getting our rates down. Even if these data aren't perfect, our CLABSI rates are unquestionably too high. Our goal is to get to zero infections—no matter how they get measured."

Dempsey continued, "Now that we have agreed that we need to use this standard definition, I think we need to talk about how we can use these data to focus our improvement efforts."

Several members of the group readily noted that it was important to routinely disseminate data at the unit level so that frontline staff would know how many infections were occurring on their units. Mary Hughes, one of the ICU nurse managers, noted, "I sometimes review the ICU quality report that includes CLABSI rates at my staff meeting, and I then post the report in the break room. However, I don't spend much time on these reports, because I can see the nurses' eyes glaze over while I'm talking. I think it's hard for them to link data expressed as an infection rate back to individual patient care. I mean, what does two infections per 1,000 line days mean in terms of the patients that they're taking care of?"

King agreed: "My staff are passionate about providing the best care possible to their patients, but a unit-level rate does not mean much to them. I think it might be more meaningful if, instead of reporting out a rate, we tried to track the number of days without infections."

Dr. Robinson eagerly responded, "That's a great idea! Not only will the staff be able to relate to the number, but it will be expressed in a way that puts the emphasis on the positive: eliminating infections."

After a little more discussion, the group agreed that the quality department would produce reports indicating "days without CLABSI infections" for each unit every month. Leaders on each unit would then be expected to share these reports to enlist their staff in support of the AMC-wide goal to get to zero infections. The group also decided that these unit-based reports, along with an aggregated report of days without infections across units, would be presented at the CLABSI work group monthly meetings. Thus, reports indicating the standard CLABSI rates of "infections per 1,000 line days" would continue to be produced and reported to the ICU leadership team so that these could be tracked over time. Finally, it was agreed that Dempsey would present these reports and data to Patterson every month to ensure the Getting to Zero campaign remained top of mind.

Clinical Bundle Implementation

In her review of the CLABSI literature, Dempsey had found that CLABSI prevention strategies were relatively straightforward from a clinical perspective. There were clear protocols for inserting and maintaining central lines, but the challenge was making sure these protocols were consistently implemented. Proper protocol for central line insertion required the physician inserting the line to adhere to strict sterile precautions, such as wearing a gown and mask, using a full drape on the patient, and practicing hand hygiene. After insertion, central line maintenance protocols were more related to nursing care and included a focus on timeliness of dressing changes, specific protocols for cleaning and accessing the line, and hand hygiene. Hospitals that had been most successful at eliminating CLABSIs had focused on making it easy for physicians, nurses, and other staff to "do the right thing, every time," and on minimizing any opportunities for error. Successful practices included use of standardized central line carts stocked with all of the materials for sterile insertion; routine use of checklists; implementation of double checks, in which nurses can stop a physician from inserting a line if protocol is not being followed; and a universal emphasis on hand hygiene.

Dempsey asked her ICU leadership team whether AMC had been following these evidence-based protocols. All of them agreed that while the AMC CLABSI prevention team had outlined guidelines for line insertion and maintenance, each unit had some flexibility as to how they implemented the practices. They all acknowledged, however, that this approach may have led to too much variation in practice and potential confusion among staff.

Dr. Robinson explained, "Some of our physicians disagree with the evidence or have found areas of the literature that are less clear, and they do not want to change their practice. They say, 'I have been putting in central lines for 20 years without a problem so why should I change now?' That said, most are willing to change if they find the evidence compelling, and if making the change is easy for them."

Hughes chimed in and noted, "Our nurses are willing to make changes if it's in the best interests of the patient, but they need to understand why the change is necessary, and then have the resources that they need to make the change effectively. Along those lines, these challenges are exacerbated when we have staff turnover or an influx of new nurses or residents who may have different approaches. Probably one of the issues we have is that we haven't been consistent in our education."

Dempsey responded: "We need to set a standard that is based on the best available evidence and make a decision that there will be one way to do things—the AMC Way—and then make sure that our physicians and unit staff have what they need to do it that way. As leaders on the unit, you need to educate your staff about the AMC Way, emphasizing why it is important to patient care, and then hold them accountable for adhering to our standard. When any person on the unit is not adhering to our standard, any other person, regardless of rank, needs to feel that she can speak up to the individual directly, or to the attending or nurse manager, to inform her that the AMC standard has not been followed. In turn, when this happens, you, as leaders, need to support and reinforce the right behavior."

After a little more discussion, the group agreed to a three-point plan for improving the consistency of practice related to central line insertion and maintenance. First, they would convene a small group of frontline physicians and nurses to develop a single set of standards for line insertion and maintenance that would become "the AMC Way." Second, they agreed to each go back to their units, review operations, and speak to the staff to identify opportunities to support and to hardwire consistent implementation of the standards. Finally, all four agreed that they would develop a systematic plan for communicating with and educating staff about the importance of infection prevention, the role of staff in preventing infections, and the AMC Way for central line insertion and maintenance.

Three weeks later, they had each worked with their respective teams to finalize standards and develop their CLABSI Prevention Plan. The next step was to roll it out on the units.

CLABSI Prevention Plan Implementation

At the next medical ICU staff meeting, King announced that they were launching a major CLABSI prevention effort on the unit. She told her staff that Patterson was upset about AMC's performance relative to other hospitals in the state, and he had challenged the ICUs to make improvements.

As she explained, "I recognize that our patient population is very sick, but I *know* we can do better. We have the best doctors and nursing staff in the state, so we should be the leaders, not the losers, in patient safety. I also know we have a lot of competing priorities, so I think we may have just taken our eye off the ball with regard to bloodstream infections. There are hospitals just like AMC that have completely eliminated CLABSIs, so I know we at AMC can too."

King unveiled a large poster proclaiming "Days Since Our Last Infection" across the top with a space to write in the appropriate number. She then noted, "We are going to put this poster in the hallway so that everyone can see it—physicians, staff, patients, and families. I am going to update it every day with a report of our current data. Unfortunately, we just had a CLABSI yesterday, so we are starting today at zero. But we can take it day by day, focusing on doing everything we can to make sure our patients don't get a CLABSI every single day, and the days will start to add up. Hopefully someday we won't even need this poster because we will no longer get infections on this unit!"

King continued, "I have asked your colleague, Ann Dillard, who has been a nurse on this unit for ten years, to be our 'CLABSI Champion.' She has already been working with me and others on the ICU management team to develop a consistent set of evidence-based guidelines that will be our standard 'AMC Way' for inserting and maintaining central lines. Our goal is to have everyone do it the same way, every time, without error."

King further explained, "Ann has been working with unit champions from the other ICUs to develop a CLABSI training blitz for all ICU nurses for next Tuesday. Meanwhile, Dr. Robinson has developed a similar event for the attendings and residents. We also plan to incorporate detailed training about the AMC Way into our new nurse orientation to make sure that anyone who comes to work on our unit learns how to work with central lines the right way, right from the start. Of course if you have any questions, or suggestions for improvement, do not hesitate to talk to Ann, Dr. Robinson, or me. We want your ideas about how we can do things better for our patients. And through all of this, the ICU leadership team will be tracking compliance with our central line insertion and maintenance protocols so that we can make sure we are doing it the right way every time."

CLABSI Prevention: The First Year

Once all of the ICU staff were trained on how to do central lines the AMC Way and staff began to modify their practices, several important changes occurred (see Exhibit II.7).

First, the physicians started including the nurses in their daily patient rounds so that the nurses could report on the status of central lines (e.g., when the dressing was last changed and any problems), and the care team could decide whether or not a patient still needed a central line.

Second, the staff quickly realized that the central line carts that were supposed to have all of the materials needed for a central line insertion the AMC Way were not consistently stocked. With the support of her manager and help from the process improvement department, Dillard convened a small group of residents and nurses to revamp the central line carts and

EXHIBIT II.7 Summary of Changes Made Involving AMC CLABSI-Prevention Initiatives

Change Made	Before Initiative	After Initiative
CLABSI prevention goal setting	• Based on benchmark comparisons to like institutions • Tracked as an ICU-based quality indicator	• Goal of zero infections based on experience of leading institutions • Included as a top priority for organization-level quality report card
Clinical bundle implementation	• General guidelines adopted based on evidence-based practice, but unit- and/or physician-level variation permitted	• Consensus process to develop evidence-informed guidelines for "the AMC Way" • Use of checklists to ensure bundle compliance every time • Routine monitoring of bundle compliance
Clinical education	• Top-down approach in which nurse manager shares clinical changes associated with CLABSI-prevention via staff meeting and/or in-servicing	• Staff-driven approach in which unit-based CLABSI champion was identified to participate in improvement efforts and support implementation; included communication and in-services to expand reach of training efforts • Input from frontline nurses routinely obtained, e.g., regarding new products, changes in policies, etc.
Reporting	• Unit-based reports of CLABSI rates (infections per 1,000 line days) shared at staff meetings	• Unit-based reports of "days since the last infection" visibly posted on the units • Celebrations and recognition for meeting major milestones, e.g., one year since the last infection • Organization-level CLABSI data routinely shared with AMC leaders; public recognition of progress and accomplishments
Other initiatives		• Interdisciplinary rounds to assess line necessity • Standardized central line cart • Unit-based CLABSI team • Visible rewards and recognition for achievement

specified processes for keeping them stocked. These newly organized carts then made inserting the lines the right way every time easy, and the right materials were always available.

Finally, the small group that developed the central line carts continued to meet and morphed into a unit-based central line task team that worked with the AMC infection control division to conduct root cause analyses when infections did occur. This empowered the members of the team further to identify opportunities for improvement, solicit feedback about line insertion and maintenance processes from frontline staff, and serve as a general resource for their peers.

As unit staff became more aware of the importance of CLABSI prevention and better understood their practices related to these infections, they became increasingly committed to the goal of eliminating CLABSIs on the unit. As promised, King updated the "Days Since Our Last Infection" number on the poster every day, right outside the nurses' station for everyone to see. And fortunately, as the practice changes began to take hold, that number kept getting larger and larger. First seven days, then ten, and then the unit had gone more than a year since its last infection. Each major milestone was marked, and the contributions of the staff were recognized with a celebration. When the unit hit one full year without an infection, the ICU leaders threw a pizza party on the unit. In addition, a friendly rivalry—or competition—between the two adult and pediatric ICUs developed. When one of the units hit a major milestone in CLABSI prevention, the others were inspired to try to beat the record. As one pediatric nurse noted, "Of course we were happy when the adult ICU hit 50 days without an infection, but then we thought to ourselves, 'If they can do it, so can we,' and we were even more committed to the work on our own unit."

The ICU managers and staff were also motivated by the fact that Patterson had added CLABSI rates as one of the three quality indicators on AMC's overall balanced scorecard. The balanced scorecard results were reported to the AMC board every quarter, and served as the basis for both manager and staff performance bonuses. Further, Patterson presented the balanced scorecard results to the hospital leadership team every month. With every success, Patterson publicly recognized the ICU managers and staff for their efforts, and praised them for their accomplishments. The ICU staff were both surprised and thrilled when Patterson showed up at their one-year celebration to personally thank them for their hard work.

Case Questions

1. What leader behaviors were most important to improving AMC CLABSI rates? At the executive level? At the unit level?
2. How was information used to facilitate improvements in CLABSI rates?
3. As an administrator at AMC, what would you be concerned about in the coming year for CLABSI prevention? How about two years from now?

Case F
Controlling Performance Management

Jacob Victory

The New Vice President

"He is not a nurse," smirked the pediatric nurse director.

"He's going to be a piece of cake," mocked the other with mischief gleaming in her eye.

They were referring to Josh Webber, their new boss who was starting that morning as the new vice president of the pediatric division. Josh was not new to the organization. He was a young and eager executive and had paid his dues working for five years as the right hand of the Visiting Nurse Service of America's (VNSA) president and CEO. Thereafter, he was promoted to operations director of the organization's highly profitable rehabilitation services division and then promoted to director of performance management, where he worked for more than a year with the pediatric division's administrator and her team to improve the division's business and clinical performance.

Josh, holding a box of files and walking confidently with his polished shoes tip-tapping on the tiles outside of his new administrative suite's entrance, had heard the exchange between the nurse directors. The comment struck Josh as odd because the two directors had worked closely with him over the last year and recent improvements in the division's operational performance had been highly praised by VNSA leadership.

"Time to don your game face, Josh!" he thought to himself. Sighing gently, Josh put on a toothy grin, turned the corner and greeted the two directors enthusiastically as he entered the suite. The nurse directors didn't miss a beat and greeted Josh with a warm, "Welcome aboard, Josh!"

The Maternal and Pediatric Service Line

The maternal and pediatric service line was only one part of the VNSA, the nation's largest for-profit home health agency.

Under the current CEO's tenure, the VNSA had become a national home care agency. It employed 30,000 nurses, rehabilitation therapists, social workers, and home health aides, and served almost 500,000 patients in six states annually. The agency earned a healthy margin on its annual $5 billion revenue base and, with a conservative management team at its helm, the VNSA was only geared to become bigger and more influential in enforcing federal long-term healthcare policy. Its many divisions and programs focused primarily on the home-bound frail elderly, especially those in the long-term care population who made up the Medicare, Medicaid, and dually eligible marketplace. At an annual growth rate of 8 to 10 percent, the VNSA was a force in the market, offering short-term, skilled nursing and professional services via its adult, pediatric, community mental health, long-term care, rehabilitation therapy, and palliative and hospice programs. It also operated a lucrative managed care company that offered myriad managed care plans to a large market base of elderly and long-term care patients; more than 200,000 members were covered under these plans.

Yet, while the organization's primary focus was on long-term care and the geriatric population, the agency's roots had been laid by its maternal and pediatric division, VNSA's first program, which had been founded more than 170 years ago. Now composed of ten pediatric programs, the division annually served more than 35,000 mothers, newborns, and children via numerous programs that focused on short-term skilled care, pediatric care management, and evidence-based preventive services and family-focused programs. Deemed the largest organization of its kind in the nation, VNSA's stated mission was to serve the most vulnerable populations, especially those who lacked access to healthcare. Almost 90 percent of the patients served lived below the poverty line and were insured by Medicaid or enrolled in Medicaid managed care plans. Most of these patients had complex illnesses and, more often than not, came from socioeconomically compromised environments. A typical patient profile included a 15-year-old mother with C-section wound care complications; a two-month-old boy with a brain tumor who recently had his left arm amputated; a 14-year-old girl with the mental capacity of a 3-year-old experiencing severe cardiac and respiratory complications and multiple rehospitalizations—and the list continued on for thousands of similar patients. VNSA's charitable care and community benefit programs were a hallmark of its mission, and the maternal and pediatric service line was at the mission's core.

With annual revenues of $50 million, the pediatric division was historically under-reimbursed and had a loss of $18 million every year. Seven of its ten programs were grant-funded, and two were funded by VNSA's board of directors' Charitable Care Benefit Fund. The program that relied on traditional insurance mechanisms for reimbursement was responsible for nearly all of the division's deficit.

Despite the annual losses, the VNSA board of directors considered this division untouchable. A subset of VNSA board members and community pediatricians also composed the pediatric division's advisory board, and these individuals and the division's chair—a full board member and an influential member of society—were key fixtures with respect to their commitment, support, and advocacy for the maternal and pediatric services the division provided to the communities it served. From a branding perspective, VNSA's executive management shared in the board's view and actively used the maternal and pediatric division in the agency's public relations efforts to market the company as one that focused on community benefit, despite its for-profit status. Moreover, the division was the lead recipient of VNSA's philanthropic endeavors. Millions of dollars were raised for the program, but not enough to reduce the deficit. Yet because VNSA was a highly disciplined agency in which most of its business leaders annually exceeded their business and clinical targets, the pediatric division stuck out like a sore thumb. In internal management meetings, executive leadership notably demanded that the division's management minimize its financial deficit and had directed a harsh eye and even harsher commentary toward the division because it had not historically met its budgeted business targets. Its clinical outcomes were average at best, although its customer satisfaction ratings were consistently among the highest of all programs in the agency.

Not surprisingly, the administrators of the pediatric division turned over frequently. In the last six years, there had been four vice presidents because the burnout rate was high. Other issues stemmed from a lack of institutional support in providing the division with adequate business oversight. The program directors in the division were either nurses or social workers who had been promoted up the ladder; these directors maintained the perspective of frontline clinicians, and focused primarily on ensuring that the sick children were served. Being labeled a "community benefit" program (a euphemism for "a program that makes no money") and watching their senior leaders leave because they were "routinely beat up on at meetings," as one nurse director put it, made the program's leaders wary of every new vice president who was brought in to lead the division. "How long will this one last?" was a frequent question.

Josh was wondering the same thing.

Who Is on Deck?

Six pairs of eyes stared at Josh. All six of his direct reports sat in front of him, one next to another. "Welcome to Josh's Leadership Assimilation," said the regional head of VNSA's organizational development (OD) human resources division. "In the next three hours you will learn about Josh, his management style, his goals, and his objectives for the next year," he continued. Standing in front of the room, Josh stared back and, being a visual person, thought that he was "looking at the living and breathing version of the division's organization chart."

The next three hours were eye-opening. The OD representative had asked the group to describe Josh. Words such as *young, a man, articulate, competitive, takes-no-prisoner type, poised, ambitious, seemingly courteous, soft-spoken, deep thinker, all-business* were only some of the terms used. Then the group was asked what they wanted to know from Josh. Most wanted to know

- how "hands-on" he planned to be in managing their divisions,
- how available he wanted them to be when he needed them,
- how he was going to manage a group of clinicians when he had no clinical training, and
- how and why he obtained his current promotion.

Only two in the group genuinely wanted to know how he was going to help them perform better, while the other four scoffed. Lorann Stutters, a director who ran two disease-based programs for adolescents, blatantly asked, "We know you've been brought here to 'fix' this division; how long do you plan to spend here before you position yourself for your next job?"

Did she really just say that? Josh thought to himself. He endured three hours of people venting about the history of the program; of questions about his intentions for the business; of sly glances that questioned his every answer; and of probing questions that had more venom than substance. Only two of the directors remained mostly quiet and asked thoughtful questions about the strategic positioning of the division.

After the meeting, Lucas Red, the OD representative leading the meeting, gave Josh a piece of paper that listed the five key impressions the directors had of Josh; this information had been collected prior to the meeting.

1. Josh is a male under 35 years of age, but he looks like he just turned 20.
2. Josh is too ambitious.
3. Josh knows how to present a complex idea in a simple, succinct way. He is a good public speaker.
4. Josh is the "golden boy," having served as the CEO's special assistant. It is obvious how he got this promotion.
5. Josh is a nonclinician; how can he possibly understand patient care issues?

"This is going to be a fun ride, Josh," he said to himself, trying to nurse his bruised ego. Josh walked back to his office, sat down, and started to draw an organizational chart.

Taking Stock

He noticed that he had six directors as direct reports, in addition to an administrative assistant. The six directors were all clinicians who ran the ten divisions; some directors ran more than one program. Each director had regional and state administrators who had managers overseeing the frontline clinicians. Regionally, there was business support staff supporting the clinical teams in each program. In turn, the vice president, along with 17 other peers, reported to the senior vice president of operations, who reported to VNSA's chief operating officer.

Josh recalled that the division was commonly referred to as a mishmash of seemingly unrelated pediatric programs. However, because his mind was always geared to compartmentalize, Josh noticed striking similarities among many of the programs. He started to outline the three themes he saw.

The largest program in terms of admissions served maternal and pediatric patients who required short-term skilled nursing, social work, rehabilitation therapies, and paraprofessional services. He labeled this first category "Short-Term, Skilled." Next, he noticed that five of the programs were focused on care management over a longer period of service (up to three years). Two of these programs focused on targeted asthma and diabetes care management and served only adolescents. The other three programs were clinical and evidence-based programs that had superb clinical and socioeconomic outcomes that exceeded city, state, and national benchmarks. Josh labeled this second category "Care Management." The other four programs focused on preventive and family-focused services, a category Josh labeled "Preventive and Family Programs." The directors who ran multiple programs fit into only one of the three categories, thus avoiding overlap.

Next, Josh listed the total numbers of patients admitted into each of the three categories and each category's revenues and deficits as a percentage of the total division's revenues and deficits. When he tallied all of the numbers, what he noticed was striking (see Exhibit II.8).

While the short-term, skilled care program served 86 percent of the total division's patients, it made up less than half of the division's revenues and represented 90 percent of the division's deficit. Compounding the problem was the fact that while the division was severely under-reimbursed, it had significant process and efficiency issues that were at the root of its high unbilled claims rates, high managed care denial and write-off rates of claims, low productivity for the nursing staff in terms of how many visits per day they each made, and relatively low process and outcomes performance on their quality scorecard indicators. As Josh was also required to manage the other programs—each with its unique set of issues, regulations, and services—he knew that he had to juggle a lot of balls. Executive management, his boss, and the advisory board to which he reported had all made polite comments about the mandated expected turnaround of the division's performance. Expectations for improving performance were thus tremendous, and the organization wanted Josh and the division to run operations, provide high-quality care to its patients,

EXHIBIT II.8

VNSA Patient Categories and Revenue

Category	% of Total Division's Patients	% of Total Division's Revenues	% of Total Division's Deficits
1. Short-term, skilled	86	46	90
2. Care management	8	29	7
3. Prevention and family	6	25	3

and improve efficiencies—and to do so only with existing resources and management staff. Josh immediately understood that he could not do all of this by himself. The million-dollar question in Josh's mind now was: "Do I have the right management team to move this mountain?"

The next day, Josh set out to answer this question. He was conscious of the positive comments that the organization's senior executives and some of his clinical staff were making behind his back because of his successes in leading other divisions—all in short time periods. Josh also recognized that most of his direct reports were threatened by his formal, business-like demeanor. Some of his directors also disliked his reputation, as he was known as a "hands-on" manager who expected his directors to not only identify the problems they were facing but to offer solutions. His complete reliance on data, facts, and transparency put off almost all of his directors because they had previously managed only via anecdotes and were traditionally not expected to be forthcoming in details, to raise management issues, or to speculate about how they'd follow up in fixing issues. Lastly, he saw the false smiles of his management staff when they spoke to him.

Despite Josh's many attempts to soothe relations, to build trust, and to focus on strategies that enhance care for patients, he knew that most of the directors were suspicious of him. The reason the last vice president of the division was moved from this division to another post within the organization had never been explained to them. As a result, they all had their theories. Josh had heard the gossip that they all accused him of "overthrowing" their friendly, harmless, and docile vice president because of his "ruthless ambition" and "connections" with the CEO. In reality, he was forced to endure this behavior because he had been forbidden by executive management to tell the directors that the last vice president had been removed by executive management because of her lack of management skills and her lack of action toward improving the poor performance of multiple programs within the division. Nevertheless, he had a job to do.

Josh decided to schedule one-on-one staff meetings every week for the next three months with each of his directors to get an understanding of their programs, their successes, and their issues regarding management, staffing, quality, business operations, and so forth. After this period he planned to transition to one staff meeting every two to three weeks with each director. Josh told everyone in advance that he expected an agenda from them prior to their staff meetings, and he welcomed their candor about any management problems during their meetings because he wanted to help them solve their problems and take their programs to the next level. He felt that the sick children his programs served deserved and needed much more.

Preliminary Meetings

At each of his first one-on-one staff meetings, Josh welcomed the director and told her that he was there to help. However, Josh also noted that he would hold each director accountable for her budgeted financial and quality targets, as well as expect the directors to be honest and open with him. He distinctly told each that he wanted total transparency with respect to her program's performance, and he made it clear that he did not punish poor performance, as long as a plan was developed and implemented to address the management issues and provided that he was updated about progress. If any of the plans detoured, Josh noted that he was there to help the directors brainstorm to solve issues. Josh's one rule was simple: "Please, do not ever put me in a position where I am surprised in a meeting—let me know what is going on in your divisions. Also, do not disagree with me in public. If you disagree with me or my decisions, take me aside and, by all means, let me know, and we'll address it. The division needs to take—and be perceived as taking—a team approach to running the care services for its patients and addressing the division's management issues." He then looked at the director in each meeting and asked directly but with a cordial smile, "How can I help you become a better manager?"

Only two directors sought assistance, one with a clinical workforce issue she was facing and one who noted that she needed to be better grounded in understanding financial statements. The other four, however, had curtly answered, "I'm fine. I don't need your help." One even said, "Why don't you stick to reviewing the dollars? We'll take care of treating the kids." Life had taught Josh that those who did not ask for help (1) were hiding something, (2) didn't know what they needed or had, or (3) were closed to a new way of thinking. He made a note of everyone's responses and politely answered that he expected a full partnership with each director moving forward.

He then asked each director to summarize her respective programs and services and to describe the main issues and performance within each, clearly stating the key business and clinical drivers of their businesses. Only the first two who initially sought his help were happy to answer him fully. The other four vaguely answered the question, despite his probing.

The two directors who had reached out definitely needed help and were happy to have someone work with them because they were hungry for guidance. The first set of meetings also clearly showed that the other four managers did not wish to improve care delivery or operations. One thing was certain: None of the four wanted to relay any information that would educate Josh about the issues they faced or Josh's own ability to lead.

Josh decided to take the high road and push the theme of transparency by being transparent about his expectations. He would treat everyone equally and expect equal work products from each. For the next three weeks, he continually repeated this sentiment to each director. Then he got to work.

Baseline Assessments

Initially, Josh asked each of his directors to identify five business drivers and up to ten clinical drivers. He wanted the information, but this was also Josh's way of testing his staff so he could assess their skill sets and their level of understanding about their respective businesses, as well as gauge their analytical abilities.

After weeks of struggle, most could not clearly identify their drivers, nor could they state what metrics or indicators would be useful to measure their drivers. Josh accepted that this was new for them and that he could not expect them to immediately address their management issues; it was clear that they needed help in identifying what was integral for each to monitor and focus on. He decided to get back to the basics and wrote a list of indicators he wanted to get his directors to sign off on. His tactic was to get the directors to think about and acknowledge the importance of the metrics he had written down.

Josh scheduled a meeting with all of the directors and asked, "How about we help each other identify what drives our respective programs? What specific business and clinical things do we rely on? What are the most important drivers needed to operate the division?"

One director shyly raised her hand and noted, "We need patients to operate our businesses."

Josh smiled, "Excellent. Let's call this business metric *admissions* or *cases*. Do you know how many admissions or cases you had last year?"

The director sheepishly responded that she did not.

"No problem," replied Josh as he wrote *admissions* on the flip chart. "We're defining metrics at this meeting so that we can begin to collect data on each driver. This will then help us to develop scorecards that will help all of us manage better. Any other things we each rely on to operate our businesses?"

Another director replied, "We rely on our billing to pay our clinicians' salaries."

Josh felt more confident as he continued to write each metric the directors noted on the flip chart. After he had listed several he noted, "Perfect. Now let's divide this up. One indicator is revenue. Another can be claims billed. Another is the denial rate, or the number of claims or dollar amounts that were denied for payment by the insurance companies. Another can be the percentage of claims written off after we appealed each denial."

Josh's questions and the directors' responses continued, but only two of his directors actually participated in the discussion; the other four merely scowled or smirked. Josh initially encouraged each director to participate, but as he had come to this meeting understanding that he did not have complete buy-in from all six directors with respect to the process, he tried to direct the conversation toward the two who were actively participating.

The meeting continued for two hours, and in this time they listed ten business drivers including census and visit volume, clinician-to-patient ratios, and nursing daily visits. On the clinical front, they came up with 15 drivers or "influencers of care," as one director called it, including rehospitalization rates for pediatric patients, documentation of high-risk infants and C-section wound care measurements, patient retention for one prevention-focused program, and immunization and breastfeeding rates. Josh also inserted a few metrics he wanted to collect, and others that he knew the CEO, COO, and senior vice president of operations wanted to have on their radar.

On a clean piece of the paper, Josh organized the business and quality metrics in the following chart, delineating a column for each indicator's target, another for actual year-to-date results, and columns for the states and regions served (see Exhibit II.9).

The meeting ended on a relatively bright note. One director enthusiastically stated, "It'll be nice to see how each of us is faring and where we need to go. I want the best for my nurses and patients!" However, the four

EXHIBIT II.9

Key Business and Quality Measures

	Target	YTD Actual	Region A	Region B
Key business measures				
Key volume metrics				
Key billing metrics				
Key financial metrics				
Key quality measures				
Key process metrics				
Key cost/utilization metrics				
Key outcomes/ diagnoses metrics				
Key patient satisfaction metrics				

directors who had silently glared at Josh during the entire meeting only raised their eyebrows and quietly walked away from the meeting. Josh walked out with one of them and asked what she thought. "You're wasting our time, Josh. I've got nurse managers to supervise," she grinned. Josh simply looked at her and wished her a good day.

The next day, Josh started to work with the programs' analyst to run the data for each metric. Running the data proved difficult for most of the indicators for several reasons: (1) the way the data were collected in the organization's databases, (2) the multiple systems used to collect the data, and (3) the varying data definitions of the indicators each system and program used.

In the following weeks, Josh and the analyst continued to run the data for each metric, by region and state, and began to develop a comprehensive baseline assessment for the division. Sometimes the data would not match because it depended on the system they used for data collection and the system they selected for reporting. As a result, it took several interim reports and multiple discussions with senior staff and finance to come to agreement about which definitions and reports to use so that they could produce a baseline assessment that everyone would agree was accurate.

The final result of the baseline showing the first quarter's results and the scorecard provided evidence that much work needed to be done. Most results were below budget or target. While it would be easy to show the staff the results, Josh knew that getting them to accept the data and then working with them to improve the results was going to be difficult.

Josh was especially apprehensive about the performance and attitude of Trudie Slivonte. Trudie was the director of the short-term, skilled care program that served the bulk of the division's patients but was the one that suffered most of the inefficiencies and financial losses. Josh always thought she "beat her chest" a little too much in bragging about her perceived sense of self-worth, expertise, and program performance. She was the one who initially smirked behind Josh's back that he was not a clinician, and later commented that he was wasting her time. Josh was hit with a double whammy: How does he address the program with the most financial and performance problems when the director is not fully on board?

Dashing to the Scorecard

The root driver of the division's performance depended indirectly on the management staff; however, the direct drivers of performance were the clinical staff—the nurses, therapists, and social workers who delivered the service. And those directly overseeing the clinical staff who made the patient visits were the individuals who could most effectively educate and influence the clinicians to improve performance. Josh got excited when he came to this realization, as he thought to himself, *This means that I don't have to rely solely on Trudie to get this done, because there are others with whom I can also work.*

Josh called Trudie into his office and with a big smile said, "Please schedule a conference call with all of the frontline managers. I'd like to work with you so we can jointly lead a discussion about the drivers of your program, its baseline performance results, and strategies to improve clinical and operational performance."

Trudie squinted. "I'm aware of the sudden interest in improvement work. But how about you don't worry about this and let me focus on it."

Josh looked at her with a grin and replied, "That sounds great. I sent you the scorecard with the baseline performance data results two weeks ago. What are the key findings from that scorecard, and what are you going to focus on when you lead the discussion without me?"

Trudie was annoyed. She knew she had no interest in letting the staff know performance results and had not read the scorecard. She replied haughtily, "I don't have time for looking at your scorecard, but I'll take care of this when I get a chance."

She started to turn and walk away but stopped in her tracks when she heard Josh firmly say, "Not exactly the ideal answer I was waiting to hear, Trudie. It isn't even part of an answer that will help us try to move forward and focus on the need to improve our results. And despite working with all of the directors for the last several months, I see no indication of your interest in leading or wanting to understand this. I expect a conference call to be arranged within the next week with all of the managers in your program; your answer makes it evident to me that I have to lead this discussion. You are welcome to attend. And moving forward, I'd appreciate your support."

Trudie stared at Josh and begrudgingly replied, "We'll schedule a meeting by next Thursday."

Over the next week, Josh and Trudie reviewed the performance scorecard for Trudie's program. The business results spoke for themselves; the quality indicators were almost all near or above targets, as shown in Exhibit II.10.

More than 25 other indicators were also listed, 10 business indicators and another 15 clinical indicators.

Josh had sent out the scorecard with these results to all regional and state managers well before the conference call. He had prepped Trudie to lead the discussion, but she lacked enthusiasm and was only minimally willing to try to understand the results. As a result, during the conference call he took the lead and explained the scorecard's purpose, the indicators, and the monthly and year-to-date results for the program as a whole. Josh then asked

EXHIBIT II.10

Sample of Key
Indicators

Sample Key Business Indicators	Metric Achieved (vs. Target)
Claims unbilled	$12M (vs. $20M annual revenues billed)
% of total managed care claims denied	>38% (vs. national benchmark of 5%)
% of total managed care claims written off	> 15% (vs. national benchmark of 6%)
Nursing daily productivity (in visits per day)	3.5 (vs. VNSA average of 6)

Sample Key Clinical Indicators	Metric Achieved (vs. Target)
Care management documentation	
High-risk infants	80% (vs. 95% target)
C-section wound care	87% (vs. 95% target)
Rehospitalization rate for pediatrics	7% (vs. 5% target)
Immunization rates	85% (vs. 90% target)
Overall patient satisfaction rate	95% (vs. 90% target)

for feedback, and the clinical managers had multiple questions for Josh and Trudie.

Most participants on the call were enthusiastic about the data, including one who remarked that the data had never been laid out so clearly—and in such detail. Others were happy to chat with Josh, as another mentioned that in the past the vice president had been "blatantly invisible" to them. Three managers asked what Josh wanted them to do with the data.

"Nothing right now," replied Josh. "My purpose is to show you the results. For the next three months, we'll have more conference calls, and prior to each, we'll share the results of the current month, and the year-to-date and previous year's data. Thereafter, we'll work together in biweekly sessions to look at the monthly trends and strategize operational improvements. Sound good?"

Collectively, they all made encouragingly positive remarks. A few noted how this would impact clinical frontline staff, to which Josh responded, "Good point. In two months, after you are all relatively comfortable with the indicators and data, I want to schedule monthly meetings with the frontline staff via conference calls."

Everyone on the call in Josh's office was eerily quiet after Josh's last comment. Trudie raised both eyebrows and said, "You mean you'd like us to pull staff from the field for a couple of hours a month and have them sit in these data-intense meetings when they could be treating patients? Are you going to waste everyone's time with this?"

Josh's face turned red. Trudie had just changed the tone of this two-hour call. He composed himself and simply said, "We pull staff from the field for monthly staff meetings, don't we? In these meetings we speak about patient care issues and process issues, but are we not also supposed to be reporting out to our clinicians about how they are performing in terms of visit productivity, patient acuity levels, and clinical results?"

One pediatric clinical manager on the call replied, "Yes, we do that."

"Then, I would suggest that it's not too much to ask to have the clinical staff in these meetings spend 30 minutes learning about our business and clinical results from a regional, state, and programmatic level, is it? I will attend each of the regional frontline group staff meetings for the next month, and I'd like 30 minutes on your agendas to share our collective results."

Trudie was fuming but contained herself and said, "What do you mean 'collective results'?"

Josh smiled and said, "The next set of scorecards will have all of the data presented by region and state and by the program as a whole."

"Just to be clear, Josh, does this mean that we're going to see each other's results?" asked one clinical manager on the phone; he sounded nervous.

Josh simply said, "Yes."

No one replied, and Josh could sense apprehension. Yet everyone signed off cordially when Josh ended the call. He looked at Trudie and stated, "In the next week, I expect to see a plan from your office that identifies the key issues in your program's scorecards and offers operational performance solutions for each of the indicators that is below target."

Trudie quietly accepted the directive and walked out of his office.

Making Progress?

In the coming months, Josh spent hours speaking directly to the frontline clinical staff and the regional managers about both the business and clinical indicators. Initially, most of the frontline staff did not understand why they were speaking directly to the vice president. Moreover, they did not understand why they were being asked to know about the business indicators specifically. In some regions, the common retort was, "Nice to 'meet you' over the phone, Josh, but we've got patients to see. You are the numbers guy and we're the clinical staff. We don't see how your business issues impact the healthcare service delivery for our patients."

Indeed, most of the clinicians he had met were of the min-dset, "You are business. I am clinical. The two do not tango."

To counter this viewpoint and to show how interrelated everything was, Josh developed a new mantra: "Think of the business and clinical areas as two hemispheres in a globe. Each half makes a whole. But understand that the clinical area drives the business side. For example, if our nurses do not increase the numbers of patients they serve each day, patients will be waiting for service. We are growing 5 percent in monthly admissions. For every patient who waits to be served, we are out of regulatory compliance to treat patients within 24 hours of referral. Additionally, each patient is tied to a number of medically necessary visits, based on their acuity and diagnoses. For each of these visits that we are not able to perform, we lose revenue. Revenue lost is tied to our ability to pay clinical and management staff to serve and oversee the treatment of services."

He gave another example to the nurses. "Most of our patients are insured by managed care companies. Each of these managed care companies expects to be asked—via a managed care report—the number of visits they will initially authorize based on the patient's medical need for services. If you do not complete this managed care report at the start of care as requested by each managed care company, we will be delivering the number of visits only on the basis of the number that you and the overseeing physician agree on for the patient's care plan. If the visits are not requested via the reports to the insurance companies, they will deny payment because they will say that we did not seek their permission to deliver the services. If you look at the scorecards I sent out, more than 40 percent of all admissions do not have authorization by the managed care companies for us to deliver the visits. This means that our denial rates are astronomical (more than 38 percent) and that revenue is not flowing into the program. Remember, if these visits were already delivered by you—our expert pediatric nurses—and we are not paid for them, that means that you are working for free. We seek to sustain the integrity of your profession and expertise by improving our business indicators."

One feisty nurse on the call interrupted: "Wait a minute. Is that why my nurse manager is always on my case for me to submit my managed care reports within a certain amount of time? I always do, but I must admit I'm late most of the time because I'm having trouble tracking down the physicians to discuss the care plan treatment and agree about the number of visits a patient needs. The reports are so long that it takes me a while to complete them. But I make the visits anyway because these patients have cancer or have messy complications from their rare congenital diseases. Do you mean that I'm contributing to that 38 percent denial rate because the insurance companies are denying payment of the visits I already delivered to my sick kids?"

"Yes," replied Josh, "but I notice that you said that you are having trouble finding the physicians and that the reports are burdensome to complete. Is this true for everyone on the call?"

Everyone started talking at once about how they were always getting the wrong physician name on their referral forms and that the managed care companies always ask for too much information in their reports. Josh took active notes during the call. In the next round of phone calls, he and the managers and clinicians came up with areas to tackle to streamline processes and improve data collection.

Over the next few months, these calls continued to produce an avalanche of issues to address. In time, Josh and the clinical managers developed another set of scorecards related to process improvement indicators and program-based and division-based dashboards that were used on a monthly basis to monitor performance. In one of his staff meetings with his directors, Josh announced that he had worked with human resources to tie the directors' annual bonuses to their respective programs' scorecard results. Most sat in silence, shocked that part of their salary was now tied to their programs' outcomes. Coupling this with the fact that the scorecards revealed each state's or region's results, by program, and that everyone—including the directors, state and regional managers, and all clinicians—were comparing themselves to each other, four of the directors became furious but kept quiet. Even after eight months of Josh leading this change, they were still not used to the level of transparency he demanded for data and reports.

What surprised (and slightly amused) Josh most was that each program, and therefore the entire division, saw its performance in most of the indicators shift in a positive direction. He learned through the grapevine that because everyone was now seeing the monthly results, friendly competition was helping to drive the performance improvements. The middle- and front-line managers—and the clinical teams—seemed to enjoy the competition more than the directors, most of whom continued to sulk about sharing the information across programs and regions. What amused Josh the most was that the directors were upset—even when their programs were improving and even when Josh and his senior team continued to get compliments from VNSA's executive management about how they'd never seen performance in the pediatric and maternal division shine so much.

Over the course of the year, Josh and his directors continued to have their one-on-one staff meetings, and he spoke monthly with the regional and state managers and clinicians about each area's performance. Eventually, one of the four directors who had scowled at the reports and the need for transparency became the improvement process's biggest promoter—this switch was likely because Josh gradually gave ownership and credit for the improvements in that area to that particular director. Nonetheless, the other three directors continued to scowl, despite their programs' successes, and they remained steadfast in refusing Josh's repeated offers to fully partner with them. The two directors who had initially given Josh no resistance had taken their respective programs to the next level in a little more than a year.

Notably, Trudie's program scored the biggest performance gains because her clinicians and managers enjoyed speaking with Josh and appreciated his continual encouragement to do better after each incremental improvement. In fact, over the course of 17 months, the program's performance skyrocketed (see Exhibit II.11).

However, while Trudie softened her demeanor and started to playfully tease Josh and, at times, rose up to his expectations, she continued to gossip behind Josh's back—comments that Josh heard but ignored. It seemed that the more Josh encouraged her to improve performance, the more she gossiped.

Over the course of the next year, Josh, the senior vice president of operations, and the vice president for finance and business operations raised the targets and budgeted numbers to drive further improvements. While the division continued to lose money because it was underfunded by its programs' grant contracts and traditional reimbursement mechanisms, its performance in terms of its operational efficiencies, budgeted expenditures, and cash flow improved significantly. Josh encouraged and continually empowered the three of his directors who supported him and who drove their staff to further success.

EXHIBIT II.11
VNSA Program
Improvements

Key Business Indicators

- 29% improvement in RN daily visits

- 1.5% managed care denial rates (down from 40%)

- 0.8% managed care write-off rates (down from 21%)

- 40% reduction in unbilled claims

- 70 percentage-point improvement in timely scheduling of visits

- 3.9% attrition of patient census (down from 11%)

- $1.8 million better than budgeted expenditures

Key Clinical Indicators

- 10% improvement in care processes documentation

- 20% improvement in immunization rates and breastfeeding rates

- 5% reduction in rehospitalization rates

During their annual performance evaluation meetings, he gave these three directors high marks on their respective performance evaluations and awarded them with the highest bonuses allowed. And while the other three directors who gave Josh the biggest headaches continued to scoff at everything Josh said and did, their programs fared well because of the performance improvement initiative. Josh fairly awarded them high praise for their program's performance, but was blunt about their behaviors, attitudes, and general mannerisms.

Before the holiday season in his third year on the job, Josh scheduled a 1:00 p.m. meeting to discuss these three resistant directors' management styles and his difficulty in managing them. He had tolerated enough, and he wanted to set the record straight. However, five minutes before the scheduled meeting, Josh received a call from his boss, the senior vice president of operations.

"I am taking you out of the division, and we're asking you to lead a multiyear initiative across the company that will consolidate divisions, streamline processes, improve efficiencies, and reduce costs. You will have no staff, but we can ask others in other divisions to unofficially work with you. Do you accept this position?" she asked. "I need your answer."

Josh was surprised by the call. It was unexpected, and he, while flattered, had other initiatives in mind for the pediatric division. He was only getting started with leading this part of the organization, even after three years on the job.

He looked up from the call and saw, at his office's doorstep, three irate directors looking at him. Trudie looked the maddest of them all. It was their signal that he was late for the 1:00 p.m. meeting.

Case Questions

1. What is your interpretation of what happened in this case? Assume for the moment that Josh was successful at improving performance and that this was why he was being transferred.
2. If you were Josh's boss, would you have advised or supervised him differently? In what ways is Josh's boss responsible for what occurred in the case study?
3. What are some strategies Josh could have implemented to obtain more buy-in from his directors? How would you have managed and responded to Trudie, in particular?
4. To which incentives do or will the six directors best respond? Whose organization is this?

5. How likely is it that the momentum Josh created in improving performance among the six directors will be lost by his successor?
6. Was Josh a success, and will he go on to other "performance improvement" triumphs at VNSA?

Short Case 7
Sparks Medical Center and the Board of Trustees

Anthony R. Kovner

Sam Phillips, chairman of Sparks Medical Center's board of trustees, wondered why hospital board meetings were so different from those at his spice company, Phillips' Flavors, Inc. The hospital board discussed the reports of various committees, reviewed accreditation and licensing reports, and listened to reports and recommendations about state regulations and reimbursement. At Phillips' Flavors, Inc., the board discussed the future of the business, what the competition was doing, and strategies to increase market share and profit margins.

Clara Burns, CEO of Sparks Medical Center, made the following recommendations to Phillips regarding more effective board meetings:

1. Board discussion should focus on the organization's mission.
2. Objectives and strategies should be established.
3. A strategy to plan and measure board performance should be developed.

Sam realized that it would be difficult to address these issues given the board structure and organization, which led to excessive amounts of meeting time spent on routine committee and management reports. The current process resulted in a full agenda and little time to deal with issues critical to the future of the medical center.

Case Questions

1. What do you recommend that Sam do now?
2. Identify constraints and opportunities that Sam will face when implementing your recommendations.

Short Case 8
Ergonomics in Practice

J. Mac Crawford and Ann Scheck McAlearney

Riverlea Rehabilitation Hospital's administrators had recently begun to notice high levels of absenteeism, workers' compensation claims, and time off from work associated with back and other injuries suffered by their workers. Staff were prone to injuries when patients lost their balance while being moved—especially when staff were required to use their own bodies to prevent patient falls. Patients, in turn, could be injured when staff were unable to secure the patients due to the overwhelming physical load or because of preexisting injuries or deficits in staff members' physical strength. Tim Montana, the administrative director, had heard that the new system of patient lifting devices planned for installation at Riverlea Hospital could effectively reduce both the number of workers' injuries and associated workers' compensation claims and absenteeism rates, but the new system was expensive. Montana believed the lift system's cost would be worth the benefits, but he wanted to make sure.

The new lift system had been designed so that patients could be placed in a harness and moved from a bed to a chair, the bathroom, or anywhere else in the room. It was meant to be used consistently, and consistent use was apparently associated with reduced risk of injury to both staff and patients.

To prove that the new lift system helped address the problems associated with the musculoskeletal injuries reported by Riverlea nursing staff, Montana enlisted a team of researchers from the local school of public health. Montana wanted to be able to provide quantifiable evidence that the new system had made a positive impact at Riverlea.

During Montana's meeting with the research team, Dr. Jason Terry, the lead environmental health services researcher, explained that the best approach to evaluating the impact of the lift system would be to undertake a longitudinal study of the health of Riverlea personnel. As Terry explained, the research team could first collect baseline information using existing injury data, then supplement these data by collecting new information about work practices, shifts, and musculoskeletal symptoms among the target workers. After installation of the new lift system hospital wide, the researchers could collect follow-up data to assess the system's efficacy.

Montana convinced the rest of Riverlea's administrative team that a research study was justified, and approved the budget request to support the investigation. Baseline data were collected before the lift system was installed, and plans for the follow-up assessment were made. However, Montana observed the implementation and initial use of the lift system at Riverlea and was concerned about the process. He and his team had seen evidence that many staff members were using the devices incorrectly, were using them intermittently, or were not using them at all. Well aware that improper use of the system would bias any research data collection process, Montana decided to ask the engineering department to check whether the lift system was operating as planned. After a week of study, the engineering personnel reported to Montana that the lifts themselves were functioning properly, so that was not the problem.

Montana next asked individual staff members for their opinions about the lift system. After only a handful of conversations, Montana realized that there were plenty of opinions about the lift system, and most of these were negative. Staff appeared unconvinced about the value of the lift system, and instead were delighted to tell Montana stories about how they had managed to "work around" the system to lift their patients in the "usual way." Montana still believed that the lift system could have a positive impact at Riverlea, but he knew that current use patterns were inconsistent and inappropriate. He knew he had to do something to intervene, but he didn't know where to start.

Case Questions

1. What options does Montana now have to convince staff to use the new lift system consistently and properly?
2. Are there appropriate metrics and goals by which to evaluate the success of the lift system implementation? What metrics should be used to meet what goals? And what is an appropriate timeline for meeting those goals?
3. What would be an appropriate role for a research team evaluating the impact of a new lift system?
4. Who should be accountable for correct adoption and use of the new lift system?
5. For a different organization considering installing a new lift system, what type of process would you propose to build staff support and buy-in for the system? Who would be the relevant stakeholders to include in planning for the new lift system's introduction?

Short Case 9
Financial Reporting to the Board

Anthony R. Kovner

Act I

At the December board meeting for Christian Health System, board member Sam Brown received the following 2008 Operating Budget Highlights from Larry Dolan, chief financial officer:

HOSPITAL 2008 OPERATING BUDGET HIGHLIGHTS

- The surplus for 2008 is projected to be approximately $640,000.

VOLUME

- The budget is based on 28,000 inpatient discharges, or 76 discharges per day. This rate is 1.6 discharges a day higher than the hospital's projections for 2007 (74.4).
- The closing of Clark Hospital and the recruitment of new physicians are expected to produce the projected growth in discharges.
- Other hospital outpatient services (emergency, ambulatory surgery) are conservatively budgeted to continue at current volumes.

REVENUE

- Total revenue is budgeted to increase by 5.7 percent:
  - Net patient service revenue is projected to increase by 7.6 percent.
  - Other revenue is budgeted to decrease by 17.8 percent, mostly due to the loss of one-time items such as donations, and a projected decrease in investment income.
  - The reduction in investment income is a product of an anticipated decline in cash and investment balances due to amounts owed to Eastern State, pension payments, and capital purchases.
- New rates were included in the budget for Medicare, Medicaid, and other payers:
  - New Medicare rates included an inpatient increase of 1.5 percent. In the 2008 rate, the city wage index decreased.
  - Medicaid rates have been budgeted at the preliminary January 2008 issued rates, which includes an adjusted trend factor of 1.88 percent.

- New negotiated rates for managed care are included in the revenue model by payer. The following are some examples of these increased rates:
  - Blue Cross: +6 percent
  - Aetna: +4 percent
  - Plan 1: +10 percent
  - Plan 2: +6 percent
  - United Medicaid: +15 percent, and Commercial: +3 percent
  - Plan 3: +5 percent
- Case-mix indexes for Medicare (1.43), Medicaid (1.38), and Plan 4 nonmaternity (1.22) are budgeted at the actual levels through October 2007.

EXPENSES

- Total expenses are budgeted at 5.8 percent above projections of 2007 spending.
- This reflects the following:
  - The expansion of the available medical/surgical acute care beds by 16, with 8 beds as of January 1, 2008, and another 8 beds as of February 29, 2008, for a total increase of 16 beds.
  - The following contractual increases:
    - RN union: 3 percent, as of January 1, 2008
    - Technical and professional union: 3 percent as of January 1, 2008, and 3 percent as of December 1, 2008
    - Security guards union: 3 percent as of January 1, 2008
    - A 3 percent salary increase for nonunion staff as of April 1, 2008
  - Supplies and other expenses were increased for inflation at a rate of 3 percent.
- Other noteworthy expense changes included in the budget:
  - Benefits: an 11.8 percent increase from projected 2007 to 2008 as a function of the increased cost of union benefits and increases to nonunion healthcare benefits
  - Physician contracted services: an 11.9 percent increase reflecting both changes in salaries and increased coverage (e.g., labor and delivery, 24/7 coverage)
  - Bad debt: a decrease of 10.4 percent from projected 2007 to 2008 as a continuation of the "Stockamp Effect" and increases in charity care

Act II

The day after the board meeting, Brown sent the following e-mail to Dolan:

To: Larry Dolan
From: Sam Brown
Re: Financial Reporting to the Board

1. The purpose of this memo is to improve the quality of financial reporting to the board so that the board can add more value to hospital performance.
2. This is not the first time I have expressed these concerns to you. I become especially frustrated around budget time. The board spends way too little time examining the budget.
3. I do not feel sufficiently informed about the choices that underlie financial performance despite 17 years of service on the board, including several years on the executive committee as chair of the performance committee and as vice chair of our Medicaid managed care plan.
4. I would like to see a plan and a commitment from you to do better.

Questions That Came to Mind from Reading Your Distributed Materials and from Listening to Your Presentation

- You made no report on last year's results in relation to what you had forecast when last year's budget was presented.
- There was no summary of or explanation of variance in the financials presented.
- What are the assumptions on which next year's budget is based? For example, what are the specifics regarding the impact on admissions of Clark Hospital's closing?
- How can we increase revenues?
- What are we doing to decrease rehospitalizations?
- What investments should we be considering to improve quality of care?
- How do our expenses compare with benchmark hospitals?
- Why can't we make greater improvements in our lengths of stay, and what would be the impact of such improvements on our operating financials?
- What is the relationship between our financials and our strategic plan?
- What is our community service budget? How do we spend these funds currently? How could we spend them better?
- You don't seem to be getting much help from the board with these matters. Is there a problem with leadership of the finance committee?
- What are our options for controlling the increase in health benefits each year?

- Where is the discussion about how Christian will meet its capital needs in the future?

Act III

Two days after his e-mail, Brown received the following e-mail reply from Dolan:

> Thanks for your thoughtful questions. Most of these issues are discussed in great detail by the finance committee. I think if you read some of the minutes from those meetings you could get a better sense of the issues that are discussed.
>
> Regarding capital, as we have said at the past several board meetings, we are in the process of refinancing our housing complex. This effort will allow us to continue to operate the housing and allow us to continue providing existing subsidies to tenants, while at the same time draw significant funds from the refinancing. We are currently estimating approximately $30 million. In addition to this we continue to explore with the state options for moving funds from our Medicaid managed care plan to Christian Health System. And as I mentioned last night, we are obtaining $5 million in TELP financing and $2.1 million in state ERDA financing. Additionally, we were able to come to final endorsement with HUD much faster than any facility in the region on our $87 million borrowing. So all in all, while the capital picture is not great, primarily due to the funding needed for our pension plan, I think we are doing better than most hospitals in the city that serve high proportions of Medicaid and uninsured patients.
>
> I also think the finance staff works very closely with the program side of the house in trying to figure out new ways to fund productive, high-quality programs. Two examples of that were discussed last night: our relationship with University Hospital and our collaboration with the family health center on rehabilitation services. Our budget process is a "bottom-up" process, with detailed discussion at the cost center level, building up to cost groups, and then up to facility wide discussion. In those discussions we review old programs for viability and quality, and consider new proposals that will enhance our strategic direction. It should also be noted that over the past four years we have met our budget targets, and enhanced quality of care throughout the facility, while working in a fiscally restrained environment that has experienced reductions in both Medicaid and Medicare reimbursements that encompass approximately 75 percent of our patients.
>
> I will continue to work with the finance committee and the board to make our financial presentations more meaningful.

Case Questions

1. What are the strengths and weaknesses of board member Brown's e-mail about health system financial reporting?
2. What are the strengths and weaknesses of Dolan's e-mail response to Brown's e-mail?
3. How would you have responded to Brown's e-mail?
4. Why didn't Dolan respond as you have recommended?

Short Case 10
Handoffs in Patient Care

Brian Hilligoss

The Emergency Department at Midwest University Medical Center

Midwest University Medical Center (MUMC) is a highly specialized tertiary referral and trauma center affiliated with a major university in the Midwest. The main hospital is a 600-bed acute care facility that receives roughly 45,000 patient admissions each year, more than half of which come through the emergency department (ED).

When physicians in the ED decide to admit a patient, they complete an admission form in the electronic medical record (EMR), designating the service to which the patient is to be admitted. They also send a page to the admitting physician on that service. The admitting physician then calls the ED physician and takes a handoff over the telephone. During this handoff, the ED physician presents the patient's case, including some relevant medical history, information about the chief complaint, and how the patient has responded to care in the ED.

To a certain extent, the handoff signifies the transfer of responsibility for the patient from the ED to the inpatient service; however, this transfer can involve considerable ambiguity at times. Sometimes physicians on the inpatient services may feel that a patient would be better served by a different service. In such cases, they may redirect the admission to another service, and the ED physician must then make a handoff to that service.

Boarding in the ED

Patients must often remain in the ED for some period of time after the hand-off—a process known as "boarding"—until an inpatient bed is available and a transport tech can move the patient to the inpatient ward. Consequently, a kind of gray zone exists during boarding in which patients may receive less attention as staff incorrectly assume that someone else is looking after them.

This problem is exacerbated by the fact that boarded patients may be physically out of sight. After the handoff conversation has happened, ED staff often move these patients into the hallways of the ED to make room for other incoming patients. ED nurses and physicians, going about their duties caring for new, incoming patients, are physically removed from the hallways where the boarded patients wait. Meanwhile, the inpatient staff are even farther away. The MUMC ED is located in the basement of the hospital, while most of the inpatient wards are located in the tower on floors 4 through 11.

Because MUMC tends to operate at or near capacity, boarding is a frequent reality, and it is not unusual for patients to remain in the ED for six or more hours after the handoff. When shift changes in the ED or inpatient services happen during these times of boarding, the risk of a patient falling off someone's radar increases.

A "New" Patient?

It was 8:35 a.m. on a bleak February morning when Dr. Anita Henderson, a hospitalist, received an urgent page from a nurse. "Orders needed for Saunders. STAT. Nausea. In pain." Dr. Henderson was perplexed: she knew of no patient by the name of Saunders. She double-checked the paper list of patients she carried in her white coat. No Saunders. She looked at the whiteboard where her service lists the names of expected new patients. No Saunders. She asked several of her colleagues—other general internal medicine physicians on the hospitalist service—if they had a patient by the name of Saunders, but no one recognized the name.

Dr. Henderson had just begun her seven-day rotation on the hospital-ist service that morning. Dr. Chris Clark had rotated off the service the prior afternoon, and now his patients were her responsibility. When she arrived at 7:00 a.m., Dr. Henderson had taken handoffs from the night float residents who had been cross-covering the patients during the night. They had reported two new admissions, but neither was named Saunders.

Whose Patient Is This?

Dr. Henderson picked up the phone and called the nurse who had sent the page. The nurse reported that Mr. Saunders was a 61-year-old male with a history of smoking, emphysema, and diabetes. He had been admitted by the

ED for shortness of breath, and had just recently arrived on the general medicine floor. The nurse said that Mr. Saunders was complaining of pain and feeling nauseated. Dr. Henderson asked who was listed as the patient's attending physician. The nurse responded, "Dr. Chris Clark."

Hearing the nurse's concern regarding the patient's condition, Dr. Henderson laid aside for the time being any further questions about how this patient came to be on her service without her knowing or receiving some kind of a handoff from another physician. She went to see the patient for herself.

After examining and interviewing Mr. Saunders, Dr. Henderson concluded that he had missed at least one dose of each of his several home medications due to his stay in the ED and that he was somewhat dehydrated. His emphysema was flaring up, and he was clearly short of breath. He was also complaining of a "funny feeling in his heart." She also learned that he had been down in the ED since the previous morning, and had spent much of the afternoon and all of the night in a bed in a crowded hallway. Dr. Henderson offered an apology to soothe the clearly irritated patient and wrote orders for his medications and for fluids.

Later, Dr. Henderson sat down and looked closely at the patient's electronic medical record. She found the name of the ED resident who had issued the admission orders the previous day and sent him a page asking him to call her. Twenty minutes later, Dr. Calvin Lee, a third-year resident in the MUMC ED, called Dr. Henderson.

Dr. Henderson: This is Anita Henderson.

Dr. Lee: Hi, Anita. It's Calvin Lee returning your page.

Dr. Henderson: Hi, Calvin. Thanks for calling me back. I wanted to ask you about a patient by the name of Saunders. Did you admit him yesterday?

Dr. Lee: Saunders? Sounds familiar. We see so many...

Dr. Henderson: He says he came in yesterday morning with shortness of breath and maybe an irregular heartbeat. He has a history of smoking and emphysema...

Dr. Lee: Oh, my gosh! Yes! Did he end up on your service?

Dr. Henderson: Yes. He just arrived, and he's not doing well. I think he missed his medications and is dehydrated. Sounds like he was boarded overnight in the ED.

Dr. Lee: Could be. We were overflowing yesterday. Still super busy down here today. So, how can I help?

Dr. Henderson: Well, I just got a page from the floor nurse saying he was on my service and needed attention, but that was the first I heard of him. I'm trying to learn more about him and also find out where the ball got dropped.

Dr. Lee: Wow, nobody handed him off to you? And he's just getting to the floor now?

Dr. Henderson: Yes.

Dr. Lee: Well, that was a big ring-around-the-rosy yesterday! Well, his EKG showed an irregular heart rhythm, so I called pulmonary because I thought the abnormal rhythm might be due to his emphysema. But pulmonary said, "Oh, no, no. We think they're two separate issues. Admit to cardiology to get the heart rate under control and we'll consult." But then, when I called cardiology and they heard about the emphysema, they were like, "No, no, no. This is a pulmonary problem, and the heart is just a side victim. This has nothing to do with us, and what are we going to do with this? And he's going to be on our service for four days recovering from emphysema, and this is ridiculous and this is not what we do." Oh my gosh! They went back and forth and had me call the hospitalist service—Dr. Clark, I think. I can't even remember how many phone calls there were. I finally told them to work it out and then call me back. But I guess they never did. When I left at 3:00 p.m., I handed the patient off to my colleague.

Handoffs Within the ED

As the conversation continued, Dr. Henderson realized that the patient had been handed off several times in the ED: first when Dr. Lee's shift ended at 3:00 p.m., and then again at subsequent shift changes at 11:00 p.m. and 7:00 a.m. From experience Dr. Henderson knew that details about patient cases tend to get lost with multiple handoffs, particularly when patients have already been officially admitted and are being boarded in the ED.

Dr. Henderson learned that Dr. Lee had listed the hospitalist service as the admitting service in the EMR because at the point when he issued the admission order, it looked most likely that neither the pulmonary service nor the cardiology service was going to take the patient and that the hospitalist service would have to take him. (At MUMC, the hospitalist service is sometimes jokingly referred to as the "service of last resort" because in cases where no other service will accept a patient, that patient is to be admitted to the hospitalist service.) Dr. Henderson knew that the EMR system requires an admitting service to be selected to start the admissions process. She also knew that because Dr. Clark was responsible for the admissions pager for the hospitalist service yesterday, the EMR system would have designated him as the attending by default.

Dr. Lee also said that when he handed the patient off to his colleague at the end of his shift, he had instructed her to update the EMR once the final decision on placement had been made and to update the involved services.

Epilogue

Dr. Henderson cared for Mr. Saunders with consultations from physicians in the pulmonary and cardiology services and discharged him home after several days.

When Dr. Clark returned to work a few days later, Dr. Henderson asked him about the patient's case. Dr. Clark told her that when he had left that evening, it was still unsettled where the patient would go, as the other services were waiting for results from additional tests. Dr. Clark said he notified the night float resident about Mr. Saunders and that the ED would call if the patient were going to be admitted to the hospitalist service.

Case Questions

1. Multiple factors contributed to the problem. Identify as many distinct factors as you can.
2. Using your list of contributing factors from question 1, develop some strategies to reduce the likelihood of a recurrence.
3. Why do hospitals permit this handoff problem to continue?
4. As a hospital administrator, what would you do if this case had occurred in your hospital?

Short Case 11
An Information Technology
Implementation Challenge

Ann Scheck McAlearney

Introduction

Geneva Health System (GHS) is a large academic medical center based in Longwood, a midsized metropolitan city in the Southwest. GHS is associated with the state university, and includes three hospitals, a medical clinic facility, a medical research complex, and affiliated primary and specialty group practices spread throughout the region. Geneva University Hospital is the main hospital campus with 500 inpatient beds and equipment and facilities that are considered state of the art. GHS is well known for its cancer and rehabilitation service lines, and it has recently expanded its cardiac service line in an attempt to keep up with the increasing demand.

Despite strong clinical services lines and an excellent reputation, GHS has been reluctant to adopt new clinical information technologies (IT) and does not have an electronic health record (EHR) system. Instead, GHS's services are mainly supported by paper-based processes and a strong team in the medical records department that has been able to expand with the health system's growth.

Assessing the Situation

Dr. Dan Johnson has just been appointed CEO of GHS. He has come to the Longwood area after serving five years as CEO of a 200-bed community hospital. Johnson's predecessor, Jeffrey Ash, had retired after serving 20 years as GHS's CEO. Johnson is a definite fan of EHR and electronic medical record (EMR) systems, and he is enthusiastic about the potential for incorporating an EMR system into GHS. In particular, he is aware of the opportunities to use an EMR system to improve Geneva's ability to provide care according to evidence-based guidelines and to capitalize on the patient safety improvements that are possible with an EMR system.

The previous CEO, however, had been decidedly "old school" and had little interest in leading the charge to put Geneva on the EMR map. Instead, Ash chose to placate the established physicians and the director of medical records, Amy Chapman. Even though he was aware that the newer physicians were all carrying PDAs and iPhones, he had no interest in rocking the proverbial boat at Geneva.

Johnson is aware of the likely resistance he will face in his efforts to introduce an EMR system throughout Geneva. He has followed some of the IT implementation literature and knows that common barriers to implementation, such as physician resistance to changes in workflow and a reluctance to use practice guidelines or "cookbook medicine," may create challenges at Geneva. He also predicts resistance from the strong and capable medical records department. Given that successful EMR implementations are associated with a reduced need for space and personnel in medical records, such changes are unlikely to be warmly received.

A Hallway Conversation

As Johnson headed to the cafeteria for a cup of coffee, he was stopped in the corridor by Chapman, who was leaving the medical records department.

Johnson: Hi, Ms. Chapman. How is everything going in medical records?

Chapman: Not well, Dr. Johnson. I heard a rumor that you were considering bringing an electronic medical record system to Geneva, and that makes me very concerned.

Johnson: Well, Ms. Chapman, nothing has been decided yet, but there is a strong push nationwide to introduce EMR systems in all hospitals, and we don't want to be left behind.

Chapman: I understand that, Dr. Johnson, but I just don't think we want to do any of this too quickly. Mr. Ash had been very consistent in his message that Geneva had no reason to be an "early adopter" of such systems. As he repeatedly said, "Let all those other health systems make the mistakes first. Then we can learn from their mistakes and make our own decision. And, in the meantime, we can keep doing well what we already do well."

Johnson: I appreciate that perspective, Ms. Chapman, but I have to admit, I am a bit more likely to push the envelope than Mr. Ash. I believe an EMR system would be a great boost for Geneva, helping us to track everything electronically and potentially helping us to reduce medical errors in the process.

Chapman: But don't we already have the ability to track everything? I'm just not sure what's wrong with paper. Our medical records team is capable and responsive. I certainly haven't heard any complaints about our ability to access patient records.

Johnson: That's true, Ms. Chapman, but I don't think that we're looking far enough ahead. As other hospitals and health systems go digital, we're going to be left behind. I truly believe we do not have a choice in this situation. It is not a matter of "whether" but "when." I think it would be in the best interests of Geneva to get this going on the sooner side so that we can take advantage of the capabilities of an EMR system as soon as possible.

Chapman: Well, Dr. Johnson, I disagree. I tend to believe, "If it ain't broke, don't fix it." And the medical records department ain't broke.

Johnson: I understand your concerns, Ms. Chapman. Thanks for sharing them with me. Would you be interested in participating in a task force charged with investigating this opportunity?

Chapman: I'm not sure I think this is much of an opportunity. But since you're asking, I guess I'll need to participate.

Johnson: Thanks so much, Ms. Chapman. I appreciate your time.

As Johnson headed back to his office, he was once more reminded that none of this was going to be easy. He was especially concerned about resistance from the physicians. Although he was a physician himself, that did little to improve his credibility when he was making a case from the "dark side" of administration. He decided to seek out Dr. Jodi Smith, the chair of internal medicine, to gauge some of the sentiments from the physicians. He headed to her office to see if he could catch her for a moment.

A Physician's Perspective

Johnson: (Knocking as he enters Dr. Smith's office) Hi, Jodi. How's everything going?

Smith: Dan. Just the person I wanted to see. I heard a rumor that you were considering an EMR for Geneva, and I wanted to make sure that it was just a rumor.

Johnson: Well, Jodi, the rumor is actually true.

Smith: But Dan! Have you been following the latest research? Despite what the vendors claim, every place that puts one of these systems in reports that it actually takes the docs *more* time to do what they used to do on paper. Even after having the system in place for a while, the docs are still spending more time doing record-keeping than before—and that is time that they used to spend caring for patients! Also, when they put in a system somewhere in Pittsburgh, the EMR system was actually associated with an *increase* in the number of medical errors!

Johnson: I have followed that research, Jodi, but I think there's a bigger picture to consider here. While it's true that EMR systems do require the physicians to spend more time entering data and so forth, there's also evidence that with an EMR the right people are entering the data—not some nonclinical person trying to decipher a physician's notes about what was done, or trying to figure out if a visit was long or short. Also, evidence is beginning to build that when EMR systems are coupled with decision-support logic, such as order sets within CPOE [computerized provider order entry] systems, this type of system can actually save time. Instead of going through multiple screens to find all the meds and tests that need to be ordered, the physician can just click on the asthma order set, for instance, and review the options there.

Smith: But what about patient-centered care? Who says that every patient is alike? For heaven's sake, what if your patient needs something different? How long does it take to find that when everything is based on a standardized order set? And how about the resident physicians? Maybe they will stop thinking about making patient-specific clinical judgments and just click the standard order set for everyone! Have you really thought this through?

Johnson: I know there are issues, Jodi, but I truly believe the future of medicine is in electronic records. I'm guessing you've been following what's going on at the national level, and there are policy folks involved making a strong push toward expansion of EMRs into outpatient settings as well. Policymakers are concerned that hospitals and physicians have been too slow to adopt these systems, which they believe will improve both patient safety and the quality of care delivered, and they are beginning to propose incentive systems to encourage adoption. As I just mentioned to Amy Chapman, the director of medical records, I don't think this is a question of "whether" any more—it's just a question of "when." Geneva is a terrific health system that should be at the forefront of medical and technological advances, not waiting to see what everyone else does.

Smith: I'll bet Ms. Chapman was thrilled with the prospect of losing control of her medical records area. I think I understand your desire to help Geneva, but I don't think you've been here long enough to appreciate how great we already are. Mr. Ash repeatedly emphasized that we didn't need to be early adopters and that we could let others make the mistakes first, and I think that makes a lot of sense. Our docs are content with paper, we have a functional and responsive medical records department, and I'm not sure I sense any burning need to be the "most wired" or anything. This isn't Boston, after all. A lot of us chose to practice here because we could do what we do best—provide excellent clinical care—without the distractions of a push to be number one in the world or something like that. I'm just not sure you can make a major change like putting in an EMR and keep everyone happy like they've been for so long here.

Johnson: I realize I haven't been here at Geneva very long, but I've been working very hard to get a sense of this place before I propose any major changes. I also realize that introducing an EMR system to a place that is completely paper-based is no easy task. At this point I know there is still considerable work to be done to better understand both Geneva and the opportunities and risks associated with implementing an EMR. However, I strongly believe the future of medicine will require the electronic capabilities associated with an EMR system, and I am not willing to watch and wait much longer. I'd like to make an EMR system implementation a major goal for the coming year, and I'd appreciate it if you would consider being on a task force to make this happen. What do you think?

Smith: I think this is crazy. I agree with Mr. Ash. We should wait and see what happens at other hospitals and health systems and learn from their mistakes. There is no reason to stick our necks out on the cutting edge of EMR system implementation. And by the way, I'm not alone in my beliefs. Lots of other physicians agree. What we do here works just fine, and the people who work here are happy doing things the way they are done now. As for your task force, I don't have the time to participate in more silly administrative meetings. I need to use my time to help ensure that the clinical care we deliver here is as good as it can be. And that requires me to use my time seeing patients and overseeing our physicians in training who are learning to be better physicians.

Johnson: Well, I'm sorry you won't be able to participate more in this initiative, but I respect your time and your priorities. Thanks so much for sharing your thoughts.

Considering the Resistance

Johnson recognized that in addition to uncovering some attitudes toward EMRs, he had learned quite a bit about Geneva's organizational culture during these exploratory conversations about EMR adoption. The predominant culture appeared comfortable clinging to the status quo, and few individuals were open to the possibility of change. He had felt strong resistance from Chapman and Smith, and knew that resistance to change was a major hurdle he would have to overcome if there was any hope that an EMR implementation process could succeed.

Yet Johnson sensed that this resistance was not merely resistance to change, but resistance to change that would result in a loss of control for the individuals involved. As he reflected on his conversations with Chapman and Smith, he thought about some of the unspoken messages they had sent. Chapman and her group felt threatened by the loss of control they would have over the medical records process. With electronic systems in place, they would no longer have a major role to play in health systems operations, and their jobs might even be at stake.

Smith's comments suggested that the physicians were uninterested in changing their practice patterns because they would lose some of their control as well. The introduction of standardized order sets and other decision-support tools could truly change the way physicians practice medicine, thus leading to less discretion for individual providers with respect to viable treatment options. As both Smith and Johnson knew, with EMRs, there would be a searchable digital trail, which could be used to monitor those providers' practice patterns. While Smith mentioned her fear that newer physicians would come to rely too much on decision-support systems and stop thinking for themselves, an unspoken fear existed that if a physician did not do what the order set had defined as the right things, they might face problems.

Johnson had to plan his next steps carefully. He knew doctors valued evidence, and he had to build a good case for moving forward with an EMR implementation. He suspected learning more about implementation successes and failures would be valuable, but he also guessed other information existed out there that he was not aware of. Johnson decided to recruit a summer resident to help him expand his search for evidence and help build the case for EMR adoption.

Case Questions

1. What types of information should the summer resident collect to build the overall evidence case for an EMR system implementation? Where should she look to find this evidence?
2. What would you suggest that Dr. Johnson say to physicians who are concerned that an EMR will limit their ability to practice patient-centered medicine and provide individualized care to each individual patient? What evidence could you seek to support your argument?
3. How would adoption of an EMR affect organizational control systems at Geneva? How would it affect individuals?
4. What could be learned from speaking with hospitals and health systems about their experiences with EMR implementation? With whom would you like to speak at these organizations?
5. What would be critical success factors associated with implementation of an EMR at Geneva? What steps would you recommend to maximize the likelihood of success?

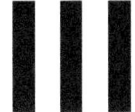
ORGANIZATIONAL DESIGN

To understand how the Professional Bureaucracy functions in its operating core, it is helpful to think of it as a repertoire of standard programs—in effect, the set of skills the professionals stand ready to use—which are applied to predetermined situations, called contingencies, [which are] also standardized.

—*Henry Mintzberg (1983)*

COMMENTARY

Understanding Organizations

Organizations are people and things combined to achieve an agreed-on goal in a changing and resource-scarce environment. Organizations have socially defined boundaries. They have a structure, a process, and outcomes. Understanding these concepts and how they relate to each other is at the core of organization theory.

Each of these basic concepts can be subdivided. *People* include workers, professionals, managers, and trustees. *Things* include long-term assets and short-term supplies. *Combination* includes dividing people and equipment into departments and a hierarchy aligned to the process of work and goals. *Resource scarcity* implies that achieving the goals of improved health must be constrained by the people and things available. The organization's *environment* can be described legally (laws governing behavior), economically (competition or monopoly), socially (how people define their work), and historically (our hospital is located where it is because that's where the donor gave us the land 100 years ago). *Goal achievement* can be estimated by measuring outcomes (patient census, mortality rates, vaccinations given). For-profit, not-for-profit, and government ownership of healthcare organizations (HCOs) relates to legal definitions and different goals; for example, long-run shareholder value maximization may be the goal of a for-profit organization. Organizations create different internal cultures. A faith-based organization may have a different vision and values than a for-profit organization, even though both may achieve their ends through the provision of high-quality care.

"I am a nurse working in the intensive care unit of Memorial Hospital." This simple statement describes an organization, its boundaries and goals, the work being done there, the technology in use, and a point in time. Another way to describe an organization is to explain its scarcities. The statement "We do what we can do best and let others do what they do best" is one way of understanding the "make or buy" managerial decisions that define the organization's boundary. "Our hospital needs computers and a food service, but we buy the former and contract out the latter because others can make and do these things better than we can."

Organizations must transform individual goals (my paycheck, my job satisfaction, my desire to help) into a unified overall goal or mission. Everyone who is a member of the organization is there because it fulfills his or her personal goals. Keeping the balance of all these personal incentives favorable over time and through changing circumstances in a way that achieves organizational goals is central to the role of management.

Understanding Organizational Design

Organizational design describes the way elements of an organization are arranged to meet the organization's goals. These elements include and affect the people and things that are combined in an organization. Mintzberg (1983, 1979) has suggested five basic types of organizational design or structure: simple, machine bureaucracy, professional bureaucracy, divisionalized firm, and "adhocracy" (Mintzberg's term for a mutually adjusting structure). These basic types represent different ways to organize work, and some ways work better than others. However, strictly causal relationships between technology and organizational design, or between environment and design, have not yet been proven.

The basic parts of Mintzberg's organizational types are the strategic apex or top managers, middle management, the technological structure (such as planners and industrial engineers), support staff (such as personnel and security), and the operating core (or workers). Each of the five types of organizational design has a different configuration of these five parts. For example, the simple organization (e.g., a doctor's office) has managers, support staff, and an operating core, but little or no technological structure or middle management.

Visually, organizational design may be depicted in an organizational chart showing relationships among these basic parts of organizations. Thus, a good organizational chart will illustrate links between and among top managers, middle management, the technological structure, support staff, and the operating core. Case G and Short Case 15 provide examples of organizational charts, but they can be considerably more complex.

The key means of organizational coordination vary according to the type of organization, and include approaches such as direct supervision, work standardization, standardization of professional skills, standardization of outputs, or mutual adjustment (Mintzberg 1983). In a simple organization, direct supervision is the key means of coordination. In a machine bureaucracy, such as a large outpatient department for the poor, work standardization is the key means of coordination. In a professional bureaucracy, such as a community hospital, standardization of professional skills is a key means of

coordinating the work. In a divisionalized firm, such as a multihospital corporation, the key means of coordination is the standardization of outputs, such
as profits or market share. Finally, in an adhocracy, work is coordinated as the
clinicians adjust on the spot to working with one another.

Work is sometimes organized according to the available physical facilities and may be influenced by an organization's history and the initial design
of its founders. For example, most doctors still are not employees of hospitals
because most physicians traditionally have been independent professionals.

According to Mintzberg (1983, 1979), work in the operating core can
be organized in one of three ways: by process or occupation (e.g., all nurses
report to the director of nursing, all physicians to their department chiefs);
by purpose or division, cutting across occupational specialties (e.g., all nurses
and physicians report to the local clinical leadership, which may be surgery,
women's health, or emergency services); or by both process and purpose, in
a matrix organization. Under this matrix method of organization, all nurses
report to the clinical leadership of the division for some activities and to the
director of nursing for others. Matrix organization solves certain coordination problems by process and by purpose but adds another layer to management, thereby increasing coordination costs. Managers must decide when to
use which form of organization and whether the benefits, if any, outweigh
the costs.

Organizational Design and Healthcare Delivery

Today, many hospitals are seen as just part of larger systems of care. Some
health systems are organized to provide a "continuum of care" including
primary care, secondary care in community hospitals, tertiary care, home
care, and long-term care all in a single market area. Such integrated delivery systems bring increased managerial challenges in planning organization
and performance measurement. Thirty years ago, a large city may have had
40 independent hospitals. Now these hospitals have either closed or merged
into a few large competing health systems or networks. These systems are
diversifying through vertical integration. Larger hospitals and health systems
are looking to purchase physician practices, and thereby employ rather than
contract with their physician providers. At the same time, industry is going
in the opposite direction. Business conglomerates with many subsidiaries and
product lines are dropping those that are not performing well and sticking to
"core competencies." Will healthcare follow this lead? Will these large integrated systems be dissolved back into their component parts?

Declining hospital occupancy rates resulting from shorter lengths of
stay and fewer admissions combined with the high fixed costs of hospitals have

fueled the competitive frenzy of the last few decades. This competition has led to many new organizational forms, and these changes are far from over. In addition, this competition has compelled closer attention to the wishes of the public and a growing emphasis on market understanding and patient satisfaction.

One new organizational form that has seen tremendous recent growth is the retail health clinic. Different ownership and operating models for these clinics have emerged, including clinics associated with a hospital or health system, those owned or operated by a drugstore retailer, and those independently financed and operated (Laws and Scott 2008). Yet this new care delivery option has raised issues around access to care for consumers, the quality of care provided by physician extenders such as nurse practitioners and physician assistants who staff the clinics, and business entities' motivations for opening and operating the clinics. While this organizational form is still new in some markets, its rapid expansion across the United States has sparked interest and controversy in both the business and policy arenas (Fenn 2008; Laws and Scott 2008; Lin 2008; Mehrotra et al. 2008; Newbold and O'Neil 2008; Paulus, Davis, and Steele 2008; Pollert, Dobberstein, and Wiisanen 2008).

Variation and Innovation in Organizational Design

Organizational variation is unending, both across the United States and around the globe. Some hospital-centered systems—such as the Hospital Corporation of America, the Voluntary Hospitals of America, or the Veterans Administration—cross healthcare markets. Health maintenance organizations (HMOs) combine the insurance function and provision of care under capitation, which is a reversal of the economic incentives of fee-for-service. Once, one could describe Kaiser-Permanente and say, "That is what HMOs are or expect to be." No longer. For example, point-of-service (POS) plans, which give enrollees a choice of care and payment levels, have become increasingly popular. Under this model, if patients use the core physicians and hospitals, they do not make copayments; if the larger preferred provider list is used, they do. The patient can go out of the network and pay even larger copayments. However, allowing patients a greater choice of providers than they would have in an HMO makes it more difficult to control quality and costs in such POS plans.

Other variations in organizational design are emerging as a result of the information revolution in healthcare. When information about patients is available electronically on a timely basis, providers may be able to make decisions about patient care alternatives without needing to be present. For instance, radiologists are now able to read films and make recommendations remotely. Surgeons can perform surgery remotely using computer-based technologies. Telemedicine is extending the reach of providers into remote and rural areas. Patients want to communicate with their providers via e-mail. Such technological innovations are encouraging HCOs to consider new approaches to delivering healthcare services that can reduce costs and improve the quality of care provided.

Process innovations are also important, as seen in the spread of techniques such as the Toyota Production System (TPS) or Lean production processes (Chalice 2007; Grunden 2008; Printezis and Gopalakrishnan 2007) and quality improvement methods such as Six Sigma (Trusko et al. 2007). In addition, there has been increasing emphasis on opportunities to apply best practices to HCOs, whether such practices are found in healthcare or outside the industry. For instance, Fred Lee's exploration of what hospitals would do differently if they were run by Disney (Lee 2004) emphasizes the importance of culture in improving the quality of service. Berry and Seltman (2008) similarly present the findings from their extensive research into the Mayo Clinic, highlighting the fundamental roles of organizational culture and shared values in delivering high-quality care.

External organizations and foundations are promoting these efforts by helping HCOs learn improvement techniques, many of which require design changes. The Boston-based Institute for Healthcare Improvement (IHI) made important strides in addressing quality improvement issues, such as the need to reduce the number of medical errors, in its 5 Million Lives Campaign from 2006 to 2008. Through its website and educational programs, IHI helps hospitals improve patient safety. Similarly, projects funded by the Robert Wood Johnson Foundation have emphasized the need to address organizational design and quality-of-care issues, such as the Urgent Matters program, which focused on the need to improve flow in hospital emergency departments to reduce overcrowding (www.urgentmatters.org), and the Expecting Success program, which explored ways of improving the quality of cardiovascular care provided in inpatient and community settings (www.expectingsuccess.org/).

Innovations in organizational design are producing improvements in care quality and reductions in healthcare costs. Within the United States, the Intermountain Healthcare system has successfully used TPS methods to reduce waste and improve efficiency while increasing the quality of the products it delivers (Jimmerson, Weber, and Sobek 2005). Similarly, results reported for Virginia Mason Medical Center of Seattle have sparked interest in both the healthcare and business communities (Spear 2005). Geisinger Health System's success has involved addressing issues such as clinical leadership, electronic health information systems implementation, and alignment of financial incentives to foster organizational innovation (Paulus, Davis, and Steele 2008). Organizational innovations overseas have produced startling results in the area of cardiac care, as demonstrated by two hospitals in India that have been able to perform open heart surgery for 10 percent of what such surgeries cost in the United States (Richman et al. 2008).

Yet healthcare in the United States remains extremely expensive and of variable quality. Barriers to change include misaligned reimbursement systems, regulatory limits on innovation, and the lack of a financial incentive system for the majority of patients to seek higher value in the care they receive. While the costs of making an international phone call, taking a transcontinental flight, or purchasing stocks are all decreasing in the United States, there is still a need for lower-cost materials, equipment, and sites of care within the healthcare system.

Organizational Design and Health

Some cost-cutting measures can be initiated with little change in the way care is organized. For example, using generic drugs and self-administered pregnancy tests and substituting physician extenders such as nurse practitioners and physician assistants for physicians save money. The next step is to "reengineer" care—or pursue "disease management" or "population health management," as it has come to be called. Reengineering care is based on answering the question, What is the best care for a defined population and how do we organize to achieve it? For example, how do we keep asthmatics out of the hospital? How do we reduce the loss from work caused by back pain? The Chronic Care Model, developed by Edward Wagner of Group Health Cooperative of Puget Sound (Bodenheimer, Wagner, and Grumbach 2002; Wagner et al. 2001; Wagner 1998), addresses the needs associated with caring for those with chronic diseases by examining the roles of primary care, care coordination, and the ability of patients to care for themselves.

From an organizational perspective, this type of approach calls for improving the organization of care and achieving measured outcomes. In addition, self-care presents another important opportunity to improve health. Asthma, diabetes, hypertension, and stress can be largely self-managed. Community coaches meeting in church basements with groups of diabetics who are trying to exercise and lose weight may be the future of healthcare focused on wellness in the community.

The Role of Management in Organizational Design

Organizations are often described at a moment in time (a photograph). They can also be described as changing over time (a movie). It is easier to describe the organization as a photograph, but the leader's task is to guide the organization over time: to envision a future preferred state and to get the organization from its present condition to that future.

Changes in organizational design, however, can be expensive and difficult to implement. It can be challenging and time-consuming to get individuals and organizations to change. Politics can also create barriers to change when powerful individuals or groups openly or covertly resist a change.

One key task of today's senior health executives is to determine which organizational design will best fit tomorrow's environment and how their organizations can get there ahead of others. This is indeed leading in uncertain times, with great rewards for the visionary who understands the environment well enough to predict correctly.

References

Berry, L. L., and K. D. Seltman. 2008. *Management Lessons from Mayo Clinic: Inside One of the World's Most Admired Service Organizations.* New York: McGraw-Hill.

Bodenheimer T., E. Wagner, and K. Grumbach. 2002. "Improving Primary Care for Patients with Chronic Illness: The Chronic Care Model." *Journal of the American Medical Association* 288: 1775–79.

Chalice, R. 2007. *Improving Healthcare Using Toyota Lean Production Methods: 46 Steps for Improvement,* 2nd ed. New York: ASQ Quality Press.

Fenn, S. 2008. "Integrating CCCs into the Hospital System." *Frontiers of Health Services Management* 24 (3): 33–36.

Grunden, N. 2008. *The Pittsburgh Way to Efficient Healthcare: Improving Patient Care Using Toyota Based Methods.* New York: Productivity Press.

Jimmerson, C., D. Weber, and D. K. Sobek II. 2005. "Reducing Waste and Errors: Piloting Lean Principles at Intermountain Healthcare." *Joint Commission Journal on Quality and Patient Safety* 31 (5): 249–57.

Laws, M., and M. K. Scott. 2008. "The Emergence of Retail-Based Clinics in the United States: Early Observations." *Health Affairs* 27 (5): 1293–98.

Lee, F. 2004. *If Disney Ran Your Hospital: 9 1/2 Things You Would Do Differently.* Bozeman, MT: Second River Healthcare Press.

Lin, D. Q. 2008. "Convenient Care Clinics: Opposition, Opportunity, and the Path to Health System Integration." *Frontiers of Health Services Management* 24 (3): 3–11.

Mehrotra, A., M. C. Wang, J. R. Lave, J. L. Adams, and E. A. McGlynn. 2008. "Retail Clinics, Primary Care Physicians, and Emergency Departments: A Comparison of Patients' Visits." *Health Affairs* 27 (5): 1272–82.

Mintzberg, H. 1983. *Structure in Fives: Designing Effective Organizations.* Englewood Cliffs, NJ: Prentice Hall.

———. 1979. *The Structuring of Organizations.* Englewood Cliffs, NJ: Prentice Hall.

Newbold, P., and M. J. O'Neil. 2008. "Small Changes Lead to Large Effects." *Frontiers of Health Services Management* 24 (3): 23–27.

Paulus, R. A., K. Davis, and G. D. Steele. 2008. "Continuous Innovation in Healthcare: Implications of the Geisinger Experience." *Health Affairs* 27 (5): 1235–45.

Pollert, P., D. Dobberstein, and R. Wiisanen. 2008. "Jumping into the Healthcare Retail Market: Our Experience." *Frontiers of Health Services Management* 24 (3): 13–21.

Printezis, A., and M. Gopalakrishnan. 2007. "Can a Production System Reduce Medical Errors in Healthcare?" *Quality Management in Healthcare* 16 (3): 226–38.

Richman, B. D., K. Udayakumar, W. Mitchell, and K. A. Schulman. 2008. "Lessons from India in Organizational Innovation: A Tale of Two Heart Hospitals." *Health Affairs* 27 (5): 1260–70.

Spear, S. 2005. "Fixing Healthcare from the Inside, Today." *Harvard Business Review* 83 (9): 78–91.

Trusko, B. E., C. Pexton, J. Harrington, and P. Gupta. 2007. *Improving Healthcare Quality and Cost with Six Sigma*. New York: FT Press.

Wagner, E. H. 1998. "Chronic Disease Management: What Will It Take to Improve Care for Chronic Illness?" *Efficient Clinical Practice* 1 (1): 2–4.

Wagner E. H., B. T. Austin, C. Davis, M. Hindmarsh, J. Schaefer, and A. Bonomi. 2001. "Improving Chronic Illness Care: Translating Evidence into Action." *Health Affairs* 20 (6): 64–78.

THE READINGS

Amer Kaissi describes how retail clinics, which have sparked interest and controversy, provide an opportunity to bridge the gap between consumers and healthcare but can create operational challenges for hospitals. A comparison between the alternative hospital-affiliated and hospital-owned retail clinic models illustrates the differences between these models, and highlights the various opportunities and challenges associated with each option.

Hospital-Affiliated and Hospital-Owned Retail Clinics: Strategic Opportunities and Operational Challenges

Amer Kaissi
From *Journal of Healthcare Management* 55 (5): 324–37

Summary

Retail clinics have experienced an exponential growth in the last few years. While the majority of retail clinics are freestanding, venture-backed companies affiliated with retail hosts, an increasing number of hospital systems have decided to develop their own retail clinics or partner with existing national companies. Using a stakeholder approach, the purpose of this article is to assess the strategic considerations behind these decisions and the operational challenges associated with them and to use the results to develop a questionnaire that can be applied in future research in a national sample of healthcare executives. We conducted eight in-depth interviews with administrative and clinical leaders in seven hospital systems across the United States that have or had a relationship with retail clinics in the last three years. Our findings show that the hospital systems' association with retail clinics involves two main models: an affiliation with retail chains that operate the clinics and ownership of the clinics with an arm's-length relationship with the retail chain. Hospital systems are engaging in these relationships for several strategic reasons: to increase market share through enhanced referrals to physician offices and hospitals, to become closer to consumers, and to experiment with nontraditional ways of delivering healthcare. Operational challenges included physician resistance and skepticism, poor financial performance, people's perception of retail clinics, staffing issues, and the newness of the business model. Six out of eight respondents thought that hospital affiliation with or ownership of retail clinics is a trend that is here to stay, although many provided caveats and stipulations. Further research is needed to provide more evidence about this emerging way of healthcare delivery.

Introduction

Retail clinics have experienced an exponential growth in the last few years; while only 63 retail clinics were in operation at the beginning of 2006, 982 clinics were operating in 2008 (Deloitte Center for Health Solutions 2008; Fottler and Malvey 2010; Rudavsky, Pollack, and Mehrotra 2009). Forecasts suggest that this explosive growth will only continue in the near future, with estimates of 6,000 clinics providing more than 50 million visits per year across the United States by 2011 (Scott 2007). While the majority of retail clinics are freestanding, venture-backed companies affiliated with retail hosts (Bohmer 2007), an increasing number of hospital systems have decided to develop their own retail clinics or partner with existing national companies (Leach 2008; Robeznieks 2007). The purpose of this article is to assess the strategic considerations behind these decisions and the operational challenges associated with them. Given that the retail clinic trend in general is relatively recent, little or no research has been done in this specific area. Therefore, this work is likely to fill a significant gap in the healthcare management literature.

Background Literature

Retail clinics are walk-in clinics located in grocery stores, drugstores, and general merchandise retailers (e.g., Walmart, Target, CVS, Walgreens). They offer a defined scope of diagnostic and treatment services for common medical conditions as well as preventive and wellness services (Fottler and Malvey 2010). Recent research suggests that the majority of retail clinic visits (90.3 percent) are for treatment of ten simple acute conditions and preventive care (Mehrotra et al. 2008). Care is usually delivered by a midlevel provider (nurse practitioner or physician assistant), and many clinics have up-front, menu-style pricing (Lin 2008). Therefore, retail clinics "represent a concept that is new to healthcare: no-frills healthcare that is offered at bargain prices" (Fottler and Malvey 2010, 3).

The main reasons driving this growth are overcrowding in emergency departments (EDs); a growing primary care physician (PCP) shortage; reduced patient access to care due to increased insurance costs; and growing consumer demands for convenience, reliability, and affordability (Fottler and Malvey 2010; Lin 2008). While the need for primary care doctors will especially peak as the first baby boomers turn 65, the American Academy of Family Physicians (2010) predicts a shortage of 40,000 family physicians by 2020.

From a patient perspective, retail clinics offer a high value proposition by addressing the frustrations of waiting patients, as no appointments are needed, evening and weekend operating hours are provided, and wait times are 15 minutes or less (Deloitte Center for Health Solutions 2008). Moreover, the clinics are located in settings that are already visited by consumers multiple times per week. Customer polls show high overall satisfaction with retail clinics (Harris Interactive 2007), and recent studies seem to support these findings (e.g., Hunter, Morreale, and Wall 2009).

Several concerns about retail clinics relating to the potential for fragmentation of care and to the possibility of compromised quality and patient safety have been raised by physician groups (Paddock 2007). However, these criticisms have not been supported by empirical evidence. In fact, recent evidence suggests that retail clinics provide similar or better quality of care at lower costs (Mehrotra et al. 2009; Rohrer, Angstam, and Furst 2009; Thygeson et al. 2008).

When the retail clinic trend first started, retailers were driving it and traditional healthcare providers such as hospital systems were not part of it. However, a number of large systems have recently started to operate their own retail clinics (Fenn 2008; Fottler and Malvey 2010; Lin 2008; Newbold and O'Neil 2008; Pollert, Dobberstein, and Wiisanen 2008). Clearly, while the systems are still not at a point of driving the movement, they are starting to play a much more important role. Of all 42 retail clinic operators in 2008, 25 were existing healthcare systems accounting for 11 percent of all the clinics (Rudavsky, Pollack, and Mehrotra 2009). Hospital systems currently have more than 120 clinics in operation, a 60 percent increase from 2008 (Deloitte Center for Health Solutions 2009).

Hospital systems are quickly seeking to take advantage of this emerging model by expanding their continuum of care and controlling referrals to their own physicians, EDs, and hospitals (Laws and Scott 2008). Building on their recognizable community brand, they are starting to compete head-to-head with the major for-profit retail clinic operators. Given that a significant number of patients are worried about staff qualifications and misdiagnoses in the retail clinic setting (Leppel 2010), hospital systems seem to be in an excellent position to ensure quality and patient safety (Lin 2008). As evidence, two of the most prestigious health systems in the United States have joined the trend. The Cleveland Clinic has lent its name to drugstore-based clinics in northeast Ohio, and the Mayo Clinic operates two clinics at a supermarket and a shopping mall in Rochester, Minnesota (Fottler and Malvey 2010).

In an influential 2006 article, Malvey and Fottler offer a stakeholder assessment that predicts the potential effects that retail clinics will have on a variety of players in the healthcare system. In their assessment (revised in the 2010 book by Fottler and Malvey), the main winners from the retail clinic movement will be the third-party payers, hospital EDs, specialist physicians, midlevel providers, urgent care clinics, employers, patients, and policymakers, whereas the main losers will be primary care physicians and medical group practices. Hospital systems are classified as potential winners or losers, depending on their ability to collaborate with, become subcontractors for, and extend services of retail clinics. We use this model as a guiding framework of this article (Exhibit III.1) and focus on one major stakeholder—hospital systems—as their relationship with retail clinics is not well explored.

Our short-term aim in this article is to answer three specific questions:

1. What are the strategic reasons behind hospital systems' ownership of or affiliation with retail clinics?

EXHIBIT III.1
Stakeholder
Model for
Retail Clinics

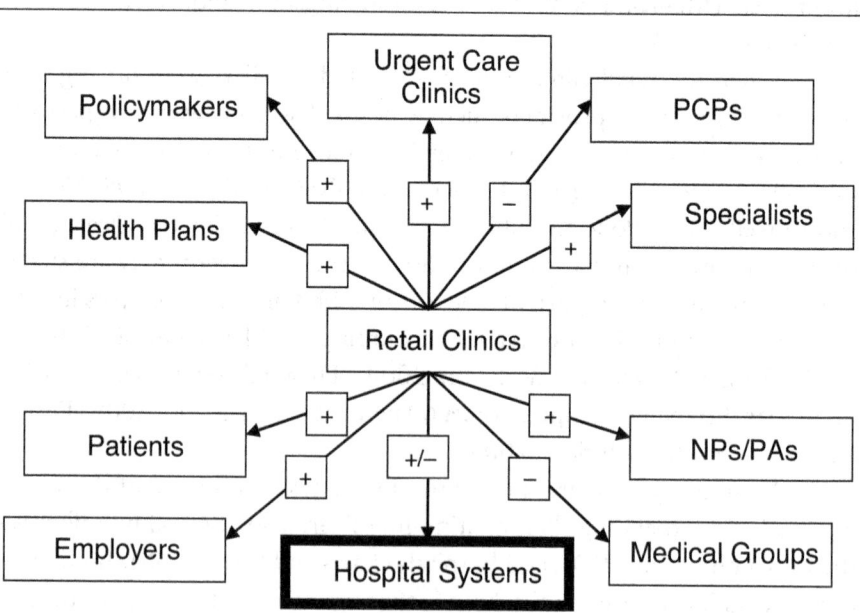

+: Denotes a winner from the retail clinic trend.
–: Denotes a loser from the retail clinic trend.
+/–: Denotes a winner/loser, depending on how the relationship evolves.
Note: NP = nurse practitioner; PA = physician assistant; PCP = primary care physician.
Source: Adapted from Malvey and Fottler (2006) and Fottler and Malvey (2010).

2. What are the operational challenges associated with these decisions?

3. Is the retail clinic trend for hospital systems a passing fad, or is it here to stay?

The long-term aim is to use the results of this study to develop a questionnaire that can be applied in future research in a national sample of healthcare executives in health systems that affiliate with or own retail clinics.

Methods

To assess hospital-affiliated or owned retail clinics, we approached (through professional relationships of the study author) nine hospital systems that had a relationship with retail clinics from 2006 to 2009. Of these, seven health systems agreed to participate, one did not answer our inquiries, and one declined to participate. One director of business development suggested that we also interview the medical director in his system, resulting in a total of eight interviews with administrative and clinical leaders in the seven systems (Exhibit III.2). The interviews were conducted by phone between July and September 2009 using structured, open-ended questions developed by the author (see "Interview Questions"). The seven

EXHIBIT III.2

Interviewees' Titles and Geographic Distribution

Interviewee's Title	Total Number of Affiliated Retail Clinics	Total Number of Owned Retail Clinics
1. Director, business development	10	—
2. Senior vice president, strategic planning	1	—
3. Vice president for clinical operations	15	4
4. Medical director of retail clinics	—	6
5. Vice president, strategic planning	6	—
6. Vice president, business development	—	5
7. Chief executive officer	—	2
8. Medical director of retail clinics*	10*	—
Total	32	17

*Represents same hospital system as interviewee 1; not included in total.

health systems represented a good mixture of owned and affiliated clinics (a total of 17 owned and 32 affiliated clinics) and operated in five states (Texas, California, Minnesota, Virginia, and Pennsylvania). The protocol used was approved by the Institutional Review Board at the author's university.

This research is qualitative in nature. Given that the phenomenon of hospital-affiliated and hospital-owned clinics is recent, we took an exploratory approach by conducting in-depth interviews. At the time of this writing, only 25 health systems in the United States own or are affiliated with retail clinics. Therefore, even though ours is a convenience sample, it still represents approximately 28 percent of US health systems. Moreover, to our knowledge, this is the first study on this specific facet of the retail clinic industry. Naturally, a valid and reliable instrument does not exist yet. In fact, that is one of the long-term goals of this study: to uncover issues and themes to develop a valid and reliable instrument that will be used in a national sample of healthcare executives in future research.

Interview Questions

1) Please describe how the relationship between your hospital system and retail clinics started:
   a. When did you start?
   b. How long did it take for the relationship to materialize?
   c. What model do you have in place?
   d. How many clinics do you have?
   e. In what areas are the clinics—affluent or underserved?
   f. What challenges did you face in implementing the partnership?
2) Strategically, why did you decide to do this?
   a. What does the clinic offer to the system?
   b. Does it help generate volume, or does it steal volume from PCPs? What benefits have you seen so far? Do they improve profits? Increase patient volumes?
   c. What does the system offer to the clinic?
   d. What does the affiliation offer to the community? Does it improve healthcare access to people who otherwise would not be able to get the care they need?
3) Does this strategy fit with your overall mission/vision/strategic plan? Would you describe it as a reactive or proactive strategy?
4) Is this trend of hospital-affiliated clinics a fad, or is it here to stay?

Findings

Models of Operations

For retail clinics that have linkages with a hospital system, the two common models of operations are (1) a partnership or affiliation between the retail chain and the hospital system and (2) full ownership of the retail clinic by the hospital system. Under the first model, the retail chain owns and operates the clinics and makes decisions about the clinics' locations and the hiring of the clinicians. The hospital system, on the other hand, provides physician supervision, marketing, and support for referrals. Under the ownership model, the hospital system owns the clinics either directly or through a separate legal entity created exclusively for this purpose. The system decides on the location of the clinics, employs the clinicians, and pays rent to the retail chain for the space provided. As explained by one medical director, "The system owns the business; we have an arms-length relationship with [the retail chain] [that] provides the space."

Regardless of the model of operations, the most important role played by the hospital system is finding a physician or physician group willing to provide supervision over the retail clinic(s). In a partnership, the retail chain typically approaches the hospital system to provide physician supervision. The hospital system then contracts with a physician group such as a primary care group or ED group. In the case of ownership, the hospital system appoints the medical director of the retail clinic(s), contracts with the physician group, and pays the physicians for their oversight.

Strategy/Fit with Mission

One of the main purposes of this research is to assess the strategic reasons behind the health systems' decision to develop/affiliate with retail clinics. Respondents mentioned several reasons: to learn about this new model of healthcare delivery, to experiment or build innovation around core businesses, to develop referrals to physicians and to the system (i.e., to increase market share), to tie the system's brand to that of a successful retail chain, and to become closer to the community. All of the respondents indicated that this strategic move fits with their existing mission and strategic plan. As one leader explained: "Strategically, from an access point of view, yes—this fits with our mission. Anytime you can go beyond your four walls, it is good." Others explained that it fits with their systems' strategies to be patient centered, "to give them care when they need it and where they need it," and to provide an alternative to the ED.

Another important issue was to assess whether these decisions were made based on thorough strategic preparations or were hastily adopted defensive or reactive strategies. The results were mixed: Half the respondents indicated that theirs was a proactive strategy, while the other half acknowledged that it was reactive. For the latter group, the main explanation given was that they needed to establish a retail clinic relationship before one of the other systems in the market did. The health system is typically approached by a retail chain that is looking for a partner, as described by one respondent: "[Retail chain] needed to partner with somebody for physicians. So they approached us first. So we said we might as well put our name on it instead of one of our competitors doing it before us." Another respondent admitted, in hindsight, that the decision was not fully thought out: "We were thinking 'Oh my God, this train is leaving the station.' It was a new hot thing, in the *Wall Street Journal*. So we jumped in with both feet without really knowing where it would end up."

The other group offered a different take on their decision. They argued that their position as market leader in owning or partnering with a retail clinic shows a willingness to try new things and is evidence of a proactive strategy. This position was best summarized by one respondent: "We are the only retail clinics in town. The grocery chain and us realized that [national retail chains] might open a retail clinic in the market. Since we opened ours, they did not. We wanted to be the first in the market."

Effect on Referrals

As described previously, one of the main motivations to develop or affiliate with a retail clinic is to develop a patient referral base to the physicians and the hospitals within the system. However, the majority of the systems in our sample were not sure whether the clinics had actually increased referrals to their PCPs or stood in direct competition with them.

An important distinction between adult and pediatric patients was made by two of our respondents: They indicated that adults seem to be using the retail clinic *instead of* the PCP, while children seem to be using it *in addition to* the pediatrician. The reason is that many adults (especially men under 40 years old) do not have a PCP relationship, and therefore in case of minor complaints, they view the retail clinic as an alternative to that relationship. As for the pediatric population, parents were still taking their children to their regular physician for common and serious complaints but were attracted to such services offered by the retail clinics as sports physicals, camp physicals, and vaccines. These can be provided after hours and as walk-ins within a relatively short period of time, rather than needing to make an appointment and wait for lengthy periods in busy pediatricians' offices.

Location and Effect on Access

In the case of an affiliation, hospital systems have little power in deciding where the clinics should be located. For some retail chains, there seemed to be no rationale behind the location of the clinics. For example, one respondent noted that "the locations depended on where the [retail stores] are; some were in affluent areas, others in financially challenged areas, just all over the place." For other retail chains, the decision was to locate the clinics only in "supersized stores" that are typically placed in densely populated areas with upper-middle-class residents who value convenience and have discretionary income.

However, when the hospital system owns the retail clinics, several criteria are behind the location decision. For some, the clinics were placed in areas in which the system did not already have a significant presence. This reason was best summarized by one respondent: "We targeted mainly moms and families, in demographic areas with significant growth."

Other systems decided to locate the clinics in different areas with various characteristics to learn about which locations constitute a better fit for retail clinics. Some clinics were located inside the primary service area, others outside of it. One interesting lesson was learned by a system that decided to locate the clinics in lower-middle-class areas: "Today we regret our decision. We should have put them in an upper-middle-class area."

Given this, determining whether the clinics were improving access to uninsured people or just improving convenience for insured ones was important. The majority of our respondents agreed with the latter rather than the former. One respondent explained, "Given that the typical visit costs $60–$70, it might be too expensive for the uninsured," and another added, "It is more a convenience for people who have health insurance, as you have to pay up front."

Operational Challenges

As highlighted in the stakeholder model, PCPs are likely to be one of the biggest losers from the retail clinic trend (Exhibit III.1). A key challenge to the development and operation of a new retail clinic, then, is the resistance of PCPs. The two main reasons behind this resistance are fear of competition and concerns about quality of care. A large number of physicians viewed retail clinics as a "radical change in medicine" that would steal their patients away. Other physicians did not view them positively because of their perceived lack of clear clinical guidelines in the care of patients. This issue was especially important in clinics that were owned by the retail chain rather than the hospital system. One medical director described this situation in detail: "I assumed that they [the clinicians staffing the clinic] were going to follow the Convenient Care Clinic Association guidelines. However, it turned out that each nurse practitioner was independent and doing their own thing, according to expertise and skills."

Some of the physicians were less resistant to the idea, as they saw the potential to increase their revenue by providing oversight to the clinics without having to deliver any clinical services. One respondent noted that in his market, physicians were offered $100 per hour to provide that supervision.

To alleviate the fear that their physicians were experiencing, many of the systems spent considerable time and energy educating them about the retail clinic model and convincing them that it does not compete with their core business. For some systems, the retail chains approached the local physician association; for others, they held long meetings with the PCPs to share the operating model with them.

Once the physicians were on board, some of the systems (especially those that own the clinics) involved them in the care provided in the clinics by copying the patients' medical charts electronically or by fax. Another approach used by one health system to appease its physicians was to develop urgent care centers adjacent to the retail clinic.

Other challenges were raised: poor financial performance, people's perception of retail clinics, staffing issues, and the newness of the business model. In terms of financial performance, the respondents clearly indicated that it is very hard for retail clinics to be profitable. One medical director explained: "The margin of profitability is very narrow. If you are seeing 25–30 patients per day then you need to hire a second clinician, which is very expensive. No one is going to make a lot of money from this business." Given these financial difficulties, it is not surprising that all the respondents reported at least one retail clinic closing or being in financial distress over the last three years.

A somewhat related challenge stems from the difficulty of changing people's perception of retail clinics, in part explaining why many clinics are still operating below capacity. A vice president at one system emphasized this point: "One of the challenges that we faced was getting people to understand what the retail clinic does. To get lay people [to] realize that they don't need to see a doctor, and that is a different mind-set."

Another important operational hurdle relates to staffing. A common theme that emerged from the interviews was the difficulty in attracting and retaining nurse practitioners who are willing to "sit in a box for ten hours" every day. Because the clinics are open so many hours of the day and can treat only limited conditions, the work of the clinicians tends to be boring and repetitive. Several systems indicated that they pay their clinicians who work in the retail clinics at a higher rate than those who work in other settings "to compensate them for their boredom and the fact that they are there all by themselves and they do everything for the patient."

The last challenge raised was that for the systems, the retail clinic model was relatively unknown, and no template was available for them to follow. One system hired a consultant with retail clinic expertise to help with the development of its retail clinics, while others contacted several systems that had already developed retail clinics in different geographic regions to learn from their experience.

A Fad, or Here to Stay?

One of the most important questions in this research is whether this trend of hospital-affiliated and hospital-owned retail clinics is a passing fad or is here to stay. Six out of eight respondents thought that the trend is here to stay, although many provided caveats and stipulations. The first reason given is that "hospitals will do anything to get patients to the hospital," and therefore this strategy seems like a reasonable investment to link patients to the system. The second reason relates to the fact that systems are becoming increasingly focused on customer needs, as customers demand convenience. Retail clinics present an opportunity for systems to engage customers "beyond the four walls of the hospital." As one respondent noted: "Increasingly, healthcare services will be provided closer to the customer via Internet or at the retail clinic." And the last reason was that some respondents viewed the retail clinic model as part of the continuing trend of hospital systems' employment of physicians.

However, these respondents stressed that while the trend is here to stay, it will take different forms. One emphasized that the clinics have to become more integrated with the rest of the system and more of an extension of the PCP offices. Another one explained that the clinics will not be designed as a significant referral source to the system, but rather as a "release valve" for busy PCP offices and overcrowded EDs. The two respondents who believed that the trend was not sustainable cited financial problems and the difficulty of changing people's perceptions as the main reasons for their belief.

Discussion

Hospital systems' association with retail clinics involves two main models: an affiliation with retail chains that operate the clinics and ownership of the clinics with an arm's-length relationship with the retail chain. In either model, the health system provides physician supervision and a trusted name that is synonymous with high-quality care, while the retail chain provides space in a high-traffic area and a well-known, household brand.

Hospital systems are engaging in these relationships for several strategic reasons: to increase market share through enhanced referrals to physician offices and hospitals, to become closer to consumers, and to experiment with nontraditional ways of delivering healthcare. However, the most common reason seems to be to beat the competition and be the market leader in this service. In this regard, a large number of systems indicated that they are launching retail clinic initiatives without adequate preparation or research. This reason might explain the poor financial performance and closing of some of the clinics, and it raises serious questions about vital resources that are wasted in the process.

Whether the retail clinics have lived up to their potential of increasing referrals is not clear, especially to PCP offices. An important question that was raised by several respondents was, if the retail clinic was not there, where would the patient have gone? Our respondents did not have a clear answer to this question. Data from Memorial Hermann Health System in Houston, Texas (a system that was not part of our sample), indicates that 25 percent of retail clinic patients would have gone to the PCP, 15 percent would have gone to an urgent care center, 30 percent would have gone to the ED, and 30 percent would not have sought care had the retail clinic not been in place (Fenn 2008). Evidence from our findings suggests that while many pediatric patients are using the clinics for niche services in addition to their regular physicians, some adults who do not have a PCP relationship are depending on the clinic as their major source of care.

Several criteria are used by the retail chain or the hospital system to guide the decision for choosing a location for the retail clinic. The majority of the clinics are intentionally placed in upper-middle-income, densely populated areas and in areas where the systems plan to grow. This is a clear indication that retail clinics are intended to increase convenience to insured patients rather than to increase access to uninsured patients. These findings seem to support recent national research that shows that areas with retail clinics have lower poverty levels, higher median incomes, and lower black percentage population and are less likely to be medically underserved than areas that do not have retail clinics (Pollack and Armstrong 2009).

Physician resistance and skepticism topped the list of operational challenges. Not surprisingly, physicians felt threatened by the competition presented by these clinics and had legitimate concerns about their quality of care. Most systems in our sample have gone to great lengths to assure their physicians that the clinics would not compete with them and to get them involved in supervising the clinics.

Several other operational challenges emerged from our interviews. Many of the retail clinics are struggling financially and closing in some markets, which explains reports suggesting that the retail clinic boom might be ending (Charatan 2008; Tu and Cohen 2008; Yee 2008). In addition, recruiting and retaining midlevel providers to work in these clinics is hard because of the nonchallenging and limited nature of their services. To deal with this issue, MeritCare Health System, in Fargo, North Dakota (a system that was not part of our sample), decided to have its retail clinic nurse practitioners work one or two days per week at a family clinic to keep them challenged and engaged (Pollert, Dobberstein, and Wiisanen 2008). Moreover, while the number of retail clinics has grown exponentially over the last few years, many people still do not understand what these clinics do and what services they offer, while others are skeptical about their quality of care (Leppel 2010).

Since the trend of hospital-affiliated or hospital-owned retail clinics has emerged only recently, little is understood about its strategic drivers and implications or its future. While the emergence of retail clinics in general, and the development of hospital system–affiliated retail clinics in particular, has been a pragmatic response to existing market conditions, the trend should be examined within a broader theoretical framework. That imitation strategies (fads and fashions) are a prominent feature of the healthcare organizational strategy landscape is well documented (Kaissi and Begun 2008). Thus, questions about the sustainability of this trend need to be answered: Is this another fad, or is it here to stay? Most of our respondents (who should not be viewed as unbiased commentators in any way) seem to believe that the trend is sustainable, because hospital systems will continue to reach out to consumers outside of the traditional inpatient care setting. But the keys to that sustainability seem to be greater integration with health systems and a better understanding of the role of the retail clinic as an access point that can alleviate the burden of PCP offices and EDs.

The main limitation of this study relates to the generalizability of the results. Our interviews constitute a selective profile of some health systems that are affiliated with or own retail clinics and should not be seen as a representative sample of all health systems that have engaged in these kinds of relationships.

Future Research and Conclusion

Hospital systems' association with retail clinics is a relatively recent trend. Therefore, many issues should be addressed in future research to answer important questions.

Given that two forms of operation predominate the trend, comparing the performance of hospital-affiliated and hospital-owned retail clinics in terms of profitability, market share, costs, and quality outcomes is important. Even within the owned-clinics category, measuring the degree of integration of these clinics with the rest of the system (through electronic medical record systems, for example) and determining whether that makes any difference in terms of their performance is important.

In addition, there is reason to believe that health systems that jump on the retail clinic bandwagon without a good understanding of the model are more likely to end up with financially struggling clinics. Therefore, future research should examine the strategic planning process that health systems use and assess whether the length of time of the process and its thoroughness make any difference in terms of the future viability and success of the clinics.

Another important unanswered question from the systems' perspective relates to whether retail clinics actually increase referrals to PCP offices and hospitals. Thorough research studies based on large samples that provide clear answers to this question may hold the key to whether more hospital systems will develop relationships with retail clinics in the near future.

Physician resistance and skepticism emerged as a main obstacle to the development of retail clinics. Assessing physicians' attitudes and feelings toward these clinics in a systematic way and providing a deep understanding of the various approaches that systems can adopt to address physician concerns will be important.

Clinicians who work at retail clinics operate in an unusual setting in which they have to provide various clinical and nonclinical services, but they may not feel challenged enough by the nature of the conditions treated in the clinics. Studies should assess the job satisfaction of midlevel providers who work in retail clinics versus other settings, as well as their compensation levels.

One major change that will most certainly affect all aspects of the healthcare system over the next decade relates to the potential effects of recent healthcare reform legislation. Given that these efforts are mainly intended to provide more access at a lower cost for patients, it will be interesting to see whether retail clinics will thrive or struggle in this new healthcare environment (Kaissi 2010).

In conclusion, our interviews provide a selective profile of hospital systems that have affiliated with or developed their own retail clinics. We found several strategic reasons for these decisions and identified important operational challenges that need to be overcome for this trend to continue. Further research is needed to provide more evidence about this emerging mode of healthcare delivery.

References

American Academy of Family Physicians. 2010. "Family Physician Workforce Reform: Recommendations of the American Academy of Family Physicians." AAFP Reprint No. 305b. Accessed July 11, 2012. www.aafp.org/online/en/home/policy/policies/w/workforce.html.

Bohmer, R. 2007. "The Rise of In-Store Clinics—Threat or Opportunity?" *New England Journal of Medicine* 356 (8): 765–69.

Charatan, F. 2008. "Walk-in Clinics at US Retail Outlets Run into Financial Problems." *British Medical Journal* 336 (7654): 1150–51.

Deloitte Center for Health Solutions. 2009. *Retail Clinics: Updates and Implications.* Washington, DC: Deloitte Center for Health Solutions.

———. 2008. *Retail Clinics: Facts, Trends and Implications.* Washington, DC: Deloitte Center for Health Solutions.

Fenn, S. 2008. "Integrating Retail Clinics into the Hospital System." *Frontiers of Health Services Management* 24 (3): 33–36.

Fottler, M. D., and D. M. Malvey. 2010. *The Retail Revolution in Health Care.* Santa Barbara, CA: Praeger.

Harris Interactive. 2007. "Most Adults Satisfied with Care at Retail-Based Health Clinics." Accessed July 11, 2012. www.harrisinteractive.com/NEWS/allnewsbydate.asp?NewsID=1201.

Hunter, L. P., A. P. Morreale, and J. H. Wall. 2009. "Patient Satisfaction with Retail Health Clinic Care." *Journal of the American Academy of Nurse Practitioners* 21 (10): 565–70.

Kaissi, A. 2010. "The Future of Retail Clinics in a Volatile Healthcare Environment." *Health Care Manager* 29 (3): 223–29.

Kaissi, A., and J. Begun. 2008. "Fads, Fashions and Bandwagons in Healthcare Strategy." *Health Care Management Review* 33 (2): 94–102.

Laws, M., and M. K. Scott. 2008. "The Emergence of Retail-Based Clinics in the United States: Early Observations." *Health Affairs* 5: 1293–98.

Leach, K. B. 2008. "As Industry Matures, Retail Clinics Seek Hospital Partners." *Texas Hospitals,* July/August: 10–11.

Leppel, K. 2010. "Factors Influencing Willingness to Use Convenient Care Clinics Among Baby Boomers and Older Persons." *Health Care Management Review* 35 (1): 13–22.

Lin, D. Q. 2008. "Convenient Care Clinics: Opposition, Opportunity, and the Path to System Integration." *Frontiers of Health Services Management* 24 (3): 3–11.

Malvey, D. M., and M. D. Fottler. 2006. "The Retail Revolution in Health Care: Who Will Win and Who Will Lose?" *Health Care Management Review* 31(3): 168–78.

Mehrotra, A., H. Liu, J. L. Adams, M. C. Wang, J. R. Lave, M. Thygeson, L. I. Solberg, and E. A. McGlynn. 2009. "Comparing Costs and Quality of Care at Retail Clinics with That of Other Medical Settings for 3 Common Illnesses." *Annals of Internal Medicine* 151: 321–28.

Mehrotra, A., M. C. Wang, J. R. Lave, J. L. Adams, and E. A. McGlynn. 2008. "Retail Clinics, Primary Care Physicians, and Emergency Departments: A Comparison of Patients' Visits." *Health Affairs* 5: 1271–82.

Newbold, P., and M. J. O'Neil. 2008. "Small Changes Lead to Large Effects." *Frontiers of Health Services Management* 24 (3): 23–27.

Paddock, K. 2007. "AMA Calls for Investigation of Retail Health Clinics." *Medical News Today.* Accessed July 11, 2012. www.medicalnewstoday.com/articles/75308.php.

Pollack, C. E., and K. Armstrong. 2009. "The Geographic Accessibility of Retail Clinics for Underserved Populations." *Archives of Internal Medicine* 169 (10): 945–49.

Pollert, P., D. Dobberstein, and R. Wiisanen. 2008. "Jumping into the Healthcare Retail Market: Our Experience." *Frontiers of Health Services Management* 24 (3): 13–21.

Robeznieks, A. 2007. "Look Who's Buying Retail." *Modern Healthcare* 37 (46): 26–28.

Rohrer, J. E., K. B. Angstam, and J. W. Furst. 2009. "Impact of Retail Walk-in Care on Early Return Visits by Adult Primary Care Patients." *Quality Management in Health Care* 1: 18–23.

Rudavsky, R., C. E. Pollack, and A. Mehrotra. 2009. "The Geographic Distribution, Ownership, Prices and Scope of Practice at Retail Clinics." *Annals of Internal Medicine* 151: 315–20.

Scott, M. K. 2007. *Health Care in the Express Lane: Retail Clinics Go Mainstream.* Oakland: California Healthcare Foundation.

Thygeson, M., K. A. Van Vorst, M. V. Maciosek, and L. Solberg. 2008. "Use and Costs of Care in Retail Clinics Versus Traditional Care Sites." *Health Affairs* 5: 1283–92.

Tu, H. T., and G. R. Cohen. 2008. "Checking Up on Retail-Based Health Clinics: Is the Boom Ending?" Issue Brief. *Commonwealth Fund* 48 (1): 1–11.

Yee, C. M. 2008. "Some Walk-in Clinics Closing After Boom." *Minneapolis Star-Tribune.* Accessed July 11, 2012. www.startribune.com/business/26850829.html.

Discussion Questions

1. How do retail clinics threaten existing HCOs? How do they threaten local physicians? How about other stakeholders? (Refer to Exhibit III.1, page 176.)

2. As CEO of a health system considering incorporating a retail clinic within the system, make a case to the board about whether the affiliation model or the ownership model makes the most strategic sense.

Recommended Reading

Christensen, C. M., J. H. Grossman, and J. Hwang. 2009. *The Innovator's Prescription.* New York: McGraw-Hill Publishers. Chapters 4 and 5 are especially appropriate.

Christensen and colleagues suggest that the hospital does two jobs: diagnosing problems and treating them. He says that no other business successfully houses the two different business models in the same unit. Solution shops for diagnosing problems need to get paid on a fee-for-service model. Value-added process activities for treating problems should be sold for a fixed price. This disruption in the hospital business model will result in more effective and efficient hospitals.

Discussion Questions

1. Do you agree with Christensen's conclusion? Why or why not?
2. What would have to take place for Christensen's disruption to take place on a wide scale?
3. If you agree with Christensen's diagnosis but not his conclusion, what other strategic alternatives can hospitals make to respond to current hospital operating problems?

Required Supplementary Readings

Berenson, R. A., T. Hammons, D. N. Gans, S. Zuckerman, K . Merrell, W. S. Underwood, and A. F. Williams. 2008. "A House Is Not a Home: Keeping Patients at the Center of Practice Redesign." *Health Affairs* 27 (5): 1219– 30.

Crabtree, B. F., P. A. Nutting, W. L. Miller, K. C. Stange, E. E. Stewart, and C. R. Jaen. 2010. "Summary of the National Demonstration Project and Recommendations for the Patient-Centered Medical Home." *Annals of Family Medicine* 8 (Suppl 1): S80–S90.

Herzlinger, R. 2000. "Market-Driven, Focused Healthcare: The Role of Managers." *Frontiers of Health Services Management* 16 (3, Special Issue).

Paulus, R. A., K. Davis, and G. D. Steele. 2008. "Continuous Innovation in Healthcare: Implications of the Geisinger Experience." *Health Affairs* 27 (5): 1235–45.

Zhou, Y. Y., M. H. Kanter, J. J. Wang, and T. Garrido. 2010. "Improved Quality at Kaiser Permanente Through E-mail Between Physicians and Patients." *Health Affairs* 29 (7): 1370–75.

Questions for the Required Supplementary Readings

1. Berenson and colleagues define and describe the "patient-centered medical home" (PCMH) and its potential to transform primary care, and Crabtree and colleagues present the results of a study evaluating the PCMH model. Based on your review of these two articles, how can the PCMH model negatively affect patient care? As administrator of a large multispecialty group practice, what challenges would you anticipate to be associated with introducing the PCMH model

to your physicians? What resources would you need to succeed in implementing this model?

2. You are asked to become the CEO of a 200-bed community hospital, one of three in your part of the city that is trying to be all things to all people. The board has asked you to focus on "what we do best." Using concepts from Herzlinger's article, what would you tell the board? Given Herzlinger's case for focused factories, what are arguments against this approach?

3. Paulus and associates describe a remarkable effort to improve care delivery and service at Geisinger Health System. What made this a successful effort? How might this approach be applied in other health systems? What would be constraints to applying this approach elsewhere?

4. What implementation and management challenges does the type of information technology option implemented at Kaiser present to other hospitals and health systems whose physicians are not employed by the organizations as they are at Kaiser Permanente?

Recommended Supplementary Readings

Arndt, M., and B. Bigelow. 2000. "The More Things Change, the More They Stay the Same." *Health Care Management Review* 25 (1): 65–72.

Bohmer, R. M. J. 2009. *Designing Care*. Boston: Harvard Business Press.

Bush, R. W. 2007. "Reducing Waste in U.S. Healthcare Systems." *Journal of the American Medical Association* 297 (8): 871–74.

Casalino, L. P., E. A. November, R. A. Berenson, and H. H. Pham. 2008. "Hospital-Physician Relations: Two Tracks and the Decline of the Voluntary Medical Staff Model." *Health Affairs* 27 (5): 1305–14.

Christensen, C. M., J. H. Grossman, and J. Hwang. 2009. *The Innovator's Prescription*. New York: McGraw-Hill Publishers. Chapters 4 and 5 are especially appropriate.

Conrad, D. A., and W. L. Dowling. 1990. "Vertical Integration in Health Services: Theory and Managerial Implication." *Healthcare Management Review* 15 (4): 9–22.

Cussell, C. K., J. M. Ludden, and G. M. Moon. 2000. "Perceptions of Barriers to High-Quality Palliative Care in Hospitals." *Health Affairs* 19 (5): 166–72.

Gamm, L., B. Kash, and J. Bolin. 2007. "Organizational Technologies for Transforming Care: Measures and Strategies for Pursuit of IOM Quality Aims." *Journal of Ambulatory Care Management* 30 (4): 291–301.

Gerteis, M., S. Edgman-Levitan, J. Daley, and T. L. Delbanco (eds.). 2002. *Through the Patient's Eyes: Understanding and Promoting Patient-Centered Care.* San Francisco: Jossey-Bass.

Glouberman, S., and H. Mintzberg. 2001a. "Managing the Care of Health and the Cure of Disease—Part I: Differentiation." *Health Care Management Review* 26 (1): 56–69, discussion 87–89.

———. 2001b. "Managing the Care of Health and the Cure of Disease—Part II: Integration." *Health Care Management Review* 26 (1): 70–84, discussion 87–89.

Goldsmith, J. 2000. "How Will the Internet Change Our Health System?" *Health Affairs* 19 (1): 148–56.

Griffith, J., and K. White. 2010. "Foundations of Excellent Care." *Reaching Excellence in Healthcare Management,* chap. 5. Chicago: Health Administration Press.

Grol, R. 2006. *Quality Development in Health Care in the Netherlands. The Commonwealth Fund.* Accessed July 11, 2012. www.commonwealthfund.org/Publications/Fund-Reports/2006/Mar/Quality-Development-in-Health-Care-in-the-Netherlands.aspx.

Hearld, L. R., J. A. Alexander, I. Fraser, and H. J. Jiang. 2008. "How Do Hospital Organizational Structure and Processes Affect Quality of Care?" *Medical Care Research & Review* 65 (3): 259–99.

Jha, A. K., J. B. Perlin, K. Kizer, and R. A. Dudley. 2003. "Effects of the Transformation of the Veterans Affairs Healthcare System on the Quality of Care." *New England Journal of Medicine* 310 (22): 1477–80.

Kilo, C. M. 1999. "Improving Care Through Collaboration." *Pediatrics* 103 (1): 384–92.

Kimberly, J. R., and E. Minvielle. 2003. "Quality as an Organizational Problem." In *Advances in Healthcare Organizational Theory,* ed. by S. S. Mick and M. E. Wyttenbach, 205–32. San Francisco: Jossey-Bass.

Lathrop, J. P. 1993. *Restructuring Healthcare: The Patient-Focused Paradigm.* San Francisco: Jossey-Bass.

Lawrence, D. 2002. *From Chaos to Care.* Cambridge, MA: Perseus.

Leatt, P., R. Baker, and J. R. Kimberly. 2005. "Organization Design." In *Healthcare Management,* 5th ed. ed. by S. M. Shortell and A. D. Kaluzny, 314–55. Albany, NY: Delmar.

McAlearney, A. S. 2004. "Hospitalists and Family Physicians: Understanding Opportunities and Risks." *Journal of Family Practice* 53 (6): 473–81.

———. 2003. *Population Health Management: Strategies to Improve Outcomes.* Chicago: Health Administration Press.

Mehrotra, A., M. C. Wang, J. R. Lave, J. L. Adams, and E. A. McGlynn. 2008. "Retail Clinics, Primary Care Physicians, and Emergency Departments: A Comparison of Patients' Visits." *Health Affairs* 27 (5): 1272–82.

Pham, H. H., J. M. Grossman, G. Cohen, and T. Bodenheimer. 2008. "Hospitalists and Care Transitions: The Divorce of Inpatient and Outpatient Care." *Health Affairs* 27 (5): 1315–27.

Robinson, J. C., and L. P. Casalino. 1996. "Vertical Integration and Organizational Networks in Healthcare." *Health Affairs* 15 (1): 7–22.

Rosenberg, C. 1987. *The Care of Strangers*. New York: Basic Books.

Rundall, T. G., S. M. Shortell, M. C. Wang, L. Casalino, T. Bodenheimer, R. R. Gillies, J. A. Schmittdiel, N. Oswald, and J. C. Robinson. 2002. "As Good as It Gets? Chronic Care Management with Nine Leading U.S. Physician Organizations." *British Medical Journal* 325 (26): 958–61.

Schweikhart, S. B., and V. Smith-Daniels. 1996. "Reengineering the Work of Caregivers: Role Redefinition, Team Structures, and Organizational Redesign." *Hospital & Health Services Administration* 41 (1): 19–36.

Scott, R. L., L. Aiken, D. Mechanic, and J. Moravcsik. 1995. "Organizational Aspects of Caring." *Milbank Quarterly* 73 (1): 77–95.

Shortell, S. M., R. R. Gillies, D. A. Anderson, K. M. Erickson, and J. B. Mitchell. 1996. *Remaking Healthcare in America*. San Francisco: Jossey-Bass.

Shortell, S. M., J. E. Zimmerman, D. M. Rousseau, R. R. Gillies, D. P. Wagner, E. A. Draper, W. A. Knaus, and J. Duffy. 1994. "The Performance of Intensive Care Units: Does Good Management Make a Difference?" *Medical Care* 32 (5): 508–25.

Smith, H. L. 1955. "Two Lines of Authority Are One Too Many." *Modern Hospitals* 84 (3): 59–64.

Villagra, V. G. 2004. "Integrating Disease Management into the Outpatient Delivery System During and After Managed Care." *Health Affairs* Web Exclusives W4 (May 19): 281–83.

Wachter, R., and L. Goldman. 2002. "The Hospitalist Movement 5 Years Later." *Journal of the American Medical Association* 287 (4): 487–94.

———. 1996. "The Emerging Role of Hospitalists in the American Healthcare System." *New England Journal of Medicine* 335 (7): 514–17.

Woolf, S. H. 2004. "Patient Safety Is Not Enough: Targeting Quality Improvements to Optimize the Health of the Population." *Annals of Internal Medicine* 140: 33–36.

Woolhandler, S., T. Campbell, and D. U. Himmelstein. 2003. "Costs of Healthcare Administration in the United States and Canada Hospitals." *New England Journal of Medicine* 349 (8): 760–75.

Zuckerman, H. S., D. W. Hilberman, R. M. Andersen, L. R. Burns, J. A. Alexander, and P. Torrens. 1998. "Physicians and Organizations: Strange Bedfellows or a Marriage Made in Heaven?" *Frontiers of Health Services Management* 14 (3): 3–34.

THE CASES

In healthcare, discussion about organizational design occurs at four levels. The first is at the patient care level. New questions are being asked: How do we organize the best care for asthma or hypertension or back pain? Answering this question requires a definition of "best," data on the population served, a team of staff members working to achieve these goals, and management support. How can the physical design of our organization improve the care and service we provide to patients? Case I, "Selling an Evidence-Based Design for Waterford Hospital" raises some of the issues associated with facilities design and its implications for patient care.

At the next level of aggregation are the issues of the design of the hospital, nursing home, and other care organizations. How do we put the component departments together? Restructuring, reengineering, downsizing, and right-sizing are the jargon terms of the moment. Case G, "Improving Organizational Development in Health Services," presents the issues associated with centralization versus decentralization at both the health system and service line levels. Case H, "The American Heart Institute," then discusses the implications of implementing a service line model for cardiac care in a university hospital. Short Case 14 addresses the challenges that are expected when transitioning from a decentralized to a centralized revenue cycle model in an academic medical center.

Across the country, hospitals, clinics, and insurers are grouping themselves together as systems of care. In an urban area where 30 separate hospitals once stood, there may now be three or four competing groups of hospitals within both regional and national health systems. The competing entities may be not-for-profit organizations, investor owned, or a mix of both. This new grouping strategy is the third level of organizational design.

One reason for these changes is the recognition that with managed care and alternative financing arrangements, we will need many fewer hospital beds than we now have. The leaders of a single hospital left out of such a system may wonder if it will be one of the hospitals that will disappear. One way these mergers occur is through the sale of a not-for-profit hospital to a for-profit group. The sale price plus the not-for-profit hospital's existing endowment are put into a nonprofit foundation. The income from this foundation's endowment is used to achieve the charitable and philanthropic goals of the original not-for-profit hospital. The hospital, now part of the for-profit organization, is run along business lines in a competitive environment.

In the rush to become one of the three or four biggest groups in the area, a health system bases its decisions about organizational design on expediency, comfort level, and speed rather than organizing to provide expeditious, excellent care. The local rush for size is of vital importance in a market oversupplied with hospitals. Any one urban hospital priced too high or of average quality can be ignored by insurance providers negotiating contracts. For such a hospital to exist, it will have to accept whatever price the insurance providers choose to offer, which will not be high. If the system is large enough and includes popular, specialized, and prestigious hospitals, all insurance providers and managed care systems must deal with it. As a result, such a system will not be a "price taker" but a "price giver." It can charge full price for its services because the insurer or HMO has no choice. Case H's development of "The American Heart Institute" is an example of a hospital's attempt to capitalize on the opportunity to focus on excellence in a particular area (cardiac care) to expand market share.

The fourth level of design is at the state or national policy level. One notable effort to change the context of healthcare delivery was the Clinton administration's unsuccessful national health plan initiative. However, the current devolution of decision making related to Medicaid from the federal to the state level will also change the context of care. Some states, such as Hawaii, Oregon, and Massachusetts, have provided interesting examples of system reform, while the state of California struggled along similar lines. Resolution of the present healthcare reform debate will undoubtedly lead to different organizational reactions, based on changes in priorities and reimbursement levels. Short Case 12 presents the case of a hospital considering the design implications of becoming an accountable care organization (ACO) in response to policy-level pressure to implement this model.

The interaction of all four of these levels of organization and system design makes healthcare delivery a most lively arena. The field is creating unprecedented opportunities for creative leadership and the organization of whole new ways of providing better care at lower cost. New business models are being introduced, such as convenient care clinics or retail clinics located in pharmacies and grocery stores, and existing organizations are challenged to respond to competition from these new sources of care.

The coordination of many different professional workers with varying skills, views of the world, perceptions of what needs to be done, and licensing statutes lies at the heart of this new design for health services organizations.

Work can be organized in many different ways in large health services organizations: by task or purpose, by facility, or by client group served. Short Case 15 describes a situation in which the organization of work can create confusion for the individual employee. Often, several different organizing principles operate in the same organization, sometimes appropriately and sometimes for historical reasons. As Clibbon and Sachs (1969) have pointed out, a laboratory is a place, obstetrics is a health condition, outpatients are people, dietary is a service, intensive care is a need, day care is a category of residential status, radiology is a group of techniques, and rehabilitation is a purpose.

The structure of many HCOs was more appropriate for conditions when those organizations were founded than it is for today. Organizational structure is determined in part by the nature of the work the organization has to do, its physical facilities, its history, and the culture of the society and of like institutions. As a result, questions about what structure would truly be best for a particular organization or service remain common. Short Case 13, about integrating rehabilitation services, raises both structural and cultural issues associated with needed changes in organizational design.

Reference

Clibbon, S., and M. L. Sachs. 1969. "Healthcare Facilities: An Alternative to Baili-wick Planning in Patient Fostering Spaces." *The New Physician* 18: 462–71.

Case G
Improving Organizational Development in Health Services

Ann Scheck McAlearney and Rebecca Schmale

Who, What, and Where?

John Shea, CEO and president of Worthington Health System (WHS), needed some time to think. He had been leading WHS for ten years, and was contemplating the legacy he wanted to leave. WHS, based in the Midwest, was composed of four hospitals, a home health company, and an ambulatory care service line (see Exhibits III.3 and III.4). The system had been formed 12 years ago when two of the local community hospitals decided to combine forces and become a health system. The two freestanding hospitals each served distinct patient populations, with 600-bed Lincoln Hospital located downtown, and 800-bed Riverview Hospital located in a nearby suburb. Rather than take the name of either hospital, the organizing group elected to create a new, neutral name for the health system, and left each individual hospital with its original name. Shea was hired soon after the system's formation so he had personally experienced most of the changes WHS had navigated.

EXHIBIT III.3
Worthington Health System Facts at a Glance

Employees	10,400
Physicians	1,800
Volunteers	2,500
Hospitals	5
Net patient revenue	$1.2 billion
Patient days	370,000
Community benefit	$37 million
Outpatient visits	1.1 million
Avg. daily census	960
Emergency room visits	260,000
Ambulatory centers	6
Home health visits	125,000

EXHIBIT III.4
Worthington Health System Facilities

Care Sites	Type	Beds	Employees
Riverview Hospital	Tertiary	800	4,600
Lincoln Hospital	Trauma	600	2,980
Graystone Memorial Hospital	Community	200	685
Mount Rising Hospital	Community	124	512
Fairland Memorial Hospital	Community	95	450
Worthington Home Care	Home health	—	440
Ambulatory care centers (6)	Health centers, urgent care, outpatient surgery	—	690

Since the formation of WHS, the rapidly changing healthcare market and shifting patient demographics had presented a series of opportunities for WHS. Shea had successfully managed the acquisition of two other local hospitals for WHS when another local system dissolved, and he had extended the reach of WHS to the adjacent county by forming a strategic alliance with Graystone Memorial Hospital (see Exhibit III.5). Additional market changes led to the formation of Worthington Home Care, and the creation of a network of ambulatory care centers that expanded the reach of WHS. WHS was financially strong, and enjoyed a positive reputation in the area, despite competition from two other health systems and several newly developed specialty hospitals.

Shea's continuing concern was the lack of "systemness" within the broad WHS system. Building community awareness of WHS as a health system

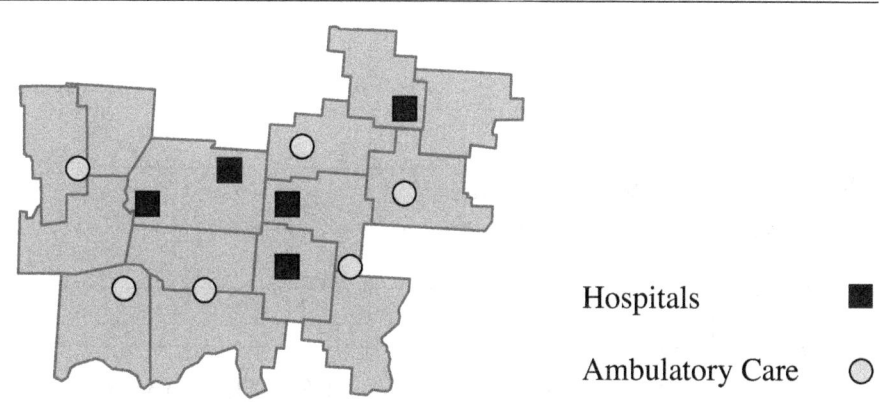

EXHIBIT III.5
Worthington
Health System
Service Area

Hospitals   ■

Ambulatory Care   ○

had taken quite some time, and patients were still primarily loyal to the original flagship hospital, Riverview, rather than to WHS. This loyalty, however, was also evident among employees. The Riverview staff identified with Riverview Hospital, not WHS, and Lincoln Hospital staff exhibited the same silo loyalty. When Shea had arrived at WHS, he was thrilled by the challenge of creating a true system with previously competing entities, but as he now reflected, he had not succeeded. He wanted his legacy to include a shift in the WHS organizational culture to one of system-focused thinking rather than entity-oriented decision making.

Several functions had been centralized in the past few years to achieve economies of scale and reduce redundancies within the system. The first functions to be centralized under the corporate umbrella were finance and supply chain. Greg Hanson, CFO, was a strong leader, and within one year, centralization saved the system more than $200 million. Some resistance to the centralization had existed, but the savings quickly made the decision difficult to dispute.

Given the current financial strength of WHS, Shea realized he had an opportunity to focus on the goal of enhancing system-focused thinking (see Exhibit III.6). Because entity culture seemed to be playing such a major role, Shea knew he must engage his employees to achieve systemness. He also knew that education, especially leadership development, could play a key role. One of Shea's goals was to advance WHS as a learning organization. This had led to two recent hires in the areas of organizational development and human resources (HR), and both Fiona Sinclair and Blake Snowdon seemed to have sensed the lack of systemness at WHS quite quickly. Shea decided to schedule a meeting with Sinclair and Snowdon to introduce his ideas.

EXHIBIT III.6
Worthington
Health System
Total Operating
Growth

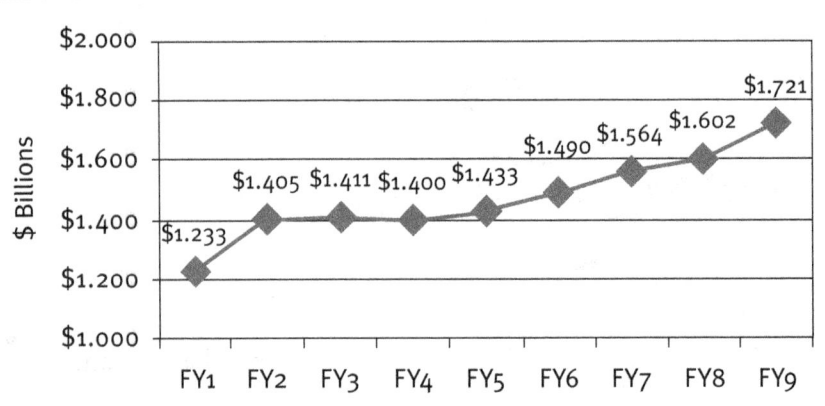

Behind the Scenes

As system vice president of organizational development, Sinclair had spent the past two months getting to know WHS and its various entities. She had come to WHS from outside the healthcare industry and had been repeatedly surprised by how "behind" she found the health system. Even basic education and training functions were still delivered at the entity level, and there was no sense of organizational identity at the system level. Yet Sinclair felt there was hope for improvement as signaled by her own recruitment and the apparent interest of the CEO.

Snowdon, director of human resources, shared Sinclair's perspective about the fragmented nature of WHS and was also struck by the seeming lack of awareness about the potential for strategic human resources management to help reduce this fragmentation (see Exhibit III.7). He had come to WHS three months ago from a smaller system based in California, and he now saw how good he had had it. Rather than a fully aligned health system that saw human resources as a strategic capability, Snowdon found WHS to be a collection of individual entities that appeared to compete among themselves for corporate-level attention. Many Riverview staff came across as arrogant because they believed they worked for the "best" hospital in the system. In contrast, Lincoln staff prized themselves on their ability to respond to the needs of the surrounding urban community, despite a largely unfavorable payer mix and staggering use of the emergency department. He hadn't yet characterized the cultures of Mount Rising or Fairland hospitals, but he felt certain they were as entrenched and individualized as those of Riverview and Lincoln.

Given their similar interests and start dates, Sinclair and Snowdon were in frequent contact. Organizationally, the department of human resources reported to the chief operating officer (COO), and Snowdon was its senior executive. The area of organizational development, however, was new for WHS, and Sinclair had been hired with the charge to create and build the department as she saw fit. She reported directly to CEO John Shea, but knew the strategic importance of close ties to human resources if she was going to be able to accomplish anything with respect to organizational development.

In Sinclair's last position she had directed the development of a corporate university to centralize training and development for the large organization. Sinclair believed this model held promise for a health system such as WHS, but was aware of the challenges associated with centralizing a previously decentralized and tightly controlled function. Coincidentally, Snowdon's last role as director of human resources for a smaller health system had involved an evaluation of the corporate university model, but that system had rejected it. Instead, Snowdon's previous role had focused on building credibility for human resources as a strategic capability of the health system. The focus was on making targeted investments in strategic human resources capabilities, such as developing hiring managers' abilities to use behavioral

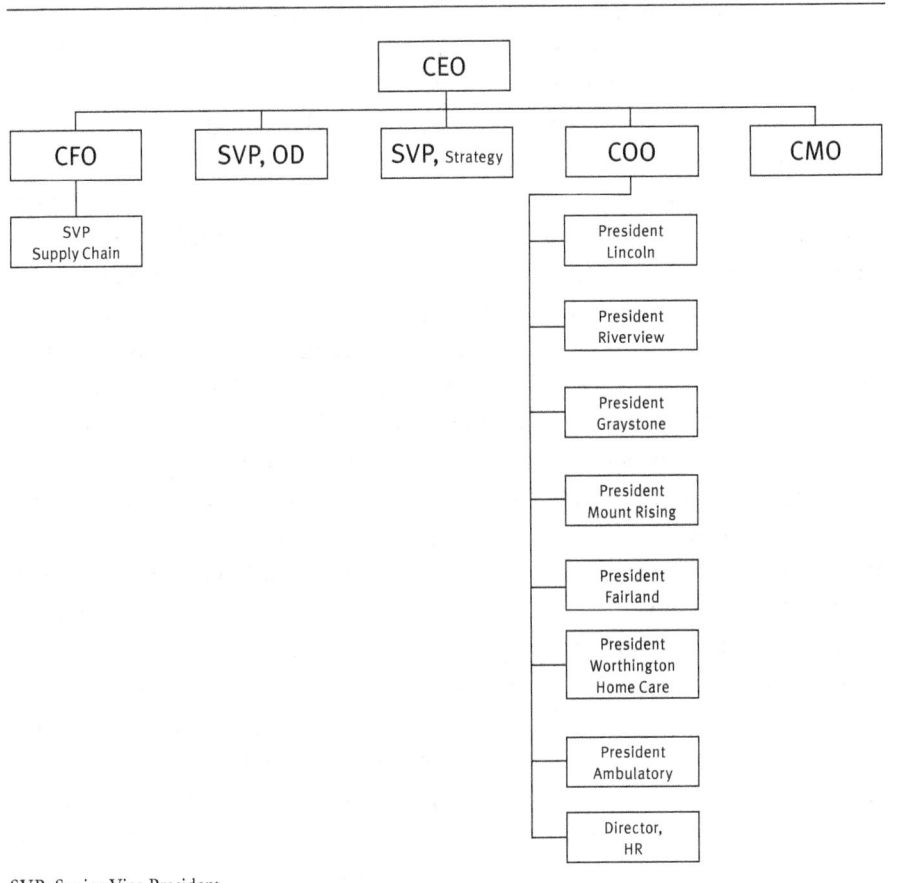

EXHIBIT III.7
Worthington Health System Organizational Chart

SVP: Senior Vice President

interviewing techniques and linking individual performance evaluations to the health system's overall performance through use of a balanced scorecard.

Getting together to prepare for their meeting with Shea, Sinclair and Snowdon discussed their initial assessments of WHS. They agreed that WHS was a disjointed collection of individual entities with little loyalty to the system, but they also agreed that a fragmented culture could change. The key, they felt, would be in centralizing the education and training function for WHS at the corporate level, but they knew this idea would be met with widespread resistance from all entities. They also knew that without the commitment and support of the CEO, a move to centralize any function within WHS would fail.

The First Meeting

Shea decided to meet with Sinclair and Snowdon in Sinclair's office, signaling his willingness to move outside the suite of executive offices to collaborate with others considered experts in their own fields. He had purposely not created an agenda for the meeting, and instead had proposed this as a "conversation" about WHS. Shea opened the meeting with the basic question, "What can we do to make WHS feel like a system?"

Neither Sinclair nor Snowdon was timid, and they had previously agreed to be completely honest and direct with Shea. They described their early observations of WHS and the component entities, and their collective assessment that there was almost nothing that bound WHS as a system other than a common logo and a centralized payroll system. Even though there were several corporate-level functions, such as strategic planning and marketing, it seemed that the individual hospitals often replicated these functions in-house to ensure entity-level control. Particularly troublesome, Sinclair and Snowdon reported, was the training and development function. Yet they noted that this also presented a tremendous opportunity to bring WHS together as a system.

While Shea knew WHS suffered from the entity-focused territoriality common to many US healthcare systems, he had been unaware of the magnitude of the problem. He was struck by the financial implications of hospital-based duplication of services. He realized that with education and training alone, duplication of training programs, evaluation processes, tracking systems, and even trainers was costing the system thousands of dollars. However, Shea was also aware that each hospital entity took training and development seriously as an entity-level capability. He knew the hospitals prided themselves on providing continuing education programs for physicians and nurses that were appropriately tailored to the hospital's perceived needs. Any move to centralize what was considered an important organizational competency would be perceived negatively and would likely be resisted. Shea knew that this issue would have to be evaluated thoroughly, and if accepted, introduced carefully.

The Charge

Shea liked the notion of centralizing the training and development function at WHS, and believed this could help him achieve his goal of transforming WHS into a cohesive system and learning organization. Yet he needed to be convinced that this approach could work, and that it would be worth the investment. He felt Sinclair and Snowdon were the appropriate individuals to lead the assessment process, and their newness within the system might help them uncover challenges or concerns less obvious to someone who had worked at WHS for a longer period.

Talking this over with Sinclair and Snowdon, Shea outlined what he would need to make his decision. First, he would need a list of the current financial and nonfinancial costs associated with decentralized training and development. While Shea knew they would not be able to cost out everything, he felt that a list and general estimate of costs could be sufficient for his purposes. Second, Shea wanted options. If, as they suspected, the centralized option was going to prove favorable, he needed to know what this could mean for WHS. Were there alternative models for centralized training and development? If so, which would be appropriate at WHS? What costs would be associated with this type of change? Further, how long would this organizational change take to implement? What would be the "value-add" of a centralized department for the entities? How could programs such as orientation, leadership development, and clinical management training reinforce a new way of thinking beyond the boundaries of each entity?

Shea asked Sinclair and Snowdon to collect the necessary data and prepare to present it to WHS senior leadership at the end of the next quarter. This would give them several months to do their background research, followed by another couple of weeks to refine their assumptions and properly frame the results of their research. Shea also offered to participate in regularly scheduled meetings so that he could remain informed about their ongoing findings and any challenges they encountered. They closed the meeting mutually energized, but Sinclair and Snowdon knew they had to get started right away.

Considering the Options

After Shea left Sinclair's office, Snowdon remained to continue the discussion with Sinclair. Their first task was to plan for the work they would have to do in the coming months. In particular, they wanted to determine the scope of the project, and try to get a sense of how to frame the alternatives.

Based on the preliminary conversations they had had with each other and their knowledge of the organizational development and training literature, they were able to outline six separate alternatives that varied based on level of centralization and magnitude of organizational changes required:

1. Centralize training and development within the existing department of human resources.
2. Centralize training and development within the new department of organizational development.
3. Centralize training and development with the creation of a new structure, a corporate university, housed with the new department of organizational development.
4. Maintain decentralized delivery of training, but centralize the development function within the existing department of human resources.
5. Outsource training and development to a third-party vendor.
6. Maintain the status quo with decentralized training and development.

Given these six alternatives, Sinclair and Snowdon's next step was to consider what information they needed to collect to assist Shea in the decision-making process. Their biggest task was to perform an organizational assessment of WHS as a whole with respect to training and development. In particular, they needed to determine what currently was going on in education, training, and development, including where these activities occurred, who or what department provided them, and how they were delivered. Within education and training, they were curious about factors such as whether any programs were offered on-line, whether some areas of the organization collaborated with others, and how clinical training and continuing education were delivered. Within development, they wanted to know if there was any formal system to track development activities, if employees in any entity or area were required to create professional development plans that could be monitored, and whether developmental programs were tied to annual performance evaluations.

Another important part of their assessment was to identify key stakeholders in the areas of training and development for each health system entity. They knew organizational politics would likely play an important role in either building support or resistance for any initiative that required a change. As a result, they needed to identify important decision makers within each entity and, ideally, recruit organizational champions who could help them with any change process.

Finally, to fully evaluate the different alternatives, they would have to develop some projections about costs associated with current operations (Alternative 6) in comparison with the five other alternatives they had outlined. Shea had recognized that there were likely nonfinancial costs associated with training and development in addition to financial costs, so they needed to consider these along with the financial and nonfinancial gains that could be accrued with each alternative.

Building the Case for Change

Shea was known for his ability to make quick decisions and then back his decisions with resource support. However, Sinclair and Snowdon knew they needed not only financial resources, but also organizational commitment to ensure success for this initiative. They were excited to move forward with their ideas about centralizing the training and development function for WHS, but they knew they needed to build their case carefully.

Case Questions

1. In addition to the several items listed in the case, what other information would need to be collected to fully evaluate the centralization–decentralization decision?
2. What should be included in developing a financial analysis of this decision?
3. What would be the nonfinancial arguments for or against centralizing training and development at Worthington Health System?
4. With whom should Sinclair and Snowdon speak when considering the impact of each alternative?
5. How might physicians and nurses be affected by the different alternatives?
6. What critical success factors would be associated with the pursuit of a centralization alternative?
7. How could a centralized organizational development department support a culture of systemness at WHS?

Case H
The American Heart Institute

Sofia V. Agoritsas and Ann Scheck McAlearney

The Case of Amanda Jones

Presenting with chest pain, 60-year-old Amanda Jones was rushed from the ambulance bay of the emergency department (ED) of East Bay University Hospital (EBUH) to the catheterization lab. The American Heart Institute

(AHI) lab team determined that Jones was experiencing an ST-segment elevation myocardial infarction (STEMI), the deadliest type of heart attack. As a result, within 30 minutes of her arrival, Jones received a percutaneous coronary intervention (PCI), but the occluded artery could not be opened.

The cardiac catheterization lab team accelerated the protocols to fast-track Jones for emergency cardiac bypass surgery with the cardiac surgeon on call. Luckily, Joseph Cusimano, MD, the chief of cardiac surgery, was available, and Jones was taken into the operating room (OR) within one hour. As time lost was a matter of life and death, it was a race against time.

Collaboration among the interdisciplinary teams of the divisions of cardiology and cardiac surgery and communication among the clinical leaders throughout the AHI were critical to Jones's survival. Fortunately for Jones, her cardiac emergency had a happy ending. She recovered and was released a week later without brain or heart damage.

What Jones didn't know, though, was that AHI was more of a virtual institute than an actual place. Although she had been seen and treated at EBUH, the collaboration and communication that occurred crossed departments, divisions, and organizational boundaries. And unfortunately, AHI's executive director Sandra Getty was not convinced that this structure always provided patients and their families with the best care and service quality they expected and deserved.

East Bay University Hospital and the American Heart Institute Cardiac Service Line

EBUH, a 700-bed teaching hospital, is one of two tertiary care facilities within True Care Health System (TCHS). EBUH is the flagship hospital for adult acute care in the health system. The other acute care hospital, True Care North, was only recently acquired by TCHS and is 20 miles away from the other four main facilities. The Children's Hospital, a psychiatric hospital, and a cancer hospital constitute the remaining three hospitals of TCHS.

AHI is the cardiac service line that spans TCHS. AHI is viewed as a leading provider and pioneer in cardiac care in the region. It is led by Dr. Barry A. Mount, an interventional cardiologist. AHI provides adult cardiac care throughout the state and includes a staff of 50 full-time employed cardiologists and eight cardiac surgeons, five of whom primarily work out of EBUH (see Exhibits III.8 and III.9). The AHI service line also includes six close-to-home cardiac outreach clinics that are part of TCHS's ambulatory care network; this network spans the suburbs around the five-hospital health system. AHI has been listed nationally by leading organizations such as Healthgrades as a top-ranking cardiac program in the United States, but it has not yet been ranked as a top program in *U.S. News & World Report*.

EXHIBIT III.8
Summary of
Cardiac Units
and FTEs
at East Bay
University
Hospital

Area	Beds	FTEs
General Cardiology—3rd Floor	50	110.5
Cardiothoracic ICU—5th Floor	15	62.3
Cardiac Intensive Care Unit—3rd Floor	10	32.75

EXHIBIT III.9
Summary
of Cardiac
Procedures and
FTEs at East
Bay University
Hospital

Area	Procedures	FTEs
Catheterization lab (main floor by ED)	5,402	84.2
Cardiac surgery (5th floor)	807	50.4
Cardiac rehabilitation (off-site)	1,810	4.1
EKG	50,125	20.2
ECHO/TEE	7,523 ECHOs/ 510 TEEs	15

The mission of AHI is to provide world-class, comprehensive cardiac care, to advance cardiac research, and to promote medical education in a fiscally responsible manner. Its vision is to become a premier center of excellence in cardiovascular medicine in the United States. Cardiology and cardiac surgery are to be coordinated in an integrated and seamless delivery system.

The AHI's goals and guiding principles are

- to foster clinical leadership and clinical expertise in high-quality cardiac care,
- to promote a patient-centered care environment and a culture of excellence,
- to develop and implement evidenced-based guidelines that are measurable and outcomes driven,
- to provide patients with appropriate education to empower them and their families to participate in their clinical decision making and self-management, and
- to create marketing initiatives that will brand the identity of AHI.

AHI Structure

AHI is, in practice, a virtual service line, requiring synergistic cooperation from all TCHS cardiac services to realize its mission and achieve its goals (see Exhibit III.10). Across AHI the involved cardiac services include general and interventional cardiology; electrophysiology; the congestive heart failure (CHF) program; cardiac rehabilitation; and cardiac surgery, including cardiac bypass surgery, the minimally invasive valve surgery program, robotics surgery, the endovascular aortic repair center, and heart transplant.

The main divisions that constitute the AHI service line are cardiology and cardiothoracic surgery. These divisions are embedded within traditional departmental structures within the departments of medicine (see Exhibit III.11) and surgery (see Exhibit III.12). As a result, budgetary control of the divisions of cardiology and cardiothoracic surgery are maintained through their departments. However, AHI service line profit and loss statements and summary of statistics reports (see Exhibit III.13) are reviewed monthly by an AHI cardiac advisory board. Furthermore, marketing activities incorporate advertising for cardiology and cardiothoracic surgery under the AHI virtual service line structure, despite the department of origin.

EXHIBIT III.10
Virtual
Organizational
Structure of
Service Line

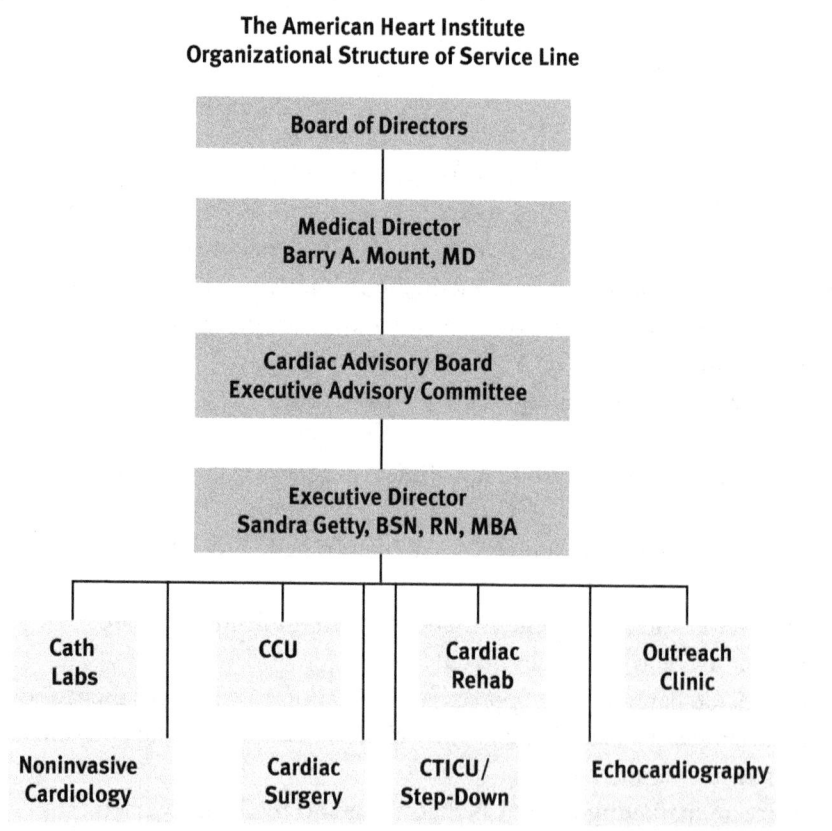

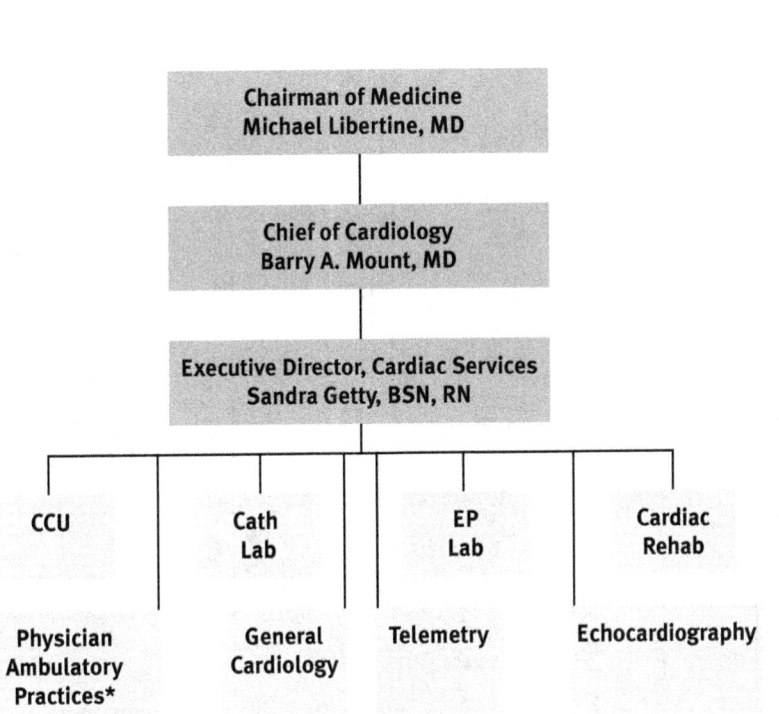

EXHIBIT III.11
Division
Organization
Structure:
Division of
Cardiology

*Physician Ambulatory Practices includes outreach clinics.

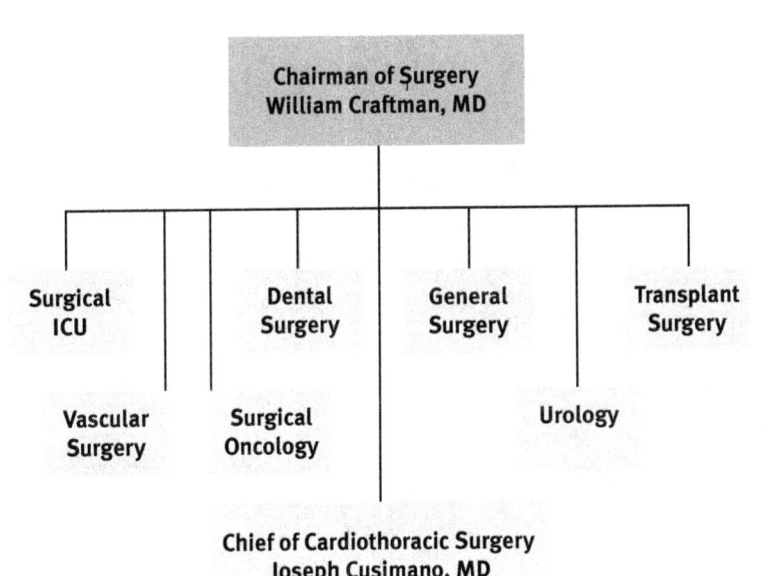

EXHIBIT III.12
Division
Organization
Structure:
Department of
Surgery

EXHIBIT III.13 Summary of Statistics (Includes East Bay University Hospital and True Care North Hospital)

The American Heart Institute
Statistical Summary
For the Month and YTD Ending March 31, 2011

	Mar-11						YTD				
	Actual	Budget	Budget Variance	Prior Month	Prior Year		Actual	Budget	Budget Variance	Prior Month	Prior Year Variance
Admissions in University Hospital											
Cardiology	348	357	−2.52%	335	310		986	1050	−6.1%	933	5.68%
Cardiac surgery	44	54	−18.52%	47	55		130	161	−19.25%	129	0.78%
	392	411	−4.62%	382	365		1116	1211	−7.84%	1062	5.08%
Patient Days											
Cardiology	1,209	1390	−13.02%	1,286	1,278		3,630	4,288	−15.35%	3703	−1.97%
Cardiac surgery	773	484	0.59711%	591	589		1,939	1,494	29.79%	1599	21.26%
Total patient days	1,982	1,874	5.76%	1,877	1,867		5,569	5,782	−3.68%	5302	5.04%
Average LOS											
Cardiology	2.96	3.41	−13.2%	3.32	3.6		3.14	3.57	−12.04%	3.42	−8.19%
Cardiac surgery	7.58	5.44	39.34%	8.21	7.18		7.79	7.58	2.77%	9.69	−19.61%
Total Weighted ALOS	3.48	3.68	5.39%	3.92	4.14		3.68	4.10	−10.27%	4.18	−11.96%

(continued)

EXHIBIT III.13 Summary of Statistics (continued)

The American Heart Institute
Statistical Summary
For the Month and YTD Ending March 31, 2011

	Mar-11					YTD				
	Actual	Budget	Budget Variance	Prior Month	Prior Year	Actual	Budget	Budget Variance	Prior Month	Prior Year Variance
Average Daily Census										
Cardiology	40	46	−13.04%	41	43	39	47	−17.02%	40	−2.5%
Cardiac surgery	26	16	62.5%	19	20	21	16	31.25%	17	23.53%
Total avg daily census	66	62	6.45%	60	63	60	63	−4.76%	57	5.26%
Other Statistics										
Cardiac caths	411	374	9.89%	401	351	1245	1175	5.96%	1102	12.98%
PTCAs/stents	118	105	12.38%	115	98	351	335	4.78%	314	11.78%
EP lab procedures	182	156	16.67%	162	143	483	442	9.28%	404	19.55%
Open heart surgeries	72	54	33.33%	51	58	172	153	12.42%	162	6.17%
Heart transplants	2	1	100.0%	0	69	4	5	−20.0%	5	−20.0%
Total	785	690	13.77%	729	719	2,255	2,110	6.87%	1,987	13.49%

Leadership Challenges for the AHI Service Line

The executive director of AHI, Sandra Getty, BSN, RN, MBA, is responsible for service line business development and serves as the liaison for cardiovascular programs. She previously worked as the nurse manager in the catheterization lab with Dr. Mount 20 years ago and played a major part in helping the division to become filmless. Since then, Getty has established an electrophysiology program, including an atrial fibrillation center and a congestive heart failure program.

In her current role she is responsible for operational leadership and review of compliance activities, coordination of operations and budget formation for all cost centers (except for cardiothoracic surgery), capital improvements, and expansion planning, including transition details. Getty has also been responsible for the acquisition and development of the community outreach centers through a series of purchases of group practices; as a result, multiple physicians are fully employed by the healthcare system. Now, she is leading on-boarding efforts for the new community physician practices, hoping to facilitate seamless transitions and maintain efficiencies in processes and care coordination.

Getty has a key responsibility to make sure that all of the programs within the cardiovascular service line are collectively marketed under the AHI brand. In addition, all the nurse managers and practice administrators in the cardiothoracic intensive care unit (CTICU), cardiac intensive care unit (CCU), and step-down and telemetry units report to her.

Recently, she led the implementation of an electronic health record system, including computerized physician order entry capability for the divisions of cardiology and cardiothoracic surgery, in both the outpatient and inpatient settings. She was also responsible for implementing the American College of Cardiology (ACC) National Cardiovascular Data Registry, and the Society of Thoracic Surgeons–approved electronic databases that had been recommended to track patient outcomes. Getty is very eager to use the new health information technologies (HIT) and systems to enable tracking of patient outcomes across the AHI service line.

By far Getty's biggest challenge is managing relationships with physician leadership and AHI faculty. The lack of cooperation among physicians, partially attributable to the currently virtual organizational structure for the AHI service line, limits her efforts to improve standardization and coordinate care across EBUH and the TCHS—despite her success implementing HIT and data registries.

Quality Improvement Challenges for the AHI Service Line

Dr. Cusimano, chief of cardiothoracic surgery, is considered a national leader in the area of cardiovascular quality improvement. He was recruited two years ago from the northeast, in part because of his reputation for quality improvement. Dr. Cusimano has been part of a consortium that includes cardiothoracic surgeons, interventional cardiologists, administrators, perfusionists, anesthesiologists, and operating room and cardiac ICU nurses; this consortium has been actively reviewing the management of cardiac disease in the region to identify quality improvement opportunities. For more than 20 years, the consortium has established and maintained registries and collectively developed ways to continuously improve the quality, effectiveness, and costs of care in delivering interventions for patients with cardiac disease. Dr. Cusimano has also played a national role in the Society of Thoracic Surgeons (STS), the national organization for cardiothoracic surgeons; with the STS, he has served as a key member of multiple executive committees.

Since coming to EBUH, Dr. Cusimano has tried to establish several multidisciplinary teams and process improvement initiatives. He strongly believes in improving patient outcomes, not just as a necessary response to increased scrutiny of programs by the state department of health but because it can also address the current AHI problems associated with outmigration of patients and decreases in patient volume. AHI is proud of its recent state-published outcomes, including 2 percent mortality in coronary artery bypass graft (CABG) surgery and a higher than 99.5 percent cath/PCI survival rate in the catheterization lab. The improvements in CABG surgery, in particular, have been particularly evident since the arrival of Dr. Cusimano. However, AHI still needs to focus on reducing mortality rates associated with valve surgeries.

Despite Dr. Cusimano's national prestige and experience with quality improvement, the current cardiothoracic surgery faculty at EBUH have not embraced the changes he has made. In fact, because all of the other EBUH surgeons were formerly trainees mentored by the current chair of surgery, Dr. Craftman, many are leery of the "new guy." Interestingly, several surgeons had noted that they believed there were already too many cardiac surgeons on staff at EBUH, so they were predictably unenthusiastic about bringing Dr. Cusimano into their group.

For the past two years, Dr. Cusimano has attempted to organize the group of cardiac surgeons. He has established multiple teaching and quality forums—including enhancing the structure, participation, and transparency of the morbidity and mortality conference meetings, and increasing clinic and didactic involvement with residents and on multidisciplinary rounds. The performance improvement meetings that review patient complications are now more structured, and processes to address opportunities for systematic solutions on the basis of root-cause analyses have been developed. In general, the tone of care quality review meetings has changed from a focus on fault-finding and berating individuals for mistakes to one of collective efforts to find opportunities for improvement.

Dr. Cusimano has also worked with Dr. Mount to develop a daily conference session for faculty from cardiology and cardiothoracic surgery during which faculty meet in the catheterization lab to review all the operative cases against recommendations from the ACC/American Heart Association guidelines prior to performing any surgeries. The objective of this multidisciplinary forum is to enhance the physicians' abilities to assess risk and determine appropriate treatments for patients in a collaborative environment. However, many of the cardiothoracic surgeons do not consistently attend the conferences, often sending a resident physician or physician assistant as their representative to present the surgical case under consideration.

In the area of HIT-facilitated clinical decision making, Getty and Dr. Cusimano recently implemented a series of inpatient order sets and evidence-based guidelines in the CTICU, step-down, and telemetry units. As a result of this process, they also decided to incorporate the division's monthly quality indicators into the AHI service line dashboard (see Exhibit III.14). Unfortunately, this level of transparency in reporting quality data has not helped improve Dr. Cusimano's reputation with his colleagues. Dr. Cusimano's lack of history with the existing faculty and weak relationships within EBUH have limited his ability to build volume and a strong referral base, thereby minimizing his own clinical productivity. As a result, the surgeons who operate the most use the newly available patient data to tout their own performance, further discounting the value of Dr. Cusimano's contributions to EBUH.

Overall, Dr. Cusimano strives to unite, motivate, and hold each of the independent cardiac surgeons accountable, but he has yet to be successful in this endeavor. One issue he has encountered is that the employment contracts of the surgeons are not uniform in structure. Dr. Cusimano has proposed to the executive administration that each physician receive a base salary and then be given an augmentation—or bonus—based on certain metrics (see Exhibit III.15). The measures would be reconciled through the department of finance on a quarterly basis. In response to this proposal, the cardiac surgeons recently met privately with the executive administration of EBUH and the chair of surgery and threatened to leave the organization. The administration's

Performance Metrics Dashboard

Quality	Baseline MTD	Current YTD	Threshold	Goal
Cardiac surgery mortality rate	4.0%	2.0%	3.0%	2.5%
AMI & congestive heart failure core measures	89.8%	90.3%	>90%	>91%
PCI risk-adjusted mortality	1.0%	0.5%	<1.0%	<1.0%

Financial Performance	MTD	YTD	YTD Budget	YTD Variance
Part A — Net income (in thousands)	$8,139	$27,112	$27,989	($877)
Part B — Net income (in thousands)	$675	$1,903	$2,105	($202)
FTE (variance)	448.4	458.3	465.5	7.2

Patient Experience	Baseline MTD	Current YTD	Threshold	Goal
Patient satisfaction	89.0%	87.5%	89.0%	90.0%

Operational Efficiency	Baseline MTD	Current YTD	Threshold	Goal
Average length of stay	3.68	4.10	4.18	4.00
Cath to CABG LOS	1.90	1.75	2.13	2.00

EXHIBIT III.14
Service Line Dashboard (Includes East Bay University Hospital and True Care North Hospital)

reaction was to increase the salaries of these surgeons because they were afraid that a large volume of surgical referrals and cases would be diverted to hospital competitors if this group of surgeons left EBUH—but this reaction clearly undermined Dr. Cusimano's individual authority within the group. Moreover, looking ahead, physicians have no direct incentive to align themselves with EBUH's or TCHS's long-term goals, and this does not bode well for future collaboration efforts.

EXHIBIT III.15 Cardiac Surgeon Compensation Model

Division of Cardiothoracic Surgery Compensation Model

Surgeon: _____   Quarter: _____

Augmentation Schedule Above Base Salary:

Goals/Measures	Weight	Threshold Performance	Target Performance	Maximum Performance
Growing the practice:				
Maintains annual clinical volume (Baseline of wRVUs).	20%	(75% likelihood) 95% of previous year	(50% likelihood) 105% of previous year	(10% likelihood) 110% of previous year
Divisional quality goals:	20%	Achieve 2 of 4	Achieve 3 of 4	Achieve 4 of 4
a. Mortality rate (CABG, valve w/CABG)				
b. Stroke rate				
c. LOS—pre-op hospital LOS (average 2 days)				
d. Tracheostomy/PEG rate				
Citizenship:	20%	Discretion of the chief	Discretion of the chief	Discretion of the chief
Discretion of the chief and based on demonstrated "teamwork" (Examples: covering other physicians when needed; attendance in departmental meetings; leadership role/volunteering for work of importance to the Division)				
Peer-reviewed articles published or nonindustry grants:				
Number	20%	1	2	3 or more
Teaching:	20%	Discretion of the chief	Discretion of the chief	Discretion of the chief
Didactic session attendance, intra-operative teaching, outpatient clinic, etc.				
TOTAL	Up to 100% of possible augmentation amount			

Additional Challenges for the AHI Service Line

Dr. Mount and the other members of the cardiac advisory board recognize that procedures have become less profitable in recent years. Increases in costs combined with high utilization of costly devices, such as drug-eluting stents and implantable cardioverter defibrillators, have contributed to this problem. Service line growth is a perpetual struggle and is influenced by a variety of factors, including shifts in patient volume from inpatient to outpatient treatments; competition across disciplines, such as cardiology, vascular surgery, and interventional radiology; and the incorporation of novel technologies, such as drug-eluting stents, that led to severe reductions in cardiac surgery volume.

In addition, these cost and growth challenges are exacerbated by additional operational and clinical issues. For instance, AHI does not have a single budget because of its design as a virtual service line. Similarly, because of the considerable variability in the particular conditions of each physician's employment contract, expectations and the level of commitment between surgeons and AHI also vary; only some of the cardiac surgeons are fully employed by the health system, and many of the contracted surgeons feel lower levels of loyalty to AHI and the health system than AHI would like to have. Finally, as is the case in most healthcare settings, internists and cardiologists follow referral patterns based on their long-lasting relationships; because many of these individuals trained as resident physicians together, they are inclined to refer to the colleagues they know rather than follow AHI criteria for ordering consults or following the on-call schedule.

Geographic limitations also pose challenges to the coordination of patients for AHI. Because the building infrastructure was built to accommodate traditional hospital departmental structures, the cardiac surgery practices, CTICU, and operating rooms are contiguous with the department of surgery and division of general surgery. However, these areas are distant (i.e., floors away) from the cardiology suites that include echocardiography, electrophysiology, the CCU, and the catheterization labs. Without centralization of services, communication between and among the various entities is complicated; this physical structure thus reinforces independent silos of activities rather than fostering collaboration throughout AHI. In addition, many of the cardiology group practices are located on different sites around campus. Way-finding for patients is confusing, and the need to improve coordination of care is further compounded.

Despite these challenges, though, the cardiac advisory board believes that a comprehensive and highly specialized heart institute that includes advanced programs will lead to profits down the road. For instance, both Drs. Mount and Cusimano believe that the division of cardiothoracic surgery needs to develop its minimally invasive valve surgery program. This need has become especially pressing as the volume of CABG surgeries performed through AHI has plateaued; it appears that many patients are being referred by community-based physicians to the competitor teaching hospital in the city rather than being sent to AHI surgeons. In comparison with the risks associated with traditional surgery, patients benefit from minimally invasive valve surgery because the breastbone is not split, the risk of infection and bleeding is lower, hospital length of stay is shorter, recovery time is accelerated, and the cosmetic result of the surgery is better. A strong minimally invasive valve surgery program at AHI would allow AHI to differentiate its product from other hospital competitors that do not offer this surgical alternative.

Strategic Planning for AHI

During the spring of 2010, the executive administration of TCHS requested that AHI conduct a strategic plan assessment for 2011–2015. Considering the market share parameters that were analyzed—including population growth, total population size, inpatient and outpatient market share, physician supply and demand, payer mix, and the Herfindhal-Hirschman Index (a measure of market concentration)—capacity for growth and market prioritization were identified as primary areas for strategic focus. Additional priorities include the following:

- Establishing a disease-based organization
- Creating an outreach team
- Building programmatic infrastructure in the congestive heart failure and electrophysiology departments
- Expanding the AHI outreach clinic network
- Expanding the cardiac rehab program
- Developing partnerships with targeted local and regional community cardiology practices
- Increasing True Care Ambulatory Network referrals to AHI physicians
- Establishing a one-stop communications office
- Using patient navigators and outreach coordinators to serve as the connectors between AHI physicians, referring community-based physicians, and patients

Results of the strategic planning process also highlighted the branding problem of the AHI and noted that much of the problem could be attributed to the virtual nature of the service line. Another problem the process identified was the cannibalization of AHI market share that was occurring in certain practices and regions because of redundancies in services offered and the substitutability of certain treatments. In some instances the planning process suggested excessive outmigration from the outreach clinics, even though they were part of the TCHS Ambulatory Network. It appeared that while the community-based cardiologists were using their affiliation with AHI to promote their own practices, they also reportedly felt disconnected from AHI and were afraid they would lose their own patients to the main AHI campus cardiologists.

Realizing the Strategic Vision: Moving from a Virtual Service Line to Bricks and Mortar?

The strategic planning process also introduced the possibility of building a freestanding cardiac hospital. The case was made that the cardiac services division was and would continue to be a pillar of revenue and contribution profits, and AHI might be able to solve some of its current problems by moving into a freestanding center. Such a center would be designed to support a comprehensive cardiac service line that included prevention, early detection, disease management, and postprocedure follow-up care. The driving forces supporting the case for developing the freestanding heart hospital included: (1) enhancing the academic stature and branding image of the cardiac service line, (2) facilitating the implementation of a more efficient clinical model, and (3) maximizing the ability of AHI to realize the value of the cardiac service line.

If this path were pursued, the freestanding facility would be expected to epitomize the image and brand of the AHI, aligning AHI with its vision and helping to promote identification of AHI as the destination center of excellence for cardiac tertiary and specialty care. As a result, community-based AHI practices would be able to focus more on general cardiac care. Centralizing specialized services in a single physical location would enable AHI to (1) design care around patient needs, (2) integrate services and knowledge, and (3) create efficiencies for disease coordination and systems processes. Costs would also be able to be managed by leveraging economies of scale and scope. It was argued that patients would be better served because all services would be centralized, and multidisciplinary advanced programs would be available in one facility. The ultimate goal was that the physical infrastructure could support programmatic development and internal physician alignment across the cardiac service line—but at a cost of $100 million.

Conclusion

At present, AHI leadership must sort out the service line situation and the alternatives ahead. Fortunately the clear consensus is that patients like Amanda Jones cannot suffer from poor service or poor care quality because of issues related to problems with misaligned incentives, poor collaboration, or inadequate coordination. Leadership realizes that it must continue to provide both clinical and nonclinical staff with the resources and education tools they need to be able to provide the best care possible. Yet introducing some of these resources and tools has proved difficult in many circumstances. Neither the employees nor the staff should get caught up in the challenges affecting the service line, but even under the most optimistic of circumstances, a new building for the AHI would not be available until 2015.

Case Questions

1. What problems and issues result from the way AHI is currently organized?
2. How are design issues exacerbated by power conflicts between and among physicians?
3. What are the issues that a new building for AHI might be able to solve? What issues might still plague AHI?
4. What would you recommend that AHI leadership do now? Who would you involve in making decisions about the future for AHI?

Case I
Selling an Evidence-Based Design for Waterford Hospital

Nathan Burt and Ann Scheck McAlearney

Campeon Health is a Midwestern healthcare system composed of five hospitals, ten affiliated hospitals, and an extensive ambulatory care network. Given favorable demographics and a strong bottom line, Campeon Health has recently decided to construct a new hospital in Waterford, a suburb of the larger Grouse Creek metropolitan area. In all, Grouse Creek currently contains three major hospital systems and a children's hospital, but despite steady population growth, new hospitals have been scarce. The Campeon Health facility would be the region's first newly constructed hospital in more than 22 years.

The Waterford suburb was considered an ideal site for the new hospital due to the wealth of the surrounding area and the growing population. In fact, Waterford boasted the highest number of children per household for the Grouse Creek metropolitan area. Contributing to the location decision was the fact that Campeon Health currently drew few patients from the Waterford area to its other hospitals because of the presence of closer competitor hospitals. Campeon's projections suggested that Waterford Hospital could draw 70 percent of its patients from among those presently receiving service outside the Campeon Health system. In addition, Campeon predicted that the new hospital would be received favorably by local physicians, including those practicing at other Campeon Health facilities. Planned to be a 90-bed community hospital, Waterford could serve as a feeder hospital for the system's large flagship hospital, Lakeside Hospital, while accommodating the preferences of physicians interested in expanding their practices to include the Waterford community.

The Charge

Prior to breaking ground for the new facility, Katherine Humphries, RN, had been appointed president of Waterford Hospital. Humphries had worked as CEO of another Campeon Health hospital for three years, and had established a strong reputation as a transformational leader. She has been charged by the board of Campeon Health and the Campeon Health CEO to lead the initiative to design, construct, staff, and operate the new community hospital in Waterford. At the present time, the Waterford Hospital site is nothing more than a field, located across the street from an existing Campeon Health ambulatory care center.

Humphries has been given relatively free rein to design the hospital. Humphries's years of experience as a registered nurse and as an operations leader have given her valuable insights into the delivery of care and ways that it can be improved. She is aware that elements of evidence-based design have been shown to improve care quality for patients and workplace climate for caregivers, and she is eager to consider this approach.

Evidence-Based Design

Evidence-based design is increasingly being used by hospitals that are trying to improve staff morale, patients' experiences, and the outcomes of care provided. Evidence-based healthcare designs are specifically used to create environments that are therapeutic, supportive of family involvement, efficient for staff performance, and restorative for workers under stress. Ultimately, evidence-based healthcare designs should result in demonstrated improvements in the organization's clinical outcomes, economic performance, productivity, customer satisfaction, and cultural measures. However, this healthcare design approach is a relatively new concept. The pool of available research and information will rarely fit a hospital's situation precisely, thus requiring critical consideration of specific design modifications and project goals.

In healthcare, the application of evidence-based design is particularly appropriate. Physicians are accustomed to practicing, at least in part, using evidence-based clinical guidelines and measures, thus the notion of applying evidence to facility design may be well received. Further, design principles focusing on the physical characteristics of facilities design that may reduce patient stress and contribute to the healing process appeal to patients and families who are likely familiar with the stressful and often frightening experiences that are common to hospital stays. Hospitals themselves have been shown to benefit economically from reduced costs and increased organizational effectiveness when applying the principles of evidence-based design (Saba and Hamilton 2006).

Evidence-based design principles include many elements of building design, several of which have been demonstrated to be effective. In particular, exposure to sunlight, access to nature through direct access or views, acuity-adaptable rooms, and decentralized nurses' stations are design elements that hold promise. For instance, studies have shown that climate and exposure to sunlight can influence the length of a patient's stay. One research group randomly assigned some bipolar patients to sunny rooms and others to rooms with less exposure to sunlight. The patients who were exposed to greater amounts of sunlight had a mean length of stay 3.67 days shorter than the control group. Similarly, patients recovering from abdominal surgery had shorter hospital stays if they had a bedside window view of nature rather than windows that looked out onto a brick wall (Ulrich et al. 2004).

Another promising feature of evidence-based design is the potential for well-designed rooms and buildings to improve clinical outcomes. In fact, the list of examples such as lower rates of acquired infections, fewer medication errors, fewer patient falls, and reduced patient stress are growing (Ulrich et al. 2004). Something as simple as placing an alcohol hand rub dispenser at the patient's bedside can yield significant improvements in practitioners' handwashing practices, thereby reducing contact infection rates. Evidence-based design can also help to reduce medication errors by focusing on care delivery elements such as lighting, environmental distractions, and workflow interruptions that may increase medication administration errors. Patient falls can also be reduced when patient rooms are well designed, and good building design can reduce noise levels, thereby reducing stress levels for patients and their caregivers (Ulrich et al. 2004).

Acuity-Adaptable Rooms

A key component of evidence-based design in hospitals is the acuity-adaptable room. While the more common universal patient room has gained popularity because of its potential to accommodate clinical needs and new technologies as future care delivery innovations are introduced, such patient rooms are still used in the traditional clinical manner, necessitating patient transfers between rooms, units, and floors when patient acuity changes. In contrast, the acuity-adaptable room is designed to accommodate a wide range of patient acuity levels, thus reducing the need to transfer patients and change the care delivery workflow (Brown and Gallant 2006).

Acuity-adaptable rooms are private rooms that are composed of a patient area, a staff area, and a family area. Evidence-based design principles are applied to the layout of acuity-adaptable rooms, thus maximizing the likelihood of care improvements to be gained from these principles. For example, a private room is quieter than a shared room, thereby potentially reducing patient and caregiver stress. Space dedicated to a family area permits social contact with family and friends to further improve the healing process (Brown and Gallant 2006). Bathrooms are situated on a headwall with rails leading to them, potentially reducing the likelihood of patient falls. In addition, the accommodation of family and friends within patient rooms on a 24-hour basis reduces the possibility of patients falling, and can also reduce patient stress.

An acuity-adaptable room design helps solve some of the problems with bottlenecks in patient flow that occur daily in most hospitals. These bottlenecks can have several negative consequences, including diversions to other hospitals or warehousing patients in hallways without adequate monitoring and nursing care. Within traditional hospitals, patient flow revolves around nursing units, which are generally organized by diagnosis type. Diagnosis type is, in turn, influenced by three factors: (1) the headwall capability to accommodate lines and gases, (2) the clinical skills of the nurse to treat different levels of acuity, and (3) the historically variable reimbursement from the Centers for Medicare & Medicaid Services (Hendrich, Fay, and Sorrells 2004). This mix of considerations about diagnosis type and nursing unit results in assignment of patients to units based on the unit's capacity to accept patients with a particular diagnosis and level of acuity. As a result, this traditional nursing unit–centric model contributes to situations where a bed may be available, but it is not the "right" bed for that particular patient. This then causes a patient flow bottleneck. Further, because many patients experience variable levels of acuity during a hospital stay, the nursing unit–centric model may also result in patients being transferred three to six times during the course of their stays (Hendrich, Fay, and Sorrells 2004). The additional coordination required by multiple transfers then increases the complexity of patient flow within the hospital and further contributes to bottlenecks. Also, as explained by Brown and Gallant (2006), "the transfer process is not a clinically benign process and has been shown to cause physiologic and psychologic distress that could lead to negative clinical outcomes." By targeting areas such as bed placement, communication, and housecleaning efficiency, slight improvements can be made within the current model of care, but a different model must be adopted to permit large gains in quality and efficiency (Hendrich, Fay, and Sorrells 2004).

A Growing Evidence Base

Improvements in clinical and patient satisfaction outcomes associated with the introduction of acuity-adaptable rooms were starting to be documented. In particular, Humphries was intrigued by two examples reported in the recent research literature where adoption of acuity-adaptable rooms had been linked to positive outcomes. These examples are described in "Examples of Acuity-Adaptable Models in US Hospitals."

Decentralized Nurse Stations

Another opportunity that has emerged out of the principles of evidence-based design is to develop decentralized nurse stations. In practice, the layout of hospitals has not changed much in decades, despite the jobs of nurses, physicians, and other caregivers having changed significantly. According to one recent study, nurses spend approximately 30 percent of their time walking around the hospital, and less than 60 percent of their time on actual patient care (Ulrich et al. 2004).

A typical nursing unit has a central nurse station with the rooms laid out in a double corridor rectangular pattern around the nurse station. This nurse station typically houses a unit clerk, provides an area for nurses to do their chart work, and accommodates the medical records of the unit's patients. A change in the layout of a floor can increase the amount of time nurses are able to be involved in direct patient care by reducing requirements for walking around. In fact, nurses working in a radial unit walk much less than nurses working in a rectangular unit (Ulrich et al. 2004). Nurses on a floor with decentralized nurse stations walk even less than those nurses working in a radial unit, as long as supplies are decentralized as well. This decentralized nurse station model thus presents many opportunities to improve the quality and efficiency of care provided, by reducing the amount of wasted time nurses spend walking around and freeing nursing time to provide direct patient care.

Examples of Acuity-Adaptable Models in US Hospitals

An Acuity-Adaptable Comprehensive Critical Coronary Care Floor at Clarian Health

Clarian Health, based in Indianapolis, Indiana, switched from a traditional model of care to an acuity-adaptable model in coronary care by building an acuity-adaptable comprehensive critical coronary care (CCCC) floor. The acuity-adaptable CCCC is capable of performing all necessary care in one room, from admission to discharge (Brown and Gallant 2006). Using a pre-post design to evaluate the success of this model, Clarian recorded two years of baseline data and then compared clinical outcomes after CCCC adoption with these baseline data.

During the baseline period, the two units that were to become the CCCC had an average of 200 intraunit transfers per month. The time spent coordinating transfers, processing paperwork, and transporting the patient was all considered to be non-value-added activity that would be better spent in direct patient care. In addition, these 200 handoffs per month elevated the risk of medical errors associated with handoffs.

After moving to an acuity-adaptable model of care, intraunit transfers were cut by 90 percent (Hendrich, Fay, and Sorrells 2004). Also noteworthy, medication errors were cut by 70 percent, likely due at least partially to the reduction in patient handoffs and transfers. Finally, patient falls decreased to a national benchmark level, and patient satisfaction increased overall (Hendrich, Fay, and Sorrells 2004).

An Acuity-Adaptable Model Implemented at Celebration Health

Celebration Health, based in Orlando, Florida, implemented an acuity-adaptable model within its new facility and saw marked improvements in clinical outcomes. In particular, patients' lengths of stay for most diagnosis-related groups (DRGs) declined significantly after introduction of the acuity-adaptable model. Comparing data with another state, Celebration Health reported that the average length of stay for five specific DRGs in its system was 5.4 days, compared with 9.5 days reported in the state of California. Thirty percent of Celebration Health patients with those five DRGs were discharged within four days. These length-of-stay improvements occurred with simultaneous reductions in nursing hours per patient day (Gallant and Lanning 2001).

Implementation Challenges

Evidence-based design options such as acuity-adaptable rooms and decentralized nurse stations have tremendous potential to improve the quality of patient care, but there are also substantial challenges associated with implementation. In particular, staffing using an acuity-adaptable model of care can be difficult. Nurses tend to practice within a specialty because they enjoy the specialty. For instance, a critical care nurse is typically very good at handling urgent situations, but often lacks the skills required to manage large numbers of patients, including providing required patient education and communicating with families. Similarly, telemetry nurses are often skilled at managing large numbers of patients, providing patient education, and dealing with patients' families, but they may lack the skills necessary to handle high-acuity patients (Brown and Gallant 2006). Critical care nurses staffed to work in an acuity-adaptable environment with decentralized nurse stations may feel uncomfortable if they do not have another critical care nurse within sight in the event that an emergency arises, or if they want to consult with another comparably trained nurse about a complex patient.

The Role of Technology

Technology can help overcome some of the challenges surrounding implementation of evidence-based design options such as acuity-adaptable rooms and decentralized nurse stations. For instance, in order for a decentralized nurse station to be successful, it must be completely independent of the central nurse station. All required supplies and technology, including computer access, must be available at the decentralized nurse station. Wireless communications, automated patient call and alarms, medication administration, and even linens must be available at the nurse station (Brown and Gallant 2006). Technology solutions can help to support these requirements, but their use has not yet been widespread.

In practice, a robust computerized physician order entry (CPOE) system can help to overcome some of the challenges presented by decentralized nurse stations. A CPOE system that is linked to all areas of the hospital can house test results and facilitate physicians' ordering of required tests and studies while also helping nurses to manage their patients effectively. While a unit clerk in a centralized nurse unit coordinates tests and studies with other departments, a CPOE system eliminates the need for this unit clerk on the nursing floor, thus reducing some of the barriers associated with adopting a decentralized nurse station model.

Technology can also help to improve communications in a decentralized nurse unit model. When patients have high acuity levels, communication between and among nurses may be problematic if nurse stations are decentralized within the hospital. However, technology can help caregivers communicate quickly and thoroughly with each other, even in a decentralized environment. For instance, new technologies such as smart beds, smart pumps, and specific clinical alarms can be adopted to improve patient monitoring and facilitate patient-related communications within this decentralized nurse unit model.

Financial Implications

Construction costs per square foot for an evidence-based design building are not much higher than for a traditional building, but increased costs should be considered. First, overall construction costs would be higher because of the modifications in architectural designs necessary to introduce sunlight within 95 percent of the building and the larger square footage required for acuity-adaptable rooms compared with traditional room sizes. From a design standpoint, introducing sunlight could be tricky for internal spaces. One solution is to build gardens within the core spaces of a building. While such gardens tend to be expensive, they do offer visible areas for community support and are often selected for their ability to contribute to the healing environment. Acuity-adaptable room sizes must be able to accommodate a large range of equipment and have space for family members. As a result, acuity-adaptable rooms may be 30 to 50 percent larger than traditional single-occupancy rooms.

Any differences in operating costs associated with an acuity-adaptable model of care are still unclear. While the skill sets required for nurses on acuity-adaptable units may be higher, those higher staff costs may be associated with shorter lengths of stay linked to improved patient well-being. A higher level of management may also be required to oversee complicated staffing needs associated with an acuity-adaptable model of care, but this may be offset by less demand for management given a higher level of skill among staff. In contrast to outstanding questions about changes in human resources costs, an evidence-based design clearly can reduce costs associated with utilities, because the availability of sunlight throughout the building will reduce electricity costs. Similarly, maintenance and supplies costs are typically reduced because of standardized equipment and supplies throughout the hospital.

Capitalizing on the Opportunity

Humphries is convinced that an evidence-based design model will be appropriate for the design of Waterford Hospital. Working with the hospital architect and contractor, Humphries has been able to outline an evidence-based design for Waterford Hospital that includes components such as acuity-adaptable patient rooms, decentralized nurse units, and liberal use of windows and open spaces to provide patients and their families with access to nature. The latest version of the architectural drawings features all private rooms for patients, with each room including a family area designed to contain a couch/bed, a refrigerator, and a separate television for the families. In addition, gardens are planned for both inside and outside the hospital, with easy access points for patients, families, and hospital staff. Staff and families will also have access to respite areas, which are spaces individuals can go to relieve stress and deal with difficult situations and decisions. Finally, all patient areas, and 95 percent of other hospital space, are designed to have access to direct or indirect sunlight.

Overall, Humphries is pleased with the preliminary plans for Waterford Hospital, but she knows she has a long way to go to convince hospital staff and physicians accustomed to working in traditional hospital environments that the evidence-based design model is sound and desirable. In fact, moving forward with an evidence-based design is risky if she does not get key stakeholders on board. She knows her next step is to build support for the application of an evidence-based design for Waterford Hospital, but she doesn't have much time.

Case Questions

1. Who are the key stakeholders who must support Humphries' vision for an evidence-based hospital design? How would you obtain their support?
2. What reactions might you predict from physicians regarding the use of evidence-based design at Waterford Hospital? How about from members of the Waterford community? The Grouse Creek community? Other local hospitals and health systems?
3. What challenges do you think Humphries and the leadership team at Waterford Hospital will face as they try to implement an acuity-adaptable model of care?

References

Brown, K. K., and D. Gallant. 2006. "Impacting Patient Outcomes Through Design: Acuity Adaptable Care/Universal Room Design." *Critical Care Nursing Quarterly* 29 (4): 326–41.

Gallant, D., and K. Lanning. 2001. "Streamlining Patient Care Processes Through Flexible Room and Equipment Design." *Critical Care Nursing Quarterly* 24 (3): 59–76.

Hendrich, A. L., J. Fay, and A. K. Sorrells. 2004. "Effects of Acuity-Adaptable Rooms on Flow of Patients and Delivery of Care." *American Journal of Critical Care* 13 (1): 35–45.

Saba, J., and K. Hamilton. 2006. "The Bottom Line on Evidence-Based Design." Presentation at American College of Healthcare Executives Congress on Healthcare Leadership, Chicago.

Ulrich, R., X. Quan, C. Zimring, A. Joseph, and R. Choudhary. 2004. Unpublished paper presented at the American Institute of Architects, Academy of Architecture for Health, virtual seminar on healing environments.

Short Case 12
System Redesign to Implement an Accountable Care Organization

David Muhlestein and Ann Scheck McAlearney

Central Health System (CHS) is the largest health system in its region and includes ten hospitals (ranging from large tertiary care centers to smaller community hospitals) located across two states in addition to 41 affiliated physician clinics, a hospice program, a home health agency, and a nursing home network. As a not-for-profit organization it has the mission of "providing the highest-quality care to all people, independent of ability to pay." Currently, the system employs 300 physicians, and 900 more are contractually affiliated with it; there are also 9,250 full-time equivalent staff. The ten CHS hospitals are autonomous in maintaining their day-to-day operations, but strategic direction and any major operational changes are led by the system's C-suite. As director of operations, you work under the chief operating officer (COO) to implement corporate strategy throughout the system.

The ACO Challenge

The COO recently informed you that the board of directors has requested a feasibility study to determine the effects on CHS if the system were to become an accountable care organization (ACO). Specifically, the board wants CHS to apply for the Medicare ACO program and to seek out similar arrangements with private insurers. Under a shared savings program, such as the program sponsored by Medicare, a baseline expenditure amount will be calculated on the basis of historical usage, and then future expenditures will be projected. If actual expenditures are less than projected expenditures, then the difference between the two (i.e., the "savings") will be partially paid to the provider, assuming certain quality benchmarks are also met. For example, if a Medicare population is projected to cost $10 million over the next year but the provider only bills for $9 million, the $1 million savings will be split between Medicare and the provider. The savings are expected to result from improved care coordination and the ACO's ability to focus on providing appropriate care.

The board would like to know what would be the best way to redesign care delivery if CHS were to become an ACO. Additionally, because the board is constantly seeking to achieve its mission and goals to provide high-quality care, it would like to know if striving to achieve the aims of an ACO (i.e., care coordination and population health management) could help them to improve care throughout CHS and at what cost.

The Current CHS Organization

CHS is a siloed healthcare system where a patient can receive specialty care that is world-class, but he is basically on his own when trying to navigate between and among the different specialties and services. Further, CHS has a competent primary care program staffed by physicians affiliated with, but not employed by, CHS; however, primary care physicians simply refer patients to specialty care services and do not follow up or monitor these referrals. The system has no central tracking of patients nor any full-time patient care coordinators; any current care coordination is provided informally by individual practitioners.

Redesigning the Health System

To become an ACO, CHS will need to monitor the care of patients from the time they enter the system, track the different services they use, and coordinate the care they receive from different providers. This will require administrative, logistic, and clinical changes. Administratively, CHS will need to develop the capabilities to communicate with patients, track patients, and convey information to providers. Clinically, CHS will need to be able to review the care provided, screen patients, ensure that appropriate preventive care is delivered, and ensure that the necessary quality-of-care benchmarks are met.

The COO recognizes that to appropriately coordinate care, fundamental changes must be made to CHS. He has suggested several potential models to organize the administrative and clinical care necessary to coordinate its patient population, and these include divisional, matrix, and parallel designs. The COO recognizes that different models will require different capital investments (primarily in information technology) and will require buy-in from different interested parties.

- *Division design.* Under a divisional model, CHS would focus administrative and clinical care coordination at each individual hospital that would be responsible for coordinating the care of patients who go to that hospital or receive their care in nearby ambulatory care settings. Hospital-level care coordinators would then be responsible to hand off patients who go to a different hospital, and they would report to a centralized office.

- *Matrix design.* With a matrix design, administrative and clinical care coordinators would be assigned to each individual hospital and would report directly to hospital management. However, they would work out of a central health system location within teams of other care coordinators who would be assigned to different hospitals, and they would additionally report to this central office.
- *Parallel design.* A parallel design would feature two separate coordination systems with one focused on administration and the other on clinical coordination. These care coordination systems could either be embedded within individual hospitals or centrally located, but both would report to the same centralized care coordinator.

The COO would like you to propose a model that will minimize the risk to CHS if becoming an ACO is not successful, while maximizing the potential upsides of becoming a more coordinated health system if care coordination succeeds at improving care quality and lowering the cost of care.

Case Questions

1. What are the strengths and weaknesses of the present system?
2. Which organizational model would you propose and why?
3. What advantages and disadvantages does the model you proposed have compared with alternative organizational structures?
4. What advantages for patient care does the proposed model provide?

Short Case 13
Integrating Rehabilitation Services into the Visiting Nurse Service of America

Jacob Victory

Over the last century, the Visiting Nurse Service of America (VNSA) has grown into a national home care entity. Serving 750,000 patients in 15 states annually and employing 25,000 nurses, therapists, social workers, and home health aides, VNSA earns a 5 percent profit margin on a $3 billion revenue base and has a conservative management team that monitors business and care quality targets. These divisions primarily serve the frail elderly, with thriving programs that focus on the homebound long-term care population, targeting the vulnerable Medicaid and dually eligible (for Medicare and Medicaid) populations. Growing at an 8 percent rate, VNSA is proud of its current market prominence and of its origins as a nursing-based home care organization.

Indeed, nurses are considered each patient's primary case coordinator, and from the CEO down to the nursing team leaders, nurses dominate the organization's culture and all levels of its decision-making processes, business strategy, resource allocation, and marketing. In fact, all divisions except rehabilitation services are headed by a nurse.

Rehabilitation Services

VNSA's rehabilitation services (rehab) division is the black sheep of the organization. It employs 3,500 physical, occupational, and speech therapists and serves about 65 percent of VNSA's patients. Rehab is considered a pseudoprogram, as it was carved out of the larger, skilled nursing–focused agency. The program reports to the vice president of operations, a clinician who is in charge of a dozen nursing-dominated programs. Yet it is an ancillary service that is not on the senior staff's immediate radar. In fact, the program is noticed only occasionally, particularly if a therapist is late in serving a VIP patient or if there is a perceived "rehab emergency" with an orthopedic patient.

VNSA patients who need rehabilitation services are primarily referred to rehab by intake nurses and nurse care coordinators. And while the organization has developed nursing teams, led by a nurse manager and clinical support staff, therapists are not integrated into these teams. Although therapists are informally invited to the team meetings, the meeting agendas are strictly nursing focused, and rehab-specific issues are never addressed. Moreover, rehab has a thin management staff. Each rehab manager supervises up to 50 therapists (each with a caseload of up to 20 patients), while each nursing manager supervises no more than ten nurses. VNSA's marketing and advertisements all focus on nurses providing care, even in scenarios in which a rehabilitation need is clearly depicted. This is, after all, a visiting nurse organization.

Jeanine Bastiane, the new rehabilitation administrator, notices these issues immediately. She has a doctorate in occupational therapy and more than 25 years of experience in running hospital, nursing home, and now home-based rehab programs. She is a fun-loving but no-nonsense leader.

She received the mandate to expand rehab and to bring the program to the next level to ensure innovation and market dominance of home-based rehabilitation services. VNSA's president accepts Bastiane's plan to bring in new management talent, and a calculated effort is planned to change the culture and mind-set of the rehab division, particularly since the program has been plagued by poor management over the past decade.

Over the next year, two directors of finance and operations are hired, as is a new clinical director who is responsible for quality improvement and staff training and education. New business, financial, quality, and workforce-related metrics are developed and monitored monthly. The clinical staff is reorganized into cohesive teams, and education and retraining sessions are designed to teach clinical best practices. Scorecards are developed to monitor outcomes and service utilization. An informal rehab-specific profit and loss statement is monitored quarterly to trend revenues and expenses.

The analysis reveals that the program has annual revenues of more than $450 million and a net profit margin of 20 percent (the next most profitable program within VNSA has a margin of 4 percent). The finance and operations directors hold the rehab managers of each state accountable for meeting targets and ensuring growth. Accountability is the new catchphrase, and 50 percent of rehab's management team resigns within seven months, complaining about how often "Big Brother" is watching. More seasoned rehab managers are immediately hired, instilling new management vigor. Though the program has been historically undernoticed, one powerful nurse executive wryly notes in a meeting, "Rehab is sure making some noise these days."

Undeniably, the noise is quite loud. The program enjoys a 22 percent growth in admissions. Bastiane persuades prominent orthopedic surgeons to refer their patients to VNSA, something the business development staff could not do. Better results than the current year are projected, and the program rates highly in employee satisfaction. Some even talk of marketing a distinct "VNSA Rehabilitation Medicine" program.

Yet, the noise is accompanied by what Bastiane calls "success woes," which ironically stem from the notable growth. The program is not getting the financial and human resources needed to sustain its growth rate.

First, although it brought in a $90 million profit for the organization, rehabilitation has no voice in how this profit is allocated. This money is put in an agencywide pool and used to subsidize the deficit-ridden programs and to fund investments in technology and new clinical programs.

Second, each therapist dictates where and when he or she will serve patients; any change in the service area that the therapists believe they "own" is met with raised eyebrows, veiled threats to leave the agency, and adamant resistance. Now, however, the productivity and service utilization of each therapist is the focus of a major quality improvement initiative, and each therapist is monitored to ensure that targeted weekly visit quotas are met (in order to meet demand). This additional focus has the frontline staff nervous and cautious.

Third, rehab does not have enough management and supervisory staff to monitor the clinicians. The added stress of assigning cases, monitoring utilization, reorganizing into teams, and focusing on quality of care and outcomes wears down an already thinly spread management staff.

Finally, executive administration requests that in addition to growth, the program develop "rehabilitation packages" to sell to managed care companies, orthopedic hospitals, and specific targeted populations such as wealthy, private-paying clientele. Without additional investment in management talent and tools to monitor growth and quality, and given the historically nurse-friendly environment at VNSA, Bastiane and her team have more than a few balls to juggle.

Bastiane chews on her pencil as she leans back in her chair. Her office is quiet—her thoughts are not.

Case Questions

1. How was rehabilitation services viewed before Bastiane was named administrator? How is this different from how it was viewed a year after her appointment?
2. What three key management challenges must Bastiane tackle first?
3. How would you advise Bastiane to better integrate rehabilitation services within VNSA?
4. How should Bastiane sell the case to obtain more financial and human resources?
5. How can she influence changing the current nursing culture to be more a clinical culture?

Short Case 14
A Department Administrator's Dilemma

David M. Kaplan

Alice Walsh had been in her role as the department administrator for the department of medicine at Central Hospital for the past ten years. Central Hospital is the largest academic medical center in the area with more than 1,135 beds, 800 full-time faculty, and 500,000 outpatient visits per year. Walsh has observed a lot of changes over the course of her three leadership transitions. Throughout all those changes, her department was able to remain autonomous and was relatively untouched—that is, until now.

Walsh was at a department administrators' meeting where the dean and chief financial officer were announcing that the faculty practice was shifting to a centralized business office model. The dean, who was also the CEO of the faculty practice plan for the organization, approved the plan mandating that all 26 departments in the faculty practice transition their independent billing operations to a centralized process controlled solely by the faculty practice organization. This change marked a major transition for all the departments within the faculty practice, especially Walsh's.

This transition came on the heels of a major consulting engagement in which the consultants identified more than $100 million in cash opportunities across all the clinical departments. The recommendation of the consultants was to develop this centralized model as a way to realize these potential opportunities. As an added advantage to this new model, the consultants outlined potential cost savings of $30 million. These savings would come in the form of staff reductions as well as system and operational efficiencies. Once the board of trustees heard about this recommendation, they strongly advised the dean to implement this model.

Walsh was used to having complete independence in doing her billing and collections. She hired and fired her own billing staff, set her own policies, and had control of her own data. Now, everything was going to change. Walsh had not thought she would ever see this day come, even though her chair, Dr. Maria Sanchez, had warned her about the possibility. Walsh remained in denial.

The department of medicine typically brings in about $60 million worth of physician receipts to the faculty practice each year. The department has eight specialty divisions that, as a whole, employ 40 faculty members and 80 support staff.

Over the next few days, Walsh developed several questions as she prepared to meet with the chief operating officer of the faculty practice, Ken Burns, who had been tasked to help the departments make this transition. Later that week, Walsh met with Burns:

Burns: Alice, how are you doing? I am sure this concept is quite a shock for you.

Walsh: Honestly, Ken, I have been struggling with this the past few days. I don't think I was mentally prepared for this transition.

Burns: I totally understand, but I think many of us saw the writing on the wall. The dean has been looking to put some tighter controls over the revenue cycle process over the past couple of years. He had a lot of concerns that departments were leaving too much cash on the table.

Once the consultants confirmed this opportunity, it was clear we would be moving in this direction.

Walsh: I understand the decision that the dean has made. If I were in his shoes, I would have probably made the same decision. That being said, I can tell you that I am very concerned about the impact this is going to have on our department. At present, we have 80 staff, 35 of whom are part of our billing staff, and they support our 40 faculty. Fifteen of these staff handle front-end registration and scheduling as well as precertification and eligibility verification for patients. Twenty of these staff handle charge entry, payment posting, and following up on accounts receivable and financial counseling of patients. What will happen to these staff and the key processes we have in place for our patients? I'm afraid this new process will create a disconnect between the faculty and the billing operation, breaking down an important connection that we strived to build.

Burns: Well, the plan, as I understand it, will be to provide a centralized pool of front desk staff and registrars who will be assigned across the faculty practice to handle the scheduling and registration for their respective suites. A centralized number will be provided to patients so that they can call for appointments in each clinical area. Faculty will be able to access their schedules at any time to see what their patient schedules look like. Any issues will be e-mailed to the physicians. Our goal is to use as many of your staff as possible in this new model. That being said, all the current staff will need to take a competency test, and, unfortunately, anyone who does not pass the test will be shifted out of the organization.

Walsh: What about the back-end billers?

Burns: A similar model will be used for the billing staff. They will be housed off-site in a cheaper space, and they will be divided by insurance groups rather than by specialties. This is so we can develop experts related to each insurance company's policies and procedures.

Walsh: Will they also have to take and pass a competency exam?

Burns: Yes.

Walsh: So what happens to our long-term, loyal employees who may be excellent at what they do, but may not be completely proficient at using the billing system? Will these people simply be dismissed?

Burns: The dean is serious about having employees who will be immediate-impact players, and while people may be good billers, if they cannot function in the new environment, then unfortunately we have no choice. That being said, perhaps there are other roles in the organization where these people could be deployed, such as patient advocates or as administrative secretaries.

Walsh: I am very saddened by this stance, but perhaps you are right and we should help these folks get placed in other practice-related positions. Another question is, how will we have access to data and reports?

Burns: An advantage of having a centralized system is that we will have the ability to generate meaningful reports based on reliable data. So we will be able to ensure that customized reports are provided on a regularly scheduled basis.

Walsh: That is good news, although I do feel that we had access to that information before this organizational shift. Ken, what is the timeline for this transition to take effect?

Burns: Good question. Right now we are in the midst of performing an overall assessment of all the departments. The plan is to complete the assessments within the next two months. Following that, the new scheduling templates and outfitting of the new space will take place within the next three to six months. The new plan will be fully implemented by the end of the year. We will be able to provide you with a comprehensive work plan with timelines in the next two to four weeks.

Walsh: What is the best way that I can remain engaged throughout this process?

Burns: I am glad you asked. I would like for you to join our work group to ensure that we remain on track, and to make sure that the interests of your large department are covered. We meet once a week, but it is a big commitment because you will be required to assist in the implementation phase—this will require additional time when we get to that phase, but that time frame is yet to be determined. Can we count on you?

Walsh: I will double-check with Dr. Sanchez, but I think this is a good idea, and it would really help me to be involved. I appreciate the invitation. This is definitely going to be a change for us as an organization, but especially for me.

Burns: I understand. Many of us share your concerns, but I think that if we work together, we can develop a plan that can work for everyone.

Walsh: I look forward to the challenge.

Case Questions

1. What is the difference between a centralized and decentralized revenue cycle model?
2. What do front-end staff and registrars do under a centralized model?
3. What do back-end billers do under a centralized model?
4. What billing model would be most effective for a department such as that described in this case and why?
5. If you were the administrator of this department, how would you react to this significant announcement? What would be your actions?

6. If you were the chief operating officer of the faculty practice plan, would you choose a different implementation plan? If so, what might that look like?
7. Do you agree with the process the dean used to implement this new model?

Short Case 15
Matrix or Mess?

Ann Scheck McAlearney

Carol is excited about her newest job change. After serving as a quality improvement (QI) manager for the past two years, she will finally be able to put her expertise in both nursing and informatics to use by taking on a new role as a clinical informaticist for the hospital. While it seemed she had been in school forever, her experience as a nurse combined with her undergraduate degree in informatics and plenty of on-the-job training in quality improvement has given her a broad perspective about how information technology could be usefully implemented to improve the quality of care provided at Valley Community Hospital.

This new job, though, while seemingly a great fit on paper, also makes Carol a bit nervous. In her prior role in QI she had reported to a single director. Her new position gave her a second boss, the director of information systems (IS) for the hospital. In a so-called matrix design, Carol reports to both directors and is responsible for satisfying them both.

In fact, the IS department as a whole is a matrixed department within the hospital. This organizational design for IS had been introduced because of the combination of functional and project responsibilities involved in each IS initiative. The functional areas of the department, such as budgeting, hiring, and training, are consistent, regardless of project. However, IS project responsibilities vary based on the nature of the project and the other hospital department(s) involved. For instance, a project to install a new drug delivery system for the hospital would have particular project-related needs associated with working with the department of pharmacy, as well as IS department needs related to staffing, accounting, and so forth. As a result, each IS manager always reports to two directors, the IS director and another hospital director, based on the clinical or other operational departments served. One prominent example Carol was aware of was that the manager of ambulatory informatics reported to both the director of IS and the director of operations for the hospital. Even the IS trainers have two bosses, as they report to the IS director and the director of education for the hospital. Exhibit III.16 shows examples of these reporting relationships, as well as where Carol's new role fits.

To Carol, this matrix arrangement for IS and QI seems to make sense given the shared goals and objectives of clinical informatics and QI within the

EXHIBIT III.16
The
Information
Systems
Department's
Matrix Design

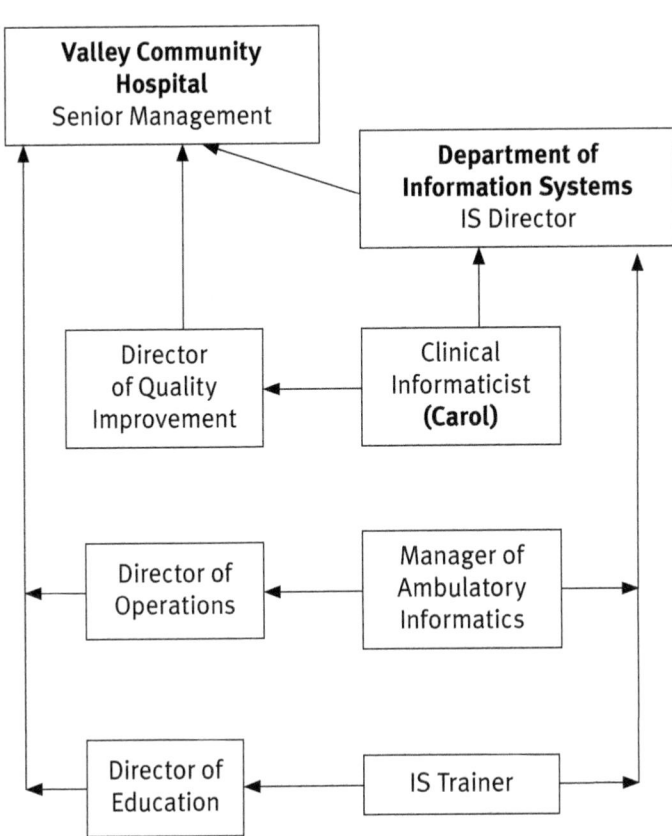

hospital. Yet she suspects issues could arise. Carol wants to make sure she is clear about each of her boss's expectations of her and her new role, but she isn't sure how to make this transition from her original single boss to a dual reporting relationship.

Case Questions

1. What issues will Carol likely face in reporting to two bosses?
2. Does the matrix organizational design make sense for this hospital's IS department, or would another design be more appropriate? What would you propose?
3. What strategies can Carol use to perform well in her new role without feeling pulled in two directions?

IV

PROFESSIONAL INTEGRATION

> In the United States, the physician is not so much part of the hospital as the hospital is part (and only one part) of the physician's practice.
> —*Eliot Freidson (1988)*

> Among the factors that have been associated with good nursing performance are: flattening of organizational structures; increased professional status for staff nurses associated with shared governance and increased autonomy over practice and the practice environment; and effective communication between nurses, physicians and administrators.
> —*Jack Needleman, Elen Kurtzman, and Kenneth Kizer (2007)*

COMMENTARY

The integration of clinician and organizational goals is one of the key challenges facing managers and clinicians in healthcare organizations (HCOs) today. The issues have become more complex as physicians increasingly are salaried by hospitals (for example, hospitalists) while nurses, in the face of a nursing shortage (at least of baccalaureate-trained nurses), are more assertive regarding pursuit of professional autonomy as more independent practitioners. Although they work together in patient care units and ambulatory care centers, physicians and nurses are educated separately (as are managers). Fragmentation of care among physicians and other clinicians is a major problem, resulting in higher costs and uneven quality.

These problems occur to a lesser degree in some large and integrated healthcare systems such as the Mayo Clinic, Geisinger Health System, and Kaiser-Permanente, among others. Progress plays out along different lines in large HCOs, where major initiatives have been developed to standardize work processes—for example, through the use of checklists.

The issue of integrating professionals and HCOs can be approached through more standard labor relations terms, where managers or clinicians negotiate contracts of work with each other. There are more than 200 different healthcare occupations, including highly trained clinicians other than physicians and nurses, such as optometrists, dentists, podiatrists, pharmacists, and physical therapists. We focus here on relations between hospitals and physicians and nurses.

Hospitals and Physicians and Nurses

A study (Health Care Advisory Board 1999) of the key drivers of physician loyalty to organizations concluded that clinical quality, efficiency, and convenient access were at the center of the physician agenda, with most hospitals not meeting physician standards for operational efficiency and staff competency. Nurses have similar concerns, as illustrated in the quote from Needleman, Kurtzman, and Kizer (2007) at the beginning of this section. Lake (2007) posits eight domains of the nursing practice environment that combine factors related to job satisfaction and professional practice. These include autonomy; a philosophy of clinical care emphasizing quality; status of nursing; empowered nursing leaders and organizational participation by nurses; recognition of and advancement based on nurse preparation and expertise; professional development; and supportive or collaborative relationships with managers, physicians, and peers.

Some goal conflict among these parties is functional. Physicians and nurses are concerned with the best possible care for their patients. Managers are concerned with the best possible care for all patients and potential patients. This conflict is functional to the extent that claims for resources to attain all the objectives can be effectively represented and adjudicated when there is trust among the parties. If there is no conflict, the result may be a lack of sufficient manager, physician, or nurse advocacy on behalf of their respective constituencies. If the divergence is too great, the result may be suboptimization, as physician and nurse objectives are achieved at the expense of hospital objectives, or vice versa. Who can be expected to pay for conflict resolutions that are acceptable to all parties? Strong leverage must exist for the interests of those who are not part of the negotiations, and development of a framework and a level of trust within which effective compromise can be achieved. The health system must also have sufficient resources when costs are twice as high as costs in most other developed countries, and yet our quality is uneven and our health outcomes are no better than those of other countries.

Physicians and nurses should expect the following from hospitals: a reasonable income and lifestyle, professional recognition, and participation in decision making (Griffith and White 2002). Of course, all workers want these working conditions; many of us cannot achieve them. What is a reasonable income anyway, relative to whose income? Some physicians and nurses can never get sufficient professional recognition. Some physicians and nurses do not want to participate in hospital (or healthcare system) decision making; others want to participate too much, given their limited skills and experience, and given certain conflicts of interest. An important part of the manager's job is managing the expectations of physicians and nurses so that they will get a clearer, more realistic view of these issues. The goal is for all parties to see and move toward a situation that benefits everyone—and not at the expense of patients or of the tax- and premium-paying public.

Market Considerations

As of 2011, larger organizations were capturing a larger share of the market, whether in hospitals, group practices, nursing homes, visiting nurse services, or health maintenance organizations and insurance companies. The size of firms selling to HCOs is increasing, including pharmaceutical and medical supply manufacturers, not to mention information hardware and software firms, outsourcing firms that include dietary and laundry services, emergency services, pharmacy and physical therapy, and management consulting firms. Professional organizations representing physicians, nurses, and other professionals do not seem to have similarly expanded their size or their market share.

The larger organizations justify their increasing share on the basis of their capability to produce superior outcomes, whether in quality of care, cost of care, or access to care. And government and insurance companies have begun to reward provider organizations on the basis of superior performance. Evidence is required to justify these claims. But certainly organizations are more likely to continue to grow and prosper when they do a better job of recruiting and retaining doctors and nurses, presumably because these organizations have systems, supporting services, and governance that result in higher-quality patient care and better service to patients.

References

Freidson, E. 1988. *Profession of Medicine: A Study of the Sociology of Applied Knowledge.* Chicago: University of Chicago Press.

Griffith, J. R., and K. R. White. 2002. *The Well-Managed Healthcare Organization,* 5th ed. Chicago: Health Administration Press.

Health Care Advisory Board. 1999. *The Physician Perspective: Key Drivers of Physician Loyalty.* Washington, DC: Advisory Board Company.

Lake, E. T. 2007. "The Nursing Practice Environment: Measurement and Evidence." *Medical Care Research and Review* 64 (2): 104S–122S.

Needleman, J., E. T. Kurtzman, and K. W. Kizer. 2007. "Performance Measurement of Nursing Care." In *Changing the U.S. Health Care System: Key Issues in Health Services Policy and Management,* ed. R. M. Andersen, T. H. Rice, and G. F. Kominski. San Francisco: Jossey-Bass.

THE READINGS

Tucker and Edmondson posit in "Why Hospitals Don't Learn from Failures" that organizational learning is an imperative so hospitals can learn from their failures. As hospitals grow larger and more complex, organizational initiatives have been undertaken to create shared databases of medical errors, focusing renewed attention on hospital processes, culture, and reporting systems. The authors conducted a detailed study of hospital nursing care processes to investigate conditions under which nurses might respond to failures they encounter in hospital operating processes. They analyzed qualitative data from 239 hours of observation of 26 nurses at nine hospitals. After completing observations, the authors conducted interviews with 12 nurses at seven of the hospital sites.

Tucker and Edmondson distinguished between first-order and second-order problem solving. The former occurs when the worker compensates for a problem by getting the supplies or information needed to finish a task that was blocked or interrupted. First-order problem solving keeps communication about problems isolated so that they do not surface as learning opportunities. Second-order problem-solving behavior occurs when the worker also takes action to address underlying causes. To learn from failures, people need to be able to talk about them without fear of ridicule or punishment. Managers have an essential role: assisting with problem-solving efforts, providing support for workers who attempt to improve their work systems, and valuing them as motivated employees.

The required supplementary readings provide context for the Tucker and Edmonson study. Carlson ("Is the Relationship Between Your Hospital and Your Medical Staff Sustainable?") and Delbecq and Gill ("Justice as a Prelude to Teamwork in Medical Centers") discuss the factors that lead to a trusting relationship between the hospital and the medical staff. Lake writes about the nursing practice environment and how it needs to be changed for better nurse–hospital relationships to occur. Griffith and White describe how the physician and nursing organizations work in large HCOs.

Why Hospitals Don't Learn from Failures: Organizational and Psychological Dynamics That Inhibit System Change

Anita L. Tucker and Amy C. Edmondson
From *California Management Review* 45 (2): 55–72.

The importance of hospitals learning from their failures hardly needs to be stated. Not only are matters of life and death at stake on a daily basis, but also an increasing number of U.S. hospitals are operating in the red.[1] Organizational learning is thus an imperative. Recent research suggests there are plenty of problems, errors, and other learning opportunities lacing these complex service organizations. In 2000, the Institute of Medicine issued a report estimating that 44,000 to 98,000 people die each year as a result of medical errors.[2] Other studies suggest, in addition, that medical errors with less serious consequences are pervasive in hospitals.[3]

Hospitals historically have relied on a dedicated and highly skilled professional workforce to compensate for any operational failures that might occur during the patient care delivery process. Great doctors and nurses, not great organization or management, have been seen as the means for ensuring that patients receive quality care. Recently, however, the medical community has responded to increased public awareness of shortcomings in healthcare delivery by calling for systematic, organizational improvements to increase patient safety. Examples of such initiatives include creating shared databases of medical errors to facilitate widespread learning from mistakes and focusing renewed attention on hospital processes, culture, and reporting systems.[4]

Front-line employees in service organizations are well positioned in these efforts to help their organizations learn, that is, to improve organizational outcomes by suggesting changes in processes and activities based on their knowledge of what is and is not working.[5] Identifying and resolving causes of problems that arise during the course of work is one method for achieving organizational learning. By catching, correcting, and removing underlying causes, front-line employees can contribute to changes that help avoid erosion of quality and customer satisfaction in the future. In this way, through initiative taking and problem solving at the front lines, organizational systems and procedures can be changed to avoid many of the most prevalent recurring problems (sometimes referred to—perhaps overly optimistically—as "low hanging fruit").

We conducted a detailed study of hospital nursing care processes to investigate conditions under which nurses might respond to failures they encounter in their hospital's operational processes by actively seeking to prevent future occurrences of similar failures. Our research suggests that, in spite of increased emphasis on these issues, hospitals are not learning from the daily problems and errors encountered by their workers. We also find that process failures are not rare but rather are an integral part of working on the front lines of healthcare delivery.

Although this study focused on hospital nurses, the lessons learned have implications for managers in other service organizations as well. The tasks carried out by nurses are knowledge-intensive, highly variable, and performed in the physical presence of customers, which heightens the worker's focus on the current customer's comfort and safety and can detract from awareness of the need to improve the organizational system through which care is delivered. These aspects are similar to work environments of other service providers who perform complex physical and mental tasks in the presence of customers, such as computer help-desk operators, repair technicians, airline crews, fire fighters, police officers, teachers, beauticians, and some customer service representatives.

Further, hospitals have many features in common with other service organizations, notably time pressure, unpredictability in the workload, the relatively low status of nurses as front-line employees, and their reliance on others for supplies and information. These features contribute both to the emergence of failures and to barriers to learning from them.

Process Failures on the Front Lines of Hospital Care Delivery

Our research identified two types of process failures—problems and errors. We define an *error* as the execution of a task that is either unnecessary or incorrectly carried out and that could have been avoided with appropriate distribution of pre-existing information. For example, we observed a patient who had been un-necessarily prepared for colonoscopy at significant expense to the hospital and discomfort to the patient before the specialist reviewed her case—revealing that the patient was not an appropriate candidate for the procedure—and cancelled it.

Hospital errors have received considerable nationwide attention re-cently; however, an emphasis on only those errors that lead to severe con-sequences such as the death of a patient has perhaps obscured the subtler phenomenon of errors that take place within the care delivery process every day—such as an unnecessary pre-operative preparation. Thankfully, most er-rors are caught and corrected before patients are harmed; however, a lack of attention to the process errors that precede more visible, consequential fail-ures may limit opportunities for organizational learning.

The second type of failure is a *problem*, which we define as a disruption in a worker's ability to execute a prescribed task because either: something the worker needs is unavailable in the time, location, condition, or quantity desired and, hence, the task cannot be executed as planned; or something is present that should not be, interfering with the designated task.[6] Examples of problems include missing supplies, information, or medications. Unlike er-rors, work process problems have received little attention in the literature or press. Like errors, problems are a valuable source of information about ways in which the system is not working.

Workers are well aware of the problems they encounter. In contrast, by definition, people are unaware of their own errors while making them. Not surprisingly, given that we observed the work processes from the viewpoint of front-line workers, the majority (86%) of the failures we observed in the care delivery process were problems rather than errors. Both kinds of failures require some kind of action for patient care to continue effectively. Whereas workers can take action to solve problems—due to their intense awareness of them—prevention of errors necessarily requires management involvement to redesign work systems in ways that make errors less likely to occur.

Research Base

In this article, we summarize findings from an in-depth study of work system failures on the front lines of care delivery in hospitals. We analyzed qualitative data from 239 hours of observation of 26 nurses at nine hospitals to develop understanding of and recommendations for organizational learning from process failures.[7] After completing the observations, we conducted interviews with twelve nurses at seven of the hospitals studied.[8]

Nursing units provide a rich context for studying problem solving. First, nurses are typically experienced and capable problem solvers because their profession requires a high level of cognitive reasoning and discretionary decision making.[9] For example, nurses coordinate patients' care with support functions such as diagnostic tests and physical and respiratory therapy, pulling together and interpreting data to recognize ominous patterns that warrant contacting physicians to intervene when a patient takes a turn for the worse. In addition, they provide direct patient care, including assessing patients' condition, administering medications, bathing and moving patients to prevent bed sores, providing treatments (e.g., blood transfusions, dressing changes), and educating patients (and their families) about their medical conditions. Nurses usually have multiple patients and meeting all of their physical and emotional needs is challenging, if not impossible. Consequently, nurses continually evaluate what needs to be done, reprioritizing their tasks to meet patients' changing needs. Second, the unpredictable nature of health care and the high level of interdependence among service-providing employees[10] (e.g., nurses, doctors, pharmacy, central supply, and laboratory) make it likely that nurses will encounter failures in the course of their day-to-day work.

With the exception of the first hospital, a community hospital actively engaged in an organizational change effort, we purposely sought hospitals with reputations for nursing excellence by asking nursing governing boards for referrals to such hospitals and by searching nursing magnet literature for hospitals nationally recognized for nursing excellence. Our goal was not gather a representative sample of hospitals, but instead to assess how excellent nursing hospitals handled service failures, while also ensuring that our findings were not biased by results from only one organization. By including multiple excellent organizations, we were able to discern that the basic pattern of problem-solving behavior was similar across these nine across hospitals, with only modest variation from site to site. These hospitals are described in Exhibit IV.1, using pseudonyms to protect their confidentiality.[11]

Failures on the Front Lines of Care Delivery

We characterized the nature of the failures we observed on the front lines of patient care delivery, and subsequently we examined nurses' responses to them. We encountered 194 failures during our observations. Problems constituted the majority (166) of these data. Nurses experienced five broad types of problems: missing or incorrect information; missing or broken equipment; waiting for a (human or equipment) resource; missing or incorrect supplies; and simultaneous demands on their time.[12] Problems were most likely to surface while nurses were preparing for patient care (88% of the problems) and/or as a result from a breakdown in information or material transfer to the nurse (91% of the problems), highlighting the boundary-crossing nature of this kind of process failures. This finding is further reinforced in interviews. Five of the twelve

Hospital	Type of Hospital	Number of Beds	Nursing Units Observed	Unionized Nurses	Observation Time (hours:min)	% of Total Observation Hours	# of Nurses Interviewed
1	Small Community	47	Intensive Care Unit	Non-Union	82:35	34%	0
2	Specialty, Urban, Teaching	98	Surgical	Non-Union	7:45	3%	0
3	Rural Community	134	Medical/ Surgical	Union	27:19	11%	2
4	Community, Private Not-for-Profit	243	Surgical and Maternity	Non-Union	34:30	14%	1
5	Community, Government	292	Oncology & Medical/ Surgical	Union	15:35	7%	3
6	Community, Government	250	Cardiac	Union	1:30	1%	1
7	Teaching, Urban	198	Oncology	Non-Union	20:30	9%	2
8	Pediatric, Teaching, Urban	163	Oncology	Union	9:11	4%	1
9	Teaching, Tertiary Care	433	Intensive Care Unit	Non-Union	40:30	17%	2
Total					239:25		12

EXHIBIT IV.1
An Overview of Hospitals Where Observation of Workers Occurred

nurses interviewed noted that although nurses should take responsibility for trying to improve how things work, many problems stem from other groups and departments. An oncology nurse commented on her perception that downstream, internal support departments were the source of many disruptions:

> "The daily problems we face are from outside of our own unit—central supply and housekeeping, for example. It is not the people on the unit. It is not what we do or don't order for our supplies. It is a system problem."

Second, we observed 28 errors, which fell into three categories: incorrect actions made by the nurse (39%), errors made by other people (18%), and unnecessary execution of tasks resulting from faulty process flows (43%). Examples of these three categories respectively include a nurse who forgot to give a patient his medications for the entire shift, nurses having to correct mistakes made by the previous shift's nurse (i.e., a patient's diet entered incorrectly in the computer system), and nurses beginning to transfer a patient to another unit before receiving information from surgeons (and in two cases, family members) that reversed the transfer decision.

Distinguishing between problems and errors highlights the different roles front-line employees can play in improvement. The relative visibility and frequency of problems, compared to errors, makes them accessible to front-line workers who are well positioned to suggest important changes that managers would not be able to identify. Second, problems carry less stigma than errors, making discussion of them less interpersonally threatening.[13] Understanding how front-line employees respond to problems is thus important for efforts to improve work systems and processes.

First-Order Problem Solving

Research on quality improvement has distinguished between two types of response to problems—short-term remedies that "patch" problems and more thorough responses that seek to change underlying organizational routines to prevent recurrence.[14] We make a similar distinction between first- and second-order problem-solving behavior in service organizations.[15] First-order problem-solving behavior occurs when the worker compensates for a problem by getting the supplies or information needed to finish a task that was blocked or interrupted. The worker does not address underlying causes, thus not reducing the likelihood of a similar problem in the future. In our research, we found that nurses implemented a short-term fix for the overwhelming majority of the failures observed, enabling them to continue caring for their patients, without taking any action to try to prevent recurrence of similar failures—that is, without prompting organizational learning. For example, an oncology floor nurse who worked on the night shift ran out of clean linen to change her patients' beds. She walked to another unit that had linen in stock and took from their supply.

At first glance, first-order problem solving seems successful: the nurse was able to obtain linen. The cost to the nurse and to the hospital was minimal; it only took a few minutes of her time and was inexpensive. Notably, this nurse did not pay for a taxi to deliver the linen from an off-site linen cleaning service, which nurses at other hospitals reported as how they often handled the problem of running out of certain supplies, including linen. Seven out of nine nurses whom we interviewed reported feeling gratified when they figured out a way to work around an obstacle enabling them to continue patient care. The nurse missing linens commented,

> "Working around problems is just part of my job. By being able to get IV bags or whatever else I need, it enables me to do my job and to have a positive impact on a person's life—like being able to get them clean linen. And I am the kind of person who does not just get one set of linen, I will bring back several for the other nurses."

Upon further reflection, it appears that first-order problem solving can be counterproductive. It keeps communication of problems isolated so that they do not surface as learning opportunities. Workers rarely inform the person responsible for the problem which prevents those people from learning that their processes could be improved. Sometimes, first-order problem solving creates new problems elsewhere, as when the above nurse took several sets of linens from another area. Moreover, considerable time (of highly paid professionals) is wasted on tasks and rework that would not otherwise be necessary. We found that, on average, 33 minutes were lost per eight-hour shift due to coping with system failures that could have been addressed and removed. Thus, first-order problem-solving behavior, ironically, can preclude improvement by obscuring the existence of problems and errors and preventing operational and structural changes that would prevent the same failures from happening again.

Our analysis identified two implicit strategies, or more colloquially, rules-of-thumb that exemplify first-order problem solving. The first rule of thumb is as follows: when you encounter a problem, do what it takes to continue the patient-care task—no more, no less. When nurses used this rule—which they did for 93% of the problems—their behavior involved securing the information or material they needed to do their jobs without probing into what caused the problem to occur. After the nurses were able to resume caring for the patient, they did not expend further effort on the incident;

that is, they neither communicated that it occurred to others nor sought to investigate or change causes. This strategy served several purposes. It allowed a nurse to meet the requirements of the current patient—a responsibility that the nurses we observed did not take lightly. It also reduced the amount of time the harried nurse spends away from patient care duties; engaging in extra activity beyond the immediate fix would be a further drain on the care current patients received.

The second rule of thumb was—when necessary for continuity of patient care—to ask for help from people who were socially close rather than from those who were best equipped to correct the problem. The second rule of thumb helped to preserve the nurse's reputation regarding his or her competence at handling the daily rigors of nursing. In addition, it allowed nurses to avoid unpleasant encounters with cantankerous physicians or managers as long as possible. At the same time, it all but precluded addressing underlying causes that might improve the system. The nurses followed this rule for 42% of the problems and deviated from it for only 7% problems (e.g., they contacted a physician or other hospital personnel rather than attempting to solve the problem on their own).[16] The appeal and power of rules of thumb upon which one can tacitly rely in a time-pressured situation may help explain the high level of consistency of nurses' responses to problems.

Second-Order Problem Solving

Second-order problem-solving behavior occurs when the worker, in addition to patching the problem so that the immediate task at hand can be completed, also takes action to address underlying causes. Second-order problem solving includes: communicating to the person or department responsible for the problem; bringing it to managers' attention; sharing ideas about what caused the situation and how to prevent recurrence with someone in a position to implement changes; implementing changes; and verifying that changes have the desired effect. Given that nurses have so little spare time for extensive second order problem-solving behavior such as tracking the problem to its source and making system changes to prevent recurrence, we categorized any behavior that called attention to the situation—thereby starting a legitimate process of inquiry into root cause which could then transpire over a period of time—as indicative of second-order problem-solving behavior. Nonetheless, only 7% of nurse responses met even these lenient criteria.

To illustrate second-order problem solving in this context, we observed an inexperienced intensive care unit (ICU) nurse transfer a two-year-old patient to the oncology floor by mistakenly leaving the sleeping child on his ICU bed rather than moving him onto the standard hospital bed in his new room, despite the protests of the oncology nurse that the highly-specialized ICU beds had to be returned. Not unexpectedly, the ICU nurse manager called the oncology unit secretary 30 minutes later, asking for the ICU bed. The oncology nurse—instead of simply returning the bed—did something that was unusual, and certainly not necessary for the immediate care of her patient. She called the ICU nurse manager, explaining, "I don't want to get anyone in trouble, but I want you to know what happened so you can talk to the nurse so that it does not happen again." In this example, the nurse took care of the immediate situation—getting the ICU bed back to the unit—and also took action to try to remove the underlying cause of the error—the new ICU nurse's mistaken belief that it was worse to move a sleeping child than to leave an ICU bed on another unit. The ICU nurse manager could then ensure that all ICU nurses were aware of this requirement. The oncology nurse's apologetic introduction, when calling the ICU to engage in system-correcting behavior, is perhaps indicative of how counter-normative such behavior can be in hospitals. Instead of being governed by tacit rules-of-thumb that everyone seems to follow without explicit decision, second-order problem solving seemed to take conscious effort.

Second-order problem solving can have positive consequences for workers and the organization. If the worker's action is successful and the problem does not recur, they will not have to face similar obstacles in the future. As a result, second-order problem solving is a way that real change is achieved. The organization can benefit from higher productivity, customer satisfaction (because service is not interrupted), and worker satisfaction (feelings of competence from improving their work systems and less frustration with completing their tasks).

Three Positive Human Resource Attributes That Prevent Learning

Why aren't hospitals—and we suspect many other service organizations as well—learning all they can from daily problems encountered by their workers? Our research suggests that it is not because problems are highly complex or difficult to solve, nor is it because nurses are unmotivated—two plausible explanations. The problems we observed, while often requiring some sort of system change for resolution, were neither ill defined nor technically challenging. Instead, they were relatively straightforward and embedded in routine processes; typical examples included missing medications, regular-diet food trays being delivered for diabetic patients, insufficient supplies, and a lack of necessary medical orders for patient care.

It is also not because nurses are uncommitted, lazy, or incompetent. The nurses studied were extremely dedicated and capable, often possessing advanced degrees and all had worked more than three years on their unit. Nine out of ten nurses whom we observed for an entire shift stayed an average of 45 minutes after their shift had ended—without extra pay—to complete their patient care duties. They ate their lunches in much less time than allotted and postponed taking personal breaks in order to provide the care they felt their patients deserved. One nurse, who worked from 7:00 A.M. until 7:00 P.M. called the unit at 4:00 A.M. after waking up, suddenly remembering something she had forgotten to tell the nurse who took over caring for her patients.

The lack of organizational learning from failures can be explained instead by three less obvious, even counterintuitive, reasons: an emphasis on individual vigilance in health care, unit efficiency concerns, and empowerment (or a widely shared goal of developing units than can function without direct managerial assistance). These three factors, while seemingly beneficial for nurses and patients alike, can ironically leave nurses under supported and overwhelmed in a system bound to have breakdowns because of the need to provide individualized treatments for patients.

First, individual vigilance—an industry norm that encourages nurses and other health care professionals to take personal responsibility to solve problems as they arise—is explicitly developed and highly valued in health care organizations. Counterintuitively, this can create barriers to organizational improvement because, in addition to encouraging individuals to be alert to things that can go wrong and to quickly take action, norms of individual vigilance encourage independence. Each caregiver thus tends to work on completing her or his own tasks without altering common underlying processes. Nurses are allowed, and even encouraged, to resolve problems independently without having to consider the impact on the system. In this way, problems of missing supplies or equipment tend to be resolved by taking the necessary items from somewhere else, hence creating another problem downstream. We found that nurses' problem-solving action tended to be directed at meeting immediate needs of patients; its scope rarely included assessing or remedying underlying causes—even when similar problems were confronted consecutively—making the chances of spurring organizational improvement and change through such efforts remote.

Second, nursing units were designed to maximize individual unit efficiency. Nursing labor is expensive and in short supply. Understandably, hospitals can ill afford to have nurses routinely working with slack resources. This staffing model leads to an organizational design where workers do not have time to resolve underlying causes of problems that arise in daily activities. Instead, nurses are barely able to keep up with the required responsibilities and are in essence forced to quickly patch problems so they can complete their immediate responsibilities. Thus, in this situation it is possible for an individual worker to be working non-stop while the content of the work technically adds little value to the customer's experience because of the amount of rework and unnecessary steps.

Third, empowerment of workers has been cited as a solution for quality and productivity problems.[17] The flip side of empowerment, however, is the removal of managers and other non-direct labor support from daily work activities, leaving workers on their own to resolve problems that may stem from parts of the organization with which they have limited interaction. Reducing the degree to which managers are available to front-line staff can be a loss for improvement efforts, especially when workers are already overburdened by existing duties. Managers tend to have a broader perspective than line workers, possess status necessary to resolve problems that cross organizational boundaries, and are capable of implementing solutions on a wider basis. This is not to say that nurses are not capable of engaging in such activities, but rather that the immediate nature of their duties precludes them from spending large amounts of time away from patient care. Without a readily available nurse manager, they are left without anyone to assist them in making these connections.

An Illusory Equilibrium Created by Responses to Process Failures

When a problem arises, a worker needs to engage in first-order problem solving merely to be able to continue his or her duties. First-order problem solving, however, does not alter the underlying conditions that gave rise to barriers to task completion, and so the failure, or one just like it, is likely to recur. This means that although the behavior appears to provide a solution, the solution, in fact, is a temporary measure. As a model of this dynamic phenomenon. Exhibit IV.2 depicts the causal relationships between these constructs.

The iterative relationship between problems (recognized by workers on the job as "barriers to task completion") and worker response (first-order problem-solving effort) is a dynamic structure of the type that researchers who study the dynamic properties of organizational systems have called a "balancing loop."[18] How it works is that the emergence of a problem (some disruption or barrier that would otherwise preclude the continuity of patient care) increases the chances (indicated by a plus sign in the thick arrow at the top of Exhibit IV.2) of a particular response—a first-order problem-solving effort. In turn, when this response successfully patches the problem, it reduces or removes the barrier (indicated by a minus sign next to the other thick arrow), allowing the caregiver to continue the patient care task.

This is a system in apparent balance. A problem shows up, action is taken, and the obstacle is gone—at least temporarily. As depicted in Exhibit IV.2, however, an increase in first-order problem solving actually reduces the likelihood that underlying causes will be addressed. First, the more effort expended in first-order problem solving, the less likely he or she is to have and take time to engage in second-order problem-solving behavior. Because first-order problem solving takes time, it can leave workers with less flexibility to investigate causes and negotiate potential countermeasures.

A more subtle mechanism through which second-order problem-solving effort is reduced is the feelings of gratification that nurses report when effectively overcoming problems on their own. One nurse expressed her satisfaction when she was able to resolve issues that were preventing her from caring for her patients, "I have a lot of job satisfaction when I go home and I feel like I did everything that a patient needed and was entitled to. Even the little things." Ironically, this rewarding feeling of competence and self-sufficiency tends to further decrease the chances of expending effort to get others involved, as needed for second-order problem solving—and so the rate of failure emergence is not reduced. This is also depicted in Exhibit IV.2,

EXHIBIT IV.2

Model of First-Order and Second-Order Problem-Solving Behavior

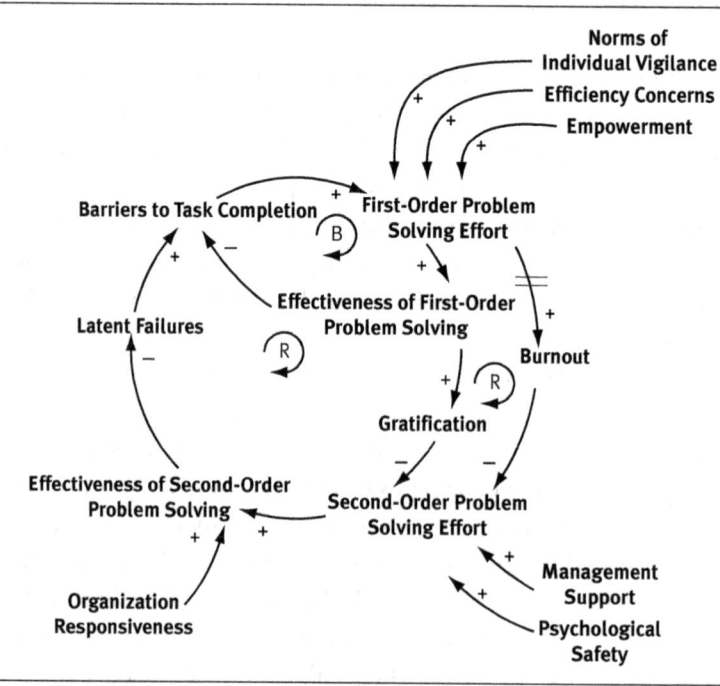

in the positive link between effective first-order problem solving and worker feelings of gratification.

In most hospitals, organizational culture and management behaviors tend to reinforce this already-robust system of individual vigilance. Seventy percent of the nurses we interviewed commented that they believed their manager expected them to work through the daily disruptions on their own. Speaking up about a problem or asking for help was likely to be seen as a sign of incompetence. As one nurse interviewed explained, "My manager is not interested in hearing about things if they are small. If I went to her with a small problem, she would say, 'Solve it yourself.' To get any attention from managers, problems have to be something that is out of your hands—something you can't solve on your own."

Further, to those directly involved, things seem to be working reasonably well. It is stressful, but basically in balance. The catch is—because first-order problem solving is time-consuming and tiring—over time, burnout begins to take its toll on the system. This time delay is represented in Exhibit IV.2 by two slash marks between first-order problem-solving effort and burnout. This symbol indicates that first-order problem-solving behavior leads to burnout—but not immediately. Frustration and exhaustion accumulate over time. Not surprisingly, worker burnout then further decreases the chances of effortful engagement in second-order problem solving (another causal arrow marked by a minus sign in Exhibit IV.2). In addition, less effort on second order problem solving means its effectiveness or ability to reduce latent failures also goes down. To illustrate this, in our study, one nurse said, "I am quite burned out as a whole with nursing. I would quit tomorrow if I could find decent work with health insurance—even for less pay."

Over time, therefore, the apparent balance of this system is revealed as illusory. Workers experience an increasing sense of frustration, exhaustion and, in some cases, leave the organization—worn out by the task of swimming upstream against an incessant tide of small, annoying problems. Across the health care delivery industry, this phenomenon is contributing to unacceptably high levels of turnover in many organizations and to widespread nursing shortages.[19]

Levers for Change

The process of developing a causal feedback model suggests the location of leverage points for change. The model shown in Exhibit IV.2 depicts first-order problem-solving behavior as a "fix that fails,"[20] that is, it illustrates the all too human response to take action expediently when things go wrong in such a way that the situation seems to improve, in the short term. Over time, however, as shown by the model, the situation gradually worsens. Thus, the power of a causal feedback model such as this is that it calls attention to variables that are well positioned for creating more fundamental, long-term change. These leverage points constitute specific ways that managers can foster organizational learning efforts by front-line workers in hospitals and other service organizations.

As the model shows, the situation can only be improved in a real rather than illusory manner through second-order problem-solving behavior. To make this happen, managerial intervention is likely to be essential. Thus, a first lever for change is management support, which can work deliberately to increase effort spent on second-order problem solving by front-line workers. This potential influence is depicted on the right side of Exhibit IV.2.

What do we mean by management support? To begin with, managers must make an effort to be regularly available for at least part of all shifts. We observed that the physical presence of managers increased the likelihood of managers being informed of problems occurring on the unit; this, in turn, allowed managers to investigate and support possible work system changes. Next, managers can counteract time pressure by providing assistance for frontline problem-solving efforts. In addition, by acting as role models of second-order problem solving, managers can teach workers to think about what could be done to prevent similar problems from occurring in the future.[21]

Second, to learn from failures, people need to be able to talk about them without fear of ridicule or punishment. Managers can help create an environment where workers feel safe taking the interpersonal risks that second-order problem-solving entails, thereby making this behavior more psychologically feasible (see Exhibit IV.2). Creating a psychologically safe work environment does not require managers be excessively warm and friendly, but instead that they invite others to express .their concerns and model fallibility by admitting their own errors.[22]

Third, managers and others in the organization must respond to initiative by following through on these suggestions and facilitating boundary-crossing improvements that help reduce the rate of problem emergence. In short, if second-order problem-solving effort does not lead to any positive changes, workers will be discouraged about spending their time on this in the future. One nurse commented, "I know nurses on our floor used to come up with suggestions for change. No one seems to listen and now no one bothers trying." Conversely, if the effort is effective (because the organization is responsive), workers' motivation to engage in second-order problem solving in the future will be strengthened. The left side of Exhibit IV.2 thus shows organizational responsiveness to nurses' attempts at second-order problem solving as a positive influence on the effectiveness of the effort.

Are these solutions feasible in the budget conscious world of health care? After all, most involve additional expenses, whether freeing up a manager to assist front-line workers with resolving failures, promoting more discussion of (and time devoted lo) tracking down causes of problems, or implementing countermeasures. Further analysis suggests that the extra expense would pay off. Although second-order problem solving requires an investment in developing both human resources and organizational routines, overtime the reduction in failures could pay for themselves. At a bare minimum, we can estimate that worker time wasted in work-arounds to cope with system failures was 8% of a shift. Even with conservative estimates, this amounts to $256,000 per year in lost nursing time for a 200-bed hospital.[23] Further, many nurses are currently "subsidizing" the hospital by working through their breaks, lunch time, and working unpaid overtime in order to make up the time they lost because of system failures and inefficiencies. This generosity backfires when nurses leave the profession due to burnout.

The savings due to reductions in patient complications could be even greater. For example, we observed one patient who stayed in the intensive-care unit for an additional night because a preparatory medication did not arrive on the floor in time and his procedure had to be delayed until the following day. Such discharge delays are extremely expensive for the hospital as they are reimbursed for a category of services provided, not by their actual costs of providing each service.[24] Moreover, many hospitals are capacity constrained, and so an extra day is a day that could have been provided to another patient.

The burden of learning from failures does not lie solely with managers. Workers must take specific actions, suggesting a list of desirable behaviors by front-line workers that differs in important ways from conventional wisdom about the ideal employee. For example, most managers would identify an ideal employee as one who can handle with ease any problem that comes along, without bothering managers or others. From an organizational learning perspective, this is questionable wisdom. The ideal employee is instead a noisy complainer, who speaks up to managers and others about the situation, thereby running the risk of being seen as someone who lacks self-sufficiency. Similarly, instead of quietly correcting others' errors without making a fuss, a frontline worker should be a nosy troublemaker, actively pointing out colleagues' mistakes. Third, the ideal employee for organizational learning does not convey an impression of flawless performance but rather openly acknowledges his or her own errors. This self-aware error-maker not only facilitates correction but also speaks up about process failure and thus contributes to a climate of openness in which others can do likewise. Finally, the ideal employee is a disruptive questioner who won't leave well enough alone. This person is constantly questioning, rather than accepting and remaining committed to, current practices. These differences are summarized in Exhibit IV.3.

Conclusions

Our study shows that it is difficult for hospital workers to use problems as opportunities for improvement. The dynamic pattern described in this article is not unique to hospitals, although it may be exaggerated in healthcare by the task variability, the extreme time pressure faced by workers, and the increasing cost pressures faced by hospitals. Other service contexts present similar features. For example, many service workers are motivated by the rewarding sense of self-sufficiency that led some of the nurses we observed to avoid reporting or getting help for fixing system failures.

Many service organizations are not learning all they can from their failures. Complex systems, like the ones used by most organizations to provide the services their customers buy, are bound to suffer from failure and poor design. Therefore, not hearing anything about what kinds of failures workers are experiencing is more likely to mean that managers are not present and receptive enough for workers. The lack of communication does not mean there are no problems. The clues managers can look for include worker frustration that input is not heard and a resigned sense that "noth-

EXHIBIT IV.3

Comparison of Traditional and Learning Views of Desirable Employee Behaviors

When the Employee Faces:	"Ideal Employee" Behaviors	Employee Behaviors Conducive to Organizational Learning
Missing materials or information	Adjust to shortcomings in materials and supplies without bothering managers or others.	*Noisy Complainer:* Remedies immediate situation but also lets the manager and supply department know when the system has failed.
Others' errors	Seamlessly corrects for errors of others— without confronting the person about their error.	*Nosy Troublemaker:* Lets others know when they have made a mistake with the intent of creating learning, not blame.
Own errors and problems	Creates an impression of never making mistakes.	*Self-Aware Error Maker:* Lets manager and others know when they have made a mistake so that others can learn from their error. Communicates openness to hearing about their errors discovered by others.
Subtle opportunities for improving the system	Committed to the current way of doing business— understands the "way things work" around here.	*Disruptive Questioner who won't let well enough alone:* Questions why do we do things this way? Is there a better way of providing the service to the patient?

ing ever changes around here." As one nurse mused, "I do not feel that my voice is heard. Often I am discouraged, so I don't input my ideas. Where would my ideas go? We are not asked for input." Over time, this leads to a sense of futile resignation that the problems are going to always be there because nothing gets resolved.

Even in the most successful service organizations, work system failures will occur. Both errors and problems can be detected and used as launching points for organizational learning and improvement by motivating changes to avoid recurrence. Frontline service providers are in the best position to discover and remove this type of work system failure. Managers have an essential role: assisting with problem-solving efforts, providing support for workers who attempt to improve their work systems, and valuing them as motivated employees. By reframing workers' perceptions of failures from sources of frustration to sources of learning, managers can engage employees in system improvement efforts that would otherwise not occur.

Acknowledgments

We wish to thank the participating hospitals and nurses and Harvard Business School's Division of Research who supported this research. We are grateful to H. Kent Bowen and Steven J. Spear for engaging the participation of two of the study sites and for advice and guidance on using observational methods to study the management of operations. Rogelio Oliva's comments were extremely helpful in clarifying our model of problem solving. Jennifer Chalfin's assistance with the model graphics is gratefully acknowledged.

Notes

1. For a report the poor financial state of hospitals in general, see for example, C. Kramer and D. Dalmand, "Ernst & Young/HCIA-Sachs Study Finds Continued Financial Woes for Hospitals on May Day," *Ernst & Young/HCIA-Sachs* [Electronic] (2001), accessed on October 8, 2002.
2. This often cited statistic comes from L.T. Kohn, J.M. Corrigan. M.S. Donaldson, "To Err Is Human: Building a Safer Health System," (Washington, D.C.: National Academy Press, Committee on Quality of Health Care in America, Institute of Medicine. 2000).
3. Many researchers have written about the pervasiveness of medical errors in hospitals. For one of the most influential studies, see L. L. Leape,

D. W. Bates, D. J. Cullen, et al, "Systems Analysis of Adverse Drug Events." *Journal of the American Medical Association.* 274/1 (1995): 35–43.

4. Both the popular press (J.P. Shapiro, "America's Best Hospitals," *U.S. News and World Report* [2000]) and the medical community (E. C. Nelson. P. B. Batalden, T. P. Huber, et al., "Microsystems in Health Care: Part I, Learning from High-Performing Front-Line Clinical Units," *Joint Commission Journal of Quality Improvement.* 28 (September 2002): 472–497] have turned their attention to flaws in the operational systems through which care is provided.

5. Sim Sitkin has argued that small failures are excellent sources of learning because they indicate that current processes can be improved upon, without causing organizations to respond defensively as large failures are likely to do, which would inhibit effective learning. S. B. Sitkin, "Learning through Failure: The Strategy of Small Losses," in L. L. Cummings and B. M. Staw, eds., *Research in Organizational Behavior.* 14 (1992): 231–266. For articles that discuss the role of front-line workers in solving operational problems, see J. P. MacDuffie, "The Road to 'Root Cause': Shop-Floor Problem-Solving at Three Auto Assembly Plants," *Management Science.* 43/4 (1997): 479–502; A. Mukherjee, M. Lapre, and L.N. Van Wassenhove. "Knowledge Driven Quality Improvement," Management Science. 44/11 (1998): S35-S49; S.J. Spear, "The Essence of Just-in-Time: Imbedding Diagnostic Tests in Work-Systems to Achieve Operational Excellence," *Production Planning & Control* (forthcoming).

6. The phenomenon of workers lacking supplies at the point and time at which they need it has been studied in depth by Steven Spear. His research into the Toyota Production System epitomized careful ethnographic observation of operating systems and the findings demonstrated the insight that this method can produce. See S. J. Spear, "The Toyota Production System: An Example of Managing Complex Social/Technical Systems: 5 Rules for Designing, Operating, and Improving Activities, Activity-Connections, and Flow-Path." unpublished doctoral dissertation. Harvard Business School, 1999.

7. For a more detailed explanation of the research methods used in this study, see A. L. Tucker, A. C. Edmondson, and S. J. Spear, "When Problem Solving Prevents Organizational Learning," *Journal of Organizational Change Management* 15/2 (2002): 122–137.

8. Given the time that had elapsed, we were unable to gain additional access to two of the hospitals.

9. The nursing literature has emphasized the importance of critical thinking, the cognitive component of nursing work. For examples, see R. Hansten and M. Washburn, "Individual and Organizational Accountability for Development of Critical Thinking," *Journal of Nursing Administration*, 29/11 (1999J): 39–45; J. L. Lee. B. L. Chang, M. L. Pearson, K. L. Kahn, and L. V. Rubenstein, "Does What Nurses Do Affect Clinical Outcomes for Hospitalized Patients? A Review of the Literature," *Health Sciences Research*, 34/5 (1999): 1011–1032; C. Taylor. 'Problem Solving in Clinical Nursing Practice," *Journal of Advanced Nursing* 26 (1997): 329–336.

10. The complications caused by the interdependence of healthcare workers are discussed in S. Glouberman and H. Mintzberg, "Managing the Care of Health and the Cure of Disease—Part 1: Differentiation," *Health Care Management Review* 26/1 (2001): 56–69.

11. The close proximity of Hospital 1 to our offices, combined with the willingness of its intensive-care unit manager to allow us extensive access, led to more hours of observations at Hospital 1 than was possible with the other institutions. In addition, Hospital 1 was the first site in which nurses were observed in this study. We thus spent considerable time at this site to develop a deep understanding of and ability to decipher hospital care processes before approaching other hospitals for access. Despite spending more time at this site than any other, however, by the end of data analysis, we were able to conclude that the incidents and behaviors observed at Hospital 1 were typical of those observed at the other eight sites. Further Hospital 1 was solidly in the 'middle of the road" in terms of both problems and nurse responses. In sum, our over-sampling of problems at this site does not pose a serious threat to the generalizability of our findings.

12. To compute inter-rater reliability for the types of problems, a random sample of ten observation days was evaluated independently by two non-nurse reviewers. The kappa statistic, which adjusts the rating downward to compensate for the probability that raters could assign items to the same category by chance, was appropriate to use in this situation. The kappa value was 0.88 for judgments about problem type, which is considered almost perfect by Landis and Koch. See J. R. Landis and G. G. Koch, "The Measurement of Observer Agreement for Categorical Data." *Biometrics,* 33 (1977): 159–174.

13. Previous research has established a positive relationship between the degree to which workers feel safe taking interpersonal risks and the amount of errors that are reported. See A. C. Edmondson, "Learning from Mistakes Is Easier Said than Done: Group and Organizational Influences on the Detection and Correction of Human Error,"

Journal of Applied Behavioral Science, 32/1 (1996): 5–28, and A. C. Edmondson, "Psychological Safety and Learning Behavior in Work Teams," *Administrative Science Quarterly,* 44/2 (1999): 350–383.

14. This pattern of simply fixing the problem rather than doing something to prevent its recurrence is also reminiscent of reactive versus preventive control, as discussed in R. H. Hayes, S. C. Wheelwright, and K. B. Clark, *Dynamic Manufacturing: Creating the Learning Organization* (New York, NY: Free Press, 1988). Similarly, John Carroll and his colleagues explore this phenomenon with regard to accident reviews undertaken by nuclear power plant employees, see J. S. Carroll, J. W. Rudolf, and S. Hatakenaka, "Learning from Experience in High-Hazard Organizations," *Research in Organizational Behavior* (forthcoming). Nelson Repenning and John Sterman contrast two types of process improvement, first-order improvement and second-order improvement, see N. Repenning and J. D. Sterman, "Capability Traps and Self-Confirming Attribution Errors in the Dynamics of Process Improvement." *Administrative Science Quarterly,* 47 (2002): 265–295.

15. Our concept of first and second-order problem solving is analogous to Argyris and Schon's notion of single and double loop learning. C. Argyris and D. Schon, *Organizational Learning; A Theory of Action Perspective* (Reading, MA: Addison-Wesley Publishing Company, 1978). It also draws from problem-solving literature in which a distinction is made between patching problems and actually removing underlying causes.

16. The reluctance to contact others about problems was common across all types and sizes of hospitals, including teaching hospitals where one might expect nurses to feel more comfortable exerting their expertise given the substantial population of inexperienced physicians-in-training and students. In fact, for the twelve instances when nurses *did* contact the source, five (42%) were from Hospital 1—a non-teaching hospital and the smallest in our sample—with another three (67% in total) from non-teaching hospitals 4 and 5. The remaining four occurred at teaching hospitals 2, 7, and 9. Furthermore, doctors were contacted immediately for only two problems, both times at community hospitals. Therefore, we conclude that reluctance to confront physicians does not systematically vary by hospital size or teaching status.

17. Linda Aiken and her colleagues found that empowerment of nurses is associated with high-quality care and low nursing turnover. L.H. Aiken,

and P.A. Patrician, "Measuring Organizational Traits of Hospitals: The Revised Nursing Work Index," *Nursing Research*, 49/3 (2000): 146–153.

18. For a detailed explanation of system dynamic models, see P. M. Senge, *The Fifth Discipline: The Art and Practice of the Learning Organization* (New York: Doubleday Currency, 1990). Two excellent articles that utilize system dynamics models to explain how organizations become trapped in self-reinforcing patterns of sub-optimal behaviors and, thus, poor performance are E. K. Keating, R. Oliva, N. P. Repenning, S. Rockart, and J. D. Sterman, "Overcoming the Improvement Paradox," *European Management Journal*, 17/2 (1999): 120–134; Repenning and Sterman, op. cit.

19. The connection between organizational factors—including the quality of hospital work processes—and the nursing shortage is discussed in R. C. Coile, Jr., "Magnet Hospitals Use Culture, Not Wages, to Solve Nursing Shortage," *Journal of Healthcare Management*, 46/4 (2001): 224–227.

20. Senge, op. cit.

21. For more on the role of the manager or a dedicated problem-solving support person in a hospital, see S. J. Spear, "Deaconess-Glover Hospital Case (B)," case no. 9-601-023, Harvard Business School, 2001.

22. For a discussion of leader behaviors associated with high psychological safety, and thus high team learning, see A. C. Edmondson, R. Bohmer, and G. P. Pisano, "Speeding Up Team Learning," *Harvard Business Review*, 79/9 (2001): 125–134.

23. Assuming average annual salary of $40,000 per nurse, the wasted nursing time is $3,200 per full-time nurse. For a 200-bed unit—the average size hospital in our sample—at 80% occupancy and a 6:1 staffing ratio operating 3 shifts per day, this amounts to $256,000 per year.

24. Industry experts estimate that it costs between $1500 and $2000 per day to keep a patient in the ICU.

Discussion Questions on Required Reading

1. What are the forces facilitating and hindering better teamwork among physicians and nurses?

2. What are the best ways to diminish process failures on the front lines of hospital care delivery?

3. What are the arguments for and against hospitals paying physicians on salary?

4. How can hospitals more effectively recruit and retain the physicians and nurses that they need?

5. How do hospital managers get better buy-in from physicians and nurses to attain hospital goals and objectives?

Required Supplementary Readings

Carlson, G. 2010. "Is the Relationship Between Your Hospital and Your Medical Staff Sustainable?" *Journal of Healthcare Management* 55 (3): 158–74.

Delbecq, A. L., and S. Gill. 1985. "Justice as a Prelude to Teamwork in Medical Centers." *Health Care Management Review* 10 (1): 45–51.

Griffith, J. R., and K. R. White. 2010. "The Physician Organization" and "Nursing." In *Reaching Excellence in Healthcare Management,* 105–28 and 129–50. Chicago: Health Administration Press.

Lake, E. T. 2007. "The Nursing Practice Environment: Measurement and Evidence." *Medical Care Research and Review* 64 (2, Suppl.): 104S–122S.

Discussion Questions on Required Supplementary Readings

1. Why don't doctors and nurses buy in more on hospital goals and strategies?
2. How does the situation differ in ambulatory care?
3. Discuss the strengths and weaknesses of hiring physicians as CEOs and nurses as chief operating officers in hospitals.
4. What is the value of nonclinician managers in supporting the work of physicians and nurses at the front lines in HCOs?

Recommended Additional Readings

Berry, L. L., and K. D. Seltman. 2008. *Management Lessons from Mayo Clinic.* New York: McGraw-Hill.

Blumenthal, D. 2002. "Doctors in a Wired World: Can Professionalism Survive Connectivity?" *The Milbank Quarterly* 80 (3): 525–46.

Bohmer, R. M. J. 2009. *Designing Care.* Cambridge, MA: Harvard Business Press.

Burns, L. R., and R. W. Mueller. 2008. "Hospital-Physician Collaboration: Landscape of Economic Integration and Impact on Clinical Integration." *The Milbank Quarterly* 86 (3): 375–84.

Christensen, C. M., J. Grossman, and J. Hwang. 2009. *The Innovator's Prescription.* New York: McGraw-Hill.

Djukic, M., and C. T. Kovner. 2010. "Overlap of Registered Nurse and Physician Practice: Implications for U.S. Health Care Reform." *Policy, Politics & Nursing Practice* 11 (1): 13–22.

Gilmartin, M. J., and T. A. D'Aunno. 2007. "Leadership Research in Health Care." *Academy of Management Annals* 1: 387–438.

Groopman, J. 2007. *How Doctors Think.* Boston: Houghton-Mifflin.

Kenney, C. 2011. *Transforming Health Care: Virginia Mason Medical Center's Pursuit of the Perfect Patient Experience.* Boca Raton, FL: CRC Press.

Steele, G. D., J. A. Haynes, D. E. Davis, J. Tomcavage, W. F. Stewart, T. R. Graf, R. A. Paulus, K. Welkel, and J. Shikles. 2010. "How Geisinger's Advanced Medical Home Model Argues the Case for Rapid-Cycle Innovation." *Health Affairs* 29 (11): 2047–53.

THE CASES

The case studies in this section emphasize the many aspects of professional integration that managers are challenged to ameliorate. First, "Where the Rubber Hits the Road: Physician–Phelps Hospital Relationships" confronts a situation in which the hospital's revenues are increasing much more slowly than its costs, while physician revenues from certain government payers have sunk precipitously lower than their costs. This situation is forcing certain physicians to look to the hospital to pay them a part-time salary in efforts to offset the decreasing third-party payments.

Second, "Getting from Good to Great: Nursing and Patient Care" focuses on two issues of great concern to the chief nursing officer. The first involves responding to pressures to seek "Magnet status" for nursing when she thinks time and energy should be directed elsewhere in empowering managers to buy into ownership of their units and to be more accountable for safety and cost performance. The second issue she faces is to proactively work with physician leaders to operationalize multidisciplinary teams to put patients first and reduce fragmentation of care.

Third, "It's a Balancing Act: Improving Clinical Operations at Blackwell Medical Center" deals with different professional integration conflicts between individual departments and the central medical school administration. The successful department of surgery is being forced to integrate its business side with other ineffective departments under the unproven managerial direction of the central dean's office. How best should the chair and his faculty practice administrator adapt to the situation?

The short cases present a range of situations in which managers have to respond to physicians who do not want to buy into a range of managerial imperatives or behaviors: complaining about nursing and clerical support, refusing to reduce capital budget demands, rejecting a hospital initiative that provides a needed service lacking in the community, and lowering excessive patient stay. A final case study deals with what should be the response of nursing and hospital leadership to staff nurse complaints that the hospital doesn't adequately "take care of our nurses."

Case J
Where the Rubber Hits the Road: Physician–Phelps Hospital Relationships

Anthony R. Kovner

As professor of healthcare management at New York University/Wagner, I was invited by Phelps Memorial Hospital Center's CEO Keith Safian to visit the hospital in 2010 and review the impact of Medicare and potential health reforms on hospital–physician collaboration.

Competitive Position of the Hospital

Phelps is a community hospital of 235 beds, operating at 70 percent occupancy. Inpatient services include medicine, surgery, psychiatry, obstetrics, pediatrics, and physical rehabilitation. Two units of mentally ill chemical-abuse patients operate at 97 percent occupancy. Pediatrics operates at 20 to 30 percent occupancy. The emergency department had 25,000 visits in 2009.

Phelps is surrounded by other hospitals and by water. Patients do not come from the west side of the Hudson River. Phelps is part of the Stellaris alliances with Northern Westchester Hospital, Lawrence Hospital Center, and White Plains Hospital Center. The region is overbedded. Phelps collaborates *and* competes with these hospitals.

Half of Phelps' discharges are from its primary service area, and 9.5 percent are from its secondary service area. For both areas, Phelps has a 29.3 percent market share. An important nonhospital competitor is the Mt. Kisco Medical Group of 150 physicians, which is located across the street from Northern Westchester Hospital, about ten miles to the northeast.

Phelps Medical Staff

The medical staff includes 470 individuals, 445 of whom are physicians. About 100 physicians admit 80 percent of the patients. Two small medical groups are the largest—the North Star group, which includes 14 primary care physicians, and the seven-person orthopedic group. The hospital lacks enough physicians with thriving practices. The medical staff is aging—40 percent of the primary care physicians are older than age 55—and the hospital has the capacity to admit more patients. The hospital salaries three obstetricians and eight internists, a family practitioner, a procedural gastroenterologist, a thoracic surgeon, and six hospitalists. Many of the directors of clinical services receive small hospital stipends; several are full-time employees.

I interviewed some key players to learn more about the situation and possibly to write a case study that would be useful for learning by physician leaders of tomorrow at Phelps Hospital.

Interview with Keith Safian, CEO

National health reform had just been passed by Congress. Mr. Safian estimates the impact on Phelps could be a negative $3.5 million each year for the next ten years. Presently, Medicare and Medicaid reimbursement to Phelps is at a rate lower than cost. Phelps operates at a 1.8 percent profit margin, while costs increased an average of 10.3 percent each year from 2007 to 2009. Phelps raises $2 to $3 million through philanthropy each year.

The hospital has physician issues. Specialists want to be paid to be on call for the ED. They want to be paid when they see indigent and Medicaid patients. They want to be paid for referring patients, although this is prohibited by law. Phelps is making some adaptations, and the CEO and the chief medical officer are considering the following options:

- The hospital has recently salaried two gastroenterologists. Voluntary cardiologists have approached the CEO about partnering to perform stress tests because reimbursement is better if these tests are done at the hospital.
- Phelps is thinking of discontinuing some outpatient mental health programs (which generate a total of 50,000 visits per year) if Medicaid cuts occur.
- The CEO does not approve of salary freezes. Phelps gave full-time employees an average 3.5 percent pay raise last year. Safian would rather cut some positions than decrease health insurance benefits.
- Phelps has started an educational program for younger physicians, the medical leaders of tomorrow. The program covers organizational and health system issues, hospital payment, and the nature of the competitive market.
- Phelps is considering building a new ambulatory surgery center on campus, although there is no pressure on operating room (OR) capacity as yet.
- Phelps has had difficulty collaborating with primary care physicians. The largest physician group has not been able to hire more primary care physicians, and they just added two specialists.

Interview with Dr. Robert Seebacher, Medical Director of Joint Replacement Services

Phelps is the only hospital where Dr. Seebacher practices. He is in a large orthopedic practice with seven partners. They now participate only in Medicare and workers' compensation. Medicare pays $1,200 for a knee operation, whereas commercial out-of-network insurance pays $22,000. Dr. Seebacher's malpractice premiums are $110,000 per year, and office overhead is 35 percent. He performs 240 joint replacements a year; he must do 100 to pay for his malpractice insurance.

Views on Medicare and Hospital Adaptation

Seebacher observes, "The United States is extremely wasteful of medical resources. For example, a 90-year-old person will find a surgeon who will do a knee or a hip replacement. So, in one year this expends more money than that person earned in her whole life. The elderly get wonderful care now, whereas 25 years ago they didn't live long enough to receive these operations. It's hard for the hospital to stop unnecessary knee replacements or take action when every gallbladder with a stone does not need to be removed."

He adds, "Many doctors do not wish to cooperate with hospital initiatives. The current payment system divides doctors from hospitals. The hospital should form partnerships with really good physicians, as they are doing, and take care of them. If the hospital is making a lot of money on a surgeon's patients and he's getting paid below his costs, the hospital should pay him a salary."

"A current problem," Seebacher observes, "is that Phelps can't get subspecialists to take call in the ED. Phelps should subsidize these physicians—for example, hand surgeons—to take call. The chief medical officer [CMO] should have more medical directors under him, and he should look for unnecessary surgery and overtreatment. Phelps should strengthen the hospitalist system, but hospitalists (and all primary care physicians) should not order 50 consults for their patients to cover themselves. There should be a more sensible focus on geriatric oversight."

Advice to the CEO

Seebacher urges that "the CEO should listen more to the CMO. The hospital should cut away from doctors whose practice patterns are poor or wasteful. Phelps should be innovative in forming relationships with physicians. Phelps should not look only at volume but also emphasize ethical and expert care. The CEO should value the high-quality physicians he has rather than search for new people. There is too much emphasis on the patients Phelps is not getting. By definition, some of these patients won't come here anyway."

Seebacher observes: "Northern Westchester Medical Center—with its all-private rooms—appeals to patients who can pay. If Phelps shrinks, the hospital could have all private rooms. Phelps has three wards full of patients who can be frightening to other patients. Patient rooms are too small. The plant has been allowed to deteriorate. Patients see 'small, tight, dingy.' We don't have the money now to change this."

Interview with Dr. Richard Peress, Director of Surgery

Dr. Peress joined the Phelps staff in 1987 and specializes in the spine and scoliosis. He performs 50 operations a year. When he started, he brought a tertiary-level approach to Westchester County. He has recently become director of surgery.

Views on Medicare and Hospital Adaptation

Dr. Peress believes the sooner Medicare collapses the better. Attempts to prop it up "won't get us where we need to go. We do what is politically expedient." Medicare has become a two-tier system—those who can afford it and those who cannot. He believes that costs will be capped for all insurers, and charging patients more will be illegal. He observes that payments for kyphoplasty (a procedure to correct spinal fractures caused by osteoporosis) were $1,500 when he started; Medicare now pays $600. The procedure takes only 20 minutes, but the operation takes an hour of the surgeon's time, and he loses money on the procedure. A plumber charges $300 an hour to unclog a toilet. For epidural injections, Dr. Peress is paid only $69 an hour, and he is putting a needle into the patient's spine.

He asks, "When does gain-sharing under Medicare become fee-splitting?" The hospital makes a lot of money on certain procedures, while the surgeon loses money. This raises questions about how the money can be more fairly distributed.

He observes that the medical staff have to change their attitudes, too. Doctors have a long history of being loners. In today's economy, the bottom line is all that counts. This is changing things for physicians. "Now all we're doing is haggling about the price." But once the hospital makes a deal with a physician, the government can't just take it away. Dr. Peress says, "I can't continue without adequate compensation."

Advice to the CEO

Dr. Peress believes that whatever decisions are made by administration, they must be worked out so that physicians also benefit. For example, hospital online documentation that provides pay-for-performance rewards to the hospital should not be accomplished on the backs of physicians. The surge of "itinerant" physicians at Phelps pains the more loyal doctors.

Dr. Peress thinks Phelps should focus on physicians with unique talents that are not universally available at neighboring hospitals. The hospital's advertisements could tout these physicians so that patients leap over competitor hospitals in surrounding counties. His practice, for example, draws from other hospitals in Orange and Dutchess counties. Dr. Peress wants Phelps to be a true regional spine center.

Physicians should make their case for gain-sharing to a joint committee, Dr. Peress says. If a physician has the talents, she should let the committee know that. Providing high-quality care—and being personable and kind—count, too. The hospital should tell the public why physicians like Dr. Peress choose to work at Phelps. He gets better support at Phelps than elsewhere—for example, nursing support in the ICU and care for his patients from board-certified subspecialists in cardiology, pulmonary, nephrology, and infectious disease, among other areas.

Dr. Peress feels the problem Dr. Lawrence Faltz, the CMO, faces is to help with the implementation and enforcement of compliance. The Stellaris computer system is a handicap because "the computer system doesn't adapt to the physicians, so we have to adapt to it."

The CEO, Mr. Safian, did what was necessary 20 years ago to get rid of the $10 million annual deficit. But Phelps cannot make money anymore just by cutting expenses. The CEO has changed, too, but austerity is not the answer. As a new initiative, Dr. Peress is leading implementation of a pain clinic in the old ED. He wants people to say positively about this and other services: "Phelps? Yeah, Phelps!"

Interview with Dr. Arthur Fass, Chief of Cardiology

Dr. Fass has been on staff at Phelps for 25 years and has been chief of cardiology since the mid-1980s. His group has three cardiologists. The hospital has two cardiology groups and a smattering of individual practitioners.

Views on Medicare and Hospital Adaptation

Dr. Fass is very concerned that, as in his private practice, hospital reimbursement is down and costs are increasing. Physicians are now talking to Phelps and other hospitals seeking to become employees. Then physicians can be guaranteed income, and physician employees become hospital employees with the hospital paying their health benefits.

Dr. Fass finds that what is important to payers is not quality or thoroughness but high volume, rushing through as many patients as possible. He observes that a financial incentive exists to refer patients not to the best physicians but according to what group they belong to.

Dr. Fass recommends that the CEO be sensitive to situations such as call in the ED. The CEO is asking physicians essentially to provide free service at 3:00 a.m.—while the hospital itself collects a fair amount of money. Physicians should be compensated in some way for this service that they are asked to provide.

Dr. Fass observes the Phelps staff includes about 100 dedicated physicians, and 20 of those are most active in providing clinical services. The hospital should only admit new physicians to their staff if they provide service primarily from a patient care rather than an economic perspective—for example, so that they can transfer patients to other hospitals for tertiary care.

Physicians should be fairly compensated for what they are asked to do, Dr. Fass believes. The CEO should sit down with neurologists, for example, and set one of them up with a good salary, office space, and staff. Not having the neurologist on call affects all doctors who then are in trouble "if their patient has an acute stroke and they can't get a neurologist."

Having a relationship with a teaching hospital would also be attractive for Phelps. This might help in attracting primary care physicians, some of whom may be tempted to set up practice in this community.

Interview with Dr. Lawrence Faltz, Chief Medical Officer

Dr. Faltz joined Phelps 15 years ago after serving as chairman of medicine and residency program director at New York/Queens for ten years. He specializes in rheumatology and internal medicine. Dr. Faltz is responsible for quality, credentialing, and physician discipline at Phelps. He is responsible for networks and academic affiliations. Dr. Faltz is active outside the hospital in the American College of Physicians, where he has held a leadership position.

Views on Medicare and Hospital Adaptation

Dr. Faltz observes that "the docs controlled the medical system up to 1980. After 1990, the payers have controlled the system." He notes that specialization raises costs. Before, the doctor waited to treat a hypertensive patient because of the risks of medications. Now there are treatments with far fewer side effects. When the patient has blood pressure of 120/80, the doctor starts controlling for hypertension. For a pneumonia patient, the physician used to get a chest X-ray and make seven visits. Now the patient sees the primary care physician every day, plus the cardiology consultant, the pulmonary consultant, and the ID consultant; he gets a chest X-ray, a CT scan, and an echo from the cardiologist. The patient now uses 30 services when he used to get eight services. All of this adds to the cost of care.

Dr. Faltz believes that physicians need to understand their obligations as members of the hospital medical staff. Some of them see being asked to be on call as a personal attack. Doctors used to build their practice by taking call. Now there are too many specialists, so it's hard to build a practice. Physicians do not get paid sufficiently, if at all, for ED visits. Managed care companies do not give physicians a fair deal, and for many physicians just being in practice means tremendous liability issues.

Lifestyle is an issue for the younger physicians. They do not see the profession as an all-encompassing lifestyle as the older physicians might have, Dr. Faltz believes. The government has to spend money on sectors other than healthcare. There is not enough money. Phelps is run as efficiently as possible. The hospital is still run as a doctors' workshop. The hospital needs more integration of physicians and hospital by service. "We need trade-offs as to where the money is going. The hospital has to accept physician governance over some hospital issues," Dr. Faltz says. Many physician leaders at Phelps lack formal education about current health policy issues. Dr. Faltz recommends that Phelps and its physicians work together to make the newly salaried physicians productive. The present reimbursement system is not conducive to this. Phelps has to figure out how best to compete with growing medical groups, such as Mt. Kisco, that are recruiting additional physicians and taking away hospital ancillary service revenues.

Regarding call in the ED, Dr. Faltz points out that (1) subspecialists do not want call but they want to keep out the competition, (2) mature practices do not need the new patient flow from the ED, and (3) primary care medical staff are unprepared to say, "if you (specialists) won't take call, we won't refer patients to you." Phelps has to move the culture. The community does not understand that when no specialist is available after hours, patients have to be transported to another hospital. Patients view that as a hospital failure, not a medical staff failure. The medical staff does not understand that the hospital and its medical staff are viewed as a single entity by the outside world. The medical staff bylaws should be changed so that physicians still have to take call even if they are 55 years old and have worked at Phelps for 20 years, which currently are grounds for exemption from call, regardless of the availability of other members of a department.

Dr. Faltz concludes: "We must see that we can't get where we want to go without each other, and we can't turn the clock back to where it was before."

I didn't have an answer to the quandary in which the hospital and its physician leaders found themselves. On one hand, neither party seems to be netting sufficient revenue to meet revenue targets. On the other hand, neither side seems to be able to work out a satisfactory method of working closer together on some kind of combined production and billing process that would meet each side's targets.

Case Questions

1. What were the financial problems facing Phelps and its medical staff in 2010?
2. What are the options for hospital initiatives and what do the physicians recommend?
3. How should the CEO proceed? Give a rationale for your recommendations.
4. What are the unresolved questions in the situation facing the CEO and the board? What are the risks in adopting your recommended strategy?
5. What do you recommend that the CEO and the CMO do to improve the situation?
6. How do you approach this case from the point of view of a younger physician? What do you expect from the hospital, and what do you think the hospital should expect from you?

Case K
Getting from Good to Great:
Nursing and Patient Care

Wilhelmina Manzano and Anthony R. Kovner

Part 1, 2007: Nursing at University Health System

The Question

"How do we get from 'good' to 'great'?" Andrea Rogers, chief nursing officer (CNO) of University Health System (UHS) asked Clark Kaplan, a nursing management consultant, in spring 2007.

UHS was a health system of five hospitals with a budget of $4 billion, located in a large eastern city and highly ranked nationally by *U.S. News & World Report.* "Of course we think we're great now. But we wish to be and to be perceived as the nation's leader in nursing," Rogers continued.

"Whatever that means," Kaplan replied. "Do you provide the best nursing care, the best patient care, or does the nursing division feature the most focused accountability with transparency of results?"

"We've kept the focus on nursing and had to deal with competing priorities. It's easy to lose sight of the main thing and 'putting patients first' when you have to plan one, three, or five years out," Rogers noted.

Strategic Planning at UHS

Kaplan had been hired to work with Rogers on strategic planning within nursing. His first task had been to try to evaluate the effectiveness of the existing process. He had chosen the following criteria for his evaluation: (1) patient and staff satisfaction, as reflected in metrics highlighting bad outcomes, such as pressure ulcers or nurse vacancy rates; (2) investment in and support for nursing by top management at UHS; and (3) focused accountability of the 200 patient care managers for patient care outcomes and nursing satisfaction. All of these metrics had to be taken into account across the five hospitals and central office that made up UHS.

Rogers began by pointing to accomplishments in strategic planning during her three years as CNO. Nursing had established a systemwide nursing board similar to the UHS medical board that sets standards of practice, governance, structure, and communication. She had also formed the Center for Professional Nursing Practice (CPNP) that includes education, research, practice, professional development, credentialing, and nursing informatics. Leadership development had become a priority, and incentive performance targets had been recently implemented for staff nurses. Under the present model, nurses can earn up to 7 percent on top of their yearly increment. The brand and reputation of nursing is very strong, within and outside UHS. The president and executive vice president of UHS support the role of nurses in taking care of patients, and UHS reports that it has invested over $30 million over the past two years to upgrade nursing.

Gerry Winograd, director of CPNP, explained the strategic planning process as follows: "We started in the summer of 2005, when we were evaluating whether to pursue Magnet status. The main areas we fell short in were staffing, recruitment and retention, cultural diversity, care models, and shared governance. UHS then had six initiatives for 2007, and nursing aligned itself with all of these initiatives: people development, quality and safety, serving the community, partnerships, financial and operating strengths, and advancing care." (See Exhibit IV.4 for a summary of the Magnet Recognition Program.)

EXHIBIT IV.4
A Summary of Program Review for the Magnet Recognition Program (from the American Nurses Credentialing Center [ANCC])

The Magnet Recognition Program was developed by the American Nurses Credentialing Center (ANCC) to recognize healthcare organizations that demonstrate nursing excellence. The program also provides a vehicle for disseminating successful nursing practices and strategies.

Recognizing high-quality patient care, nursing excellence, and innovations in professional nursing practice, the Magnet Recognition Program provides consumers with the ultimate benchmark to measure the quality of care that they can expect to receive. When *U.S. News & World Report* publishes its annual showcase, "America's Best Hospitals," being an ANCC Magnet organization contributes to the total score for quality of inpatient care (ANCC 2012). ANCC is one of only a few organizations providing outside data to inform the ranking process. In the 2010 listing, eight of the top ten medical centers (80 percent) featured in the prestigious Honor Roll were Magnet-recognized organizations. In the Children's Hospital Honor Roll, six of the top eight (75 percent) were ANCC Magnet recognized.

The Magnet Recognition Program is based on quality indicators and standards of nursing practice as defined in the revised third edition of the American Nurses Association *Nursing Administration: Scope & Standards of Practice* (2009). The "Scope and Standards for Nurse Administrators" and other foundational documents form the base on which the Magnet environment is built. The Magnet designation process includes the appraisal of qualitative factors in nursing. These factors, the "Forces of Magnetism," were first identified through research done in 1983.

The full expression of the "Forces" embodies a professional environment guided by a strong visionary nursing leader who advocates and supports development and excellence in nursing practice. As a natural outcome of this, the program elevates the reputation and standards of the nursing profession.

The Magnet application and appraisal process is designed to bring recognition to a healthcare organization's attainment of standards of excellence in nursing. It is also a rewarding and valuable educational experience for an organization seeking focus and direction for growth and development. The process is thorough and long, demanding widespread participation from the applicant organization's nurses. Healthcare organizations find the journey to be a revealing self-assessment—creating multiple opportunities for organizational advancement, team building, and enhancement of individual professional self-esteem.

Top nursing leadership now meets quarterly. This leadership group, approximately 15 people, includes nursing vice presidents and CPNP staff. With respect to shared governance, UHS has developed a means by which staff nurses can participate actively in the decision-making process for patient care. The model adapted was "patient-centered care," and dialogue is now directed at the unit level concerning what staff nurses want. (See Exhibit IV.5 for the UHS division of nursing's Mission, Vision, and Philosophy Statement.)

Perspectives About the Strategic Planning Process

Ms. Winograd is the facilitator of the strategic planning process, coordinating stakeholders and resources. She has been in the position for seven years. Two program directors assist her: one focuses on education and practice, and the other deals with practice and with obtaining Magnet status. The nursing department leaders have mixed feelings about the costs and benefits of obtaining the Magnet designation. Some argue that Magnet status is not a reliable and valid measure of quality of patient care, while others view Magnet status as worth obtaining even at high cost because of perceptions in the field and for competitive reasons. According to Ms. Winograd, the most important priority for nursing in 2007 is recruitment and retention, which she says is highly dependent on nurse manager performance. Also, the division places a high priority on increasing the time the nurse spends at the bedside, as this leads to increased professional satisfaction and better patient care.

Ella White, VP for patient services at the North Division, suggests that the value added from centralized strategic planning for the nursing division is that "we get and give advice on best practices, collaborate, and support each other. In my job, I don't get much strategic or reflective time. Everything is a crisis, and we are always at meetings." White adds that rather than beefing up the centralized QA office, a higher priority should be to create decentralized quality and safety data analyst positions. Quality and safety at UHS are centralized at the system level and across disciplines under the supervision of a physician. White needs a person dedicated to quality at North Division who works with nurse managers at the unit level, to do the "think" work and the "look" work. The other person she needs is a safety person (to do analysis of hygiene and identification and administration of medications). White argues that her administrative support is too light as a result of UHS prioritizing heavy investments at the bedside, adding capital equipment (e.g., ultrasounds on units for insertion of lines in ICUs, cooling blankets) and technology. Volume has increased, acuity has heightened, and patient turnover is quicker. The state regulators, she says, want to "suck the profits out of healthcare." White concludes that strategic planning is a good, solid process in nursing at UHS but could be improved. As she notes, "We weigh, rank, and come back to the 'main thing,' but there are too many things on our list, too many priorities."

- The **mission** of the department of nursing is to provide the highest-quality patient-centered care by promoting a culture of caring, empathy and safety; educating our patients and families by utilizing evidence-based practice; and promoting professional nursing development and advancement.

- The **vision** is to be one of the nation's leaders in nursing.

- The **values** are:
  - Practice
  - Quality, safety, and outcomes
  - Research
  - Education
  - Service excellence

- The **philosophy** of nursing at UHS is driven by the organization's vision and strategic goals, and the department of nursing's goals and values. It encompasses the intent of the ANA Code of Ethics for Nurses, ANA Standards of Practice, the State Practice Act, and regulatory standards, while keeping pace with the changing healthcare market.

  The philosophy recognizes that nursing care is organized around the needs of the patient, that quality outcomes and patient satisfaction are measures of the delivery systems, and that the multidisciplinary team approach is fundamental to the practice model.

  The department of nursing supports professional nursing practice within the departments and specialties wherever nursing is practiced within UHS.

The professional nursing practice philosophy at UHS ensures the following:

- The nurse assesses the patient and family for specific care needs to meet optimal outcomes.

- The nurse identifies the amount, degree, and level of nursing care needed to achieve those outcomes and manages the nursing resources to meet those needs.

- The nurse recognizes the contributions of other disciplines as an integral part of patient care delivery.

- The nurse provides every patient and family with complete and understandable information about care and after-care through individual contracts, group programs, and multimedia materials.

(continued)

EXHIBIT IV.5

The Mission,
Vision, and
Philosophy
Statement of
the Department
of Nursing
(continued)

The nursing organization is service oriented and strives to meet the needs of patients across the continuum of care in a culturally sensitive manner by assessing, planning, and communicating those needs to patients, families, and other professionals. This approach is holistic in scope and respectful of patients' rights. It allows for the sharing of information that fosters patient participation in decision making.

The nursing organization cultivates a climate in which staff mature professionally in the pursuit of advancement and excellence in nursing practice. The department of nursing offers learning experiences and provides role models to nursing students at all levels. On-site education for staff is supported through staff development and accredited continuing education programs.

Inherent in this philosophy is a recognition of the needs of the community by nursing's involvement in strategic planning efforts and participation in program development. It also recognizes the need for nurses to speak on community and professional issues that are within their field of competence or interest and to assist in promoting public involvement in health by defining and clarifying issues.

The department of nursing remains committed to maintaining a collaborative, multidisciplinary relationship with other health and administrative professionals. Provisions are made for the collection and evaluation of data and the development of interdisciplinary performance improvement processes in the belief that systematic inquiry will lead to improved care, efficient use of nursing time and resources, and positive patient outcomes.

White suggests that the Mission, Vision, and Philosophy Statement (Exhibit IV.5) is too wordy. She believes that the statement should instead read something similar to, "We want every nurse to be engaged and focus on 'it's all about the patient.' Nursing has got to do better. Nursing has got to raise the bar. Nursing needs to be clear about expectations. Nursing needs to understand better how we can get there. Nursing leadership will partner with staff nurses and help them achieve the UHS goal. But all nurses need to show up, participate, contribute, and be engaged in the process."

Shirley Apple, service line manager in oncology, South Division, is one of four service line directors. Her units include medical and surgical oncology (72 beds), outpatient infusion (25 chairs), radiation oncology, nurse walk-in clinics with fellows, and a few nurses who give chemotherapy to patients not on a unit. Apple has been in her job for 12 years.

Apple participates in strategic planning in the following ways. She attends the local practice council of 10 or 12 staff. Each staff member nominates two of the nurses who serve on this council. They meet 30 times a year. About 20 percent of their meeting time is spent on strategic planning. Apple also attends monthly nurse leadership meetings for the South Division, and these meetings are attended by approximately 30 nurse leaders. This group also spends about 20 percent of its time on strategic planning.

Apple attends South Division nursing meetings as well on a division "relation-based" initiative with six other unit leaders. These nurse managers focus on raising patient satisfaction scores, using a primary nursing care philosophy. After the recent implementation of this initiative on the seven units, Press-Ganey patient satisfaction scores rose significantly from the 70s to the 80s. The different divisions of UHS have chosen different ways to accomplish patient care goals. These ways are becoming more data and research driven. Children's uses a family-centered model. West Division uses the Planetree model. North Division uses a bedside strategy. Apple observes, "This all involves a lot of hard work, and it takes a lot of time to reorganize work."

Apple would like to see a way to make nursing staff more autonomous, increase professionalism, encourage personal growth, and improve management. In oncology, nurses attend education programs organized by the clinical nurse specialists and the nurse educator. Annually, 15 to 20 nurses attend the National Congress on Oncology Nursing for four days. When they return to UHS, nurses make presentations to staff and present seminars on what they have learned. Oncology nurses are incented to achieve oncology certification (the current certification rate is 10 percent among the 80 nurses).

Nursing leadership wants to empower patient care directors. But Apple asks, "Does medical leadership want this goal too?" She would like senior nursing leadership to better appreciate the amount of work that patient care and service line directors do to achieve new goals after the leadership makes decisions. For example, nursing leadership initiated an anonymous, online survey on how staff nurses felt about working in the hospital; the survey took 20 to 25 minutes for each nurse to complete. During the same week that Apple had to make sure the staff nurses completed the survey, she also had to see that all nurses got their flu shots, perform evaluations for 110 people, and implement all of these special initiatives in addition to her regular work. Apple concludes, "We don't have the support we need to get the work done." But she hastens to add, "The new initiatives to put patients first do make our work so exciting!"

Part 1 Case Questions

1. How is professional integration related to nursing division performance?
2. Why doesn't professional integration have a higher priority within the strategy planning process of the nursing division?
3. What would be a rationale for giving higher priority to professional integration in the nursing division?
4. Areas of possible integration include:
   a. Among the nursing departments in the five hospitals of UHS
   b. Between doctors and nurses in the individual hospitals
   c. Between nursing and finance in the individual hospitals
   Discuss opportunities for improving professional integration in these three areas.

Part 2, 2011: The Nursing Division at UHS: The End of the Beginning?

Professional Integration Progress

"What has happened in the last four years?" Andrea Rogers, CNO of UHS, asked herself, resuming her dialogue with Clark Kaplan, a nursing management consultant, in the spring of 2011. "The health system has done a lot of work responding to challenges—market share, engaging physicians in different service lines, planning a response to healthcare reform. We have more data. Our financial condition is stable, and last year was our best operating year in the past five years.

"In nursing, we looked at the hospital's strategic goals and asked how we can support them. We have 4,800 nurses on staff today. Our three- to five-year plan has become an eight- to ten-year plan. How do we transform care at the bedside by looking at practice? How do we care for patients safely and compassionately? How can we educate nurses at the bedside? Staff nurses must understand the context underlying what we're asking them to do.

"At the same time, key issues remain:

1. Workforce issues—recruiting, retaining, and determining the right amount of staffing. The data we get are not consistent or standardized, most notably from the National Database of Nursing Quality Indicators. These data are not risk adjusted.
2. How do we partner with schools of nursing so that nurses are receiving the right educational preparation for the future? We are now affiliated

with 21 schools of nursing. More than 1,000 nursing students were placed here last year. We seem to agree with the schools so far on what we need to do, but not on how we do it.

3. How do we respond to quality mandates from external agencies, such as The Joint Commission? We lack the infrastructure to educate and consistently implement quality metrics. The information we get is nine months after the fact. We are not always that ready nor that well equipped to respond for different reasons.

4. Financial constraints—We are asking questions about productivity and value. Can we do more in nursing for what we spend?"

Pursuing Magnet Status

Clark was intrigued. "Where are you now about pursuing Magnet status?" he asked. "I've never been convinced about its scientific validity."

Rogers responded: "I'm not sure about the benefits for the costs involved. It's become a business proposition for the people who run the Magnet program. Unfortunately, national rankings include Magnet status as one component now. Here, the health system board recently asked us, 'Are we going to be designated?' We can stack up on performance metrics or surpass other hospitals that have been designated to have Magnet status. I believe that nursing needs to move away from nursing-centric thinking and reward team performance. Only 5 percent of US hospitals have Magnet status, and the top five nationally ranked hospitals all have Magnet status. Interestingly, the Magnet people don't publicize a list of those hospitals that have lost the designation. Here, I know the union will be opposed to some of the changes that we would have to make to obtain Magnet status. You know, UHS has invested more than $52 million in the past few years to hire more nurses."

The Challenge of Accountability

"For me," Rogers continued, "a particularly important issue now is patient care director accountability for unit performance. We're not there yet. We have top performers who buy in, and their unit outcomes show it. Yet the larger pool of patient care directors needs to understand what it means to run a service and take ownership as if this were a business. We need agreement about roles, responsibilities, partnerships, and infrastructure that support such accountabilities. And here, for some patient directors, their span of control is too wide for them to reasonably be accountable for all staff performance—more than 100 staff nurses report to them."

Physician–Nurse Relationships

Clark interjected again. "How about the relationships between physicians and nurses? Are physicians a key barrier in empowering patient care directors to take accountability for unit performance?"

Rogers paused before replying. "We've seen tremendous improvement over the years at UHS with respect to the relationship between physicians and nurses. This starts at the top with the attitudes of the clinical chiefs and directors of service. I've met with each of them to find out what they needed from nursing. One thing that helps is our Physician Recognition Awards, given by physicians' nursing partners. We have great teamwork in the operating room and labor and delivery, where we have improved communication and handoffs. In general I think that physicians feel they need nurses, and they are more involved and aware. These physician–nurse partnerships are supported by the governing board, the CEO, and the medical leadership. The leaders don't just talk about it; they also do things to support nurses. I guess I would say that the culture at UHS has definitely changed."

Looking Ahead

Rogers continued, "Our goals for the next three years focus on improving nursing practice, especially by continuing to review relevant and current practice and patient safety. Next, we are attempting to stabilize and right-size the workforce. We wish to improve morale where we have a union and improve trust of staff nurses in our other hospitals so that they do not feel that they need union representation. We will also continue to keep an eye on nurse competencies to make sure staff keep up with the latest technology. A third goal is keeping up with information technology. Healthcare is so far behind other sectors, such as the financial sector. How do we get IT to support the nurse? More specifically, how can we use IT to reduce the amount of time nurses spend walking around as opposed to at the bedside? At the same time, nurses have to let go of past practice, and do their work in a different way as IT is implemented to support them."

Current Nursing Division Performance Metrics

Rogers concluded, "The key metrics we now use in evaluating nursing division performance are (1) recruitment and retention rates and turnover rates of new graduates, (2) educational preparation of workforce and certification,

(3) diversity demographics given the populations that we serve, and (4) relevant quality indicators such as rates of hospital-acquired ulcers, falls with and without serious injuries, urinary tract infections, and ventilator-associated pneumonia. We also look carefully at the new HCAHPS measures on patients' perceptions of care, such as nurse responsiveness, explanation of procedures, pain management, and cleanliness."

Part 2 Case Questions

1. How, if at all, would you change the Mission, Vision, and Philosophy Statement to place higher priority on professional integration?
2. What changes in the environment have important implications for the priority of professional integration within the nursing division?
3. What do you recommend that Rogers do about UHS acquiring Magnet status?
4. What should Rogers do to focus on patient care director accountability for unit performance?

References

American Nurses Association (ANA). 2009. *Nursing Administration: Scope & Standards of Practice*. Silver Spring, MD: ANA.

American Nurses Credentialing Center (ANCC). 2012. "Magnet Recognition Program® in the News." Accessed September 10. www.nursecredentialing.org/ Headlines/MagnetRecognitionProgramintheNews.aspx.

Case L
It's a Balancing Act: Improving Clinical Operations at Blackwell Medical Center

Anthony R. Kovner

Pedro Santana is the departmental administrator for the department of surgery at Blackwell Medical Center, one of three large academic medical centers in Eastern City.

At Blackwell there are two lines of authority—the hospital line and the school of medicine line. The hospital is profitable. The department of surgery operates under the medical school, where there are separate lines for faculty practice and managed care contracts. The chief of surgery, Dr. Will Blinick, reports to the dean of the school of medicine and the president and CEO of the medical center.

The medical center has 19 clinical departments and 12 nonclinical departments. The department of surgery, which has 45 full-time and 85 voluntary attending faculty, is one of the largest and fastest-growing departments in the school. Since 2006, the department has added 15 surgeons. The medical center subsidizes them at an annual rate of $7.9 million each year. This support is used to offset physician salaries and cover operating overhead, such as ancillary staff malpractice and programmatic expenses.

The Chief's Priorities for the Departmental Administrator

Dr. Blinick's priorities for Santana are financial: growth in practice revenues and ensuring the fiscal health of the department. The dean of the school of medicine sets financial targets for the chairs. Surgery targets for 2009 are revenues of $31 million, net collection rate of 85 percent, accounts receivable days of 80 or less, and operating within budget.

Santana's Challenges in Meeting Financial Targets

The following are the department's four biggest challenges for 2009:

1. *Space.* The dean is constantly urging the chair to recruit more surgeons, but the department has no place to house them. Practice space is full, and new recruits need clinical space. The department has no effective process for space allocation.
2. *Net collection rate (NCR) target.* The NCR target is based on a national benchmark. Practicing in New York presents different challenges that make achieving this target difficult to reach. Two-thirds of the department's practice revenue comes from seven surgeons who do not participate in insurance plans. While these physicians generate more revenue because they are nonparticipating, their accounts receivable take longer to collect and negotiate. To meet the NCR target, the department must change its strategy, such as considering writing down its charges or inputting contractual allowances sooner, which might negatively impact its revenue potential.
3. *Recruitment issues.* While the department has a standard recruitment process for bringing a new physician on board, the nuances are different

on a case-by-case basis. Specifically, the process for obtaining funding and space to support each recruit is not standardized or timely. In addition, the department has no system to track the necessary approvals for all aspects of the recruitment process. This lack of organization creates frustration for the department and for the person being recruited. The medical center is working to develop a more standardized process.

4. *Managed care systems.* The department has no mechanism in place to find out in real time whether the managed care companies are paying appropriately. As a result, Santana does not know the revenue opportunities that surgery is missing (such as over- or underpayments by insurance companies). The centralized managed care office holds the details of managed care contracts, and it will not share these details with the department of surgery or with any department.

Challenges as Viewed by the Department of Surgery

Dr. Mike McKenzie, the associate chief of surgery, suggests that the chief of surgery wears four hats: clinical, academic, research, and administrative. In an uncertain time, he is trying to grow all missions, which are different from each other and not consistent. "It's a balancing act," he says.

McKenzie suggests, "We need at least 50 percent more staff to do what we're supposed to be doing, and we have already grown 40 percent over the past few years. With one-third less space, we've doubled our visits. We had an agreement with attending surgeons that we would not expand space beyond these walls. But times have changed, management has changed, and we have new leadership. Full-timers now admit 70 percent of the patients, whereas we used to admit 30 percent of the patients. We need to reconsider our options." Exhibit IV.6 shows the surgery department's areas of growth.

According to McKenzie, "The hospital views our department as a savior. The medical school has seen tremendous growth in revenues. Our practice plan belongs to the school, as a wholly owned subsidiary. Now we're working on customer service and quality. The faculty practice administration wants centralization; we think we can do it better. Our strategy is to keep demonstrating how good we are."

The chief of surgery, Dr. Blinick, spends 30 percent of his time in clinical practice and 70 percent on departmental affairs, clinical best practice, education, research, and business and development. His three goals for 2009 are (1) clinical excellence, (2) medical and surgical advancement, and (3) generating a profit. He says these goals are aligned with the goals of the hospital and the medical school. Management is the central instrument that allows the chief to operationalize these goals seamlessly and effectively.

Dr. Blinick indicates that the hospital and the school support the department financially and help in developing administrative strategy. As examples, they provide legal support to develop contracts and marketing support through advertising. Dr. Blinick says that Santana is doing a spectacular job. "His priorities are in order, and he's moving the ball down the court. Santana manages people well, creates a positive environment, and is a hard worker."

EXHIBIT IV.6
Surgery: Areas
of Growth

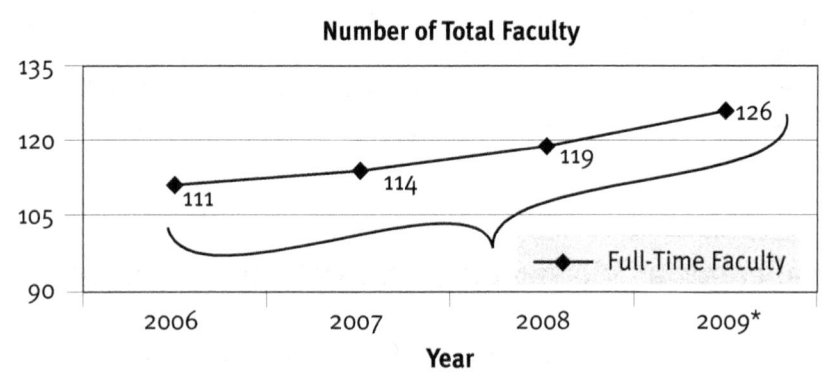

*Projected
Source: Department of A&P Files.

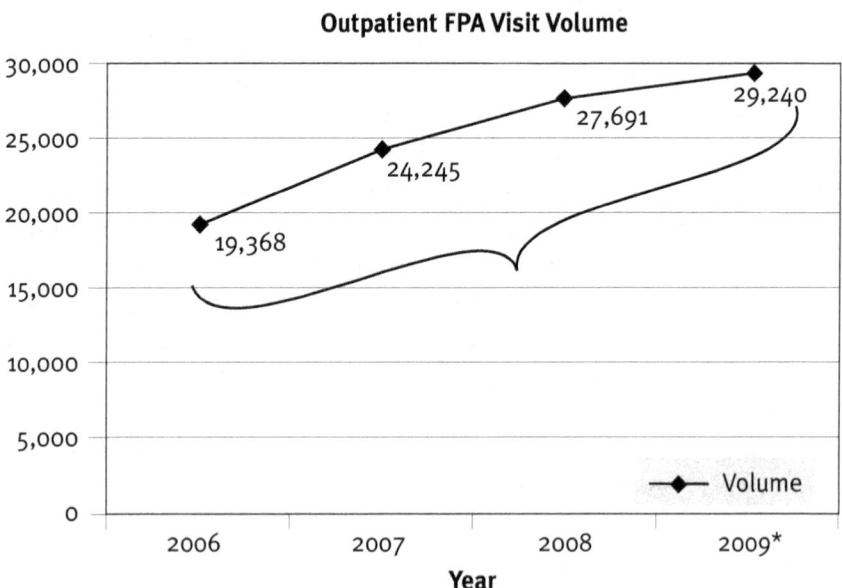

*Projected
Source: IDX.

EXHIBIT IV.6
Surgery:
Areas of
Growth
(continued)

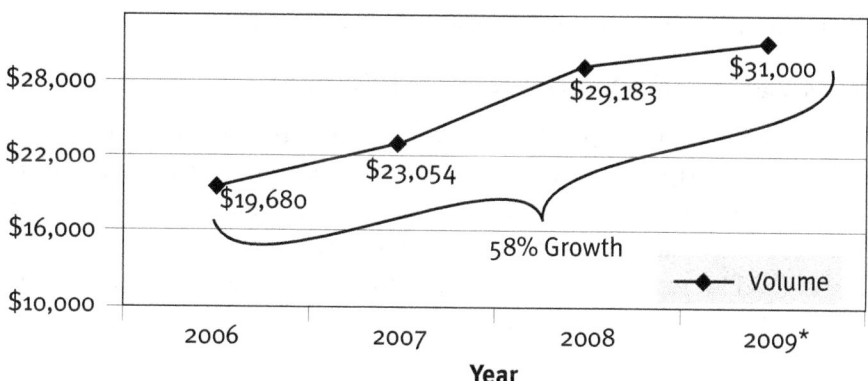

Contribution Margin (all faculty)

- 2006: $48
- 19%
- 2007: $57
- 11%
- 2008: $63
- 5%
- 2009*: $66
- 38% Growth

Legend: ◆ Contribution Margin

Year

*Projected
Source: TSI.

FPA Gross Receipts (in millions)

- 2006: $19,680
- 2007: $23,054
- 2008: $29,183
- 2009*: $31,000
- 58% Growth

Legend: ◆ Volume

Year

*Projected
Source: FPA Scorecard/IDX.

The Medical School's View

Dr. Bruce Percy is associate dean for operations at the medical center and VP for school of medicine operations. He was formerly dean of the dental school. According to Dr. Percy, none of the departmental administrators report to him—they report to their respective chiefs. "We have to get things changed by consensus." He also does not have any reporting line to the medical center faculty practice administration (FPA). His current time is spent as follows: 30 percent on contracts, offers, and business plans; 30 percent on departmental work for clinical and nonclinical departments; 20 percent on faculty compensation; and 20 percent on research, budgeting, compliance, and human resource activity.

Percy's goals for 2009 are as follows: (1) raising the level and education of departmental administrators, (2) reducing costs and keeping the school fiscally prudent by breaking even, and (3) establishing a voice in the FPA.

Percy's View of the Department of Surgery

Percy says that while the department is doing well overall, "they [surgery] have decided the compensation of certain surgeons without sufficiently involving us [the medical school], so the school loses a lot of money because the incentives were based on relative value units rather than on the relationship between revenues and expense. Also, many of the surgeons get 50 percent of the receipts, while the corresponding overhead for them is way over 50 percent. The formula doesn't make sense to us, and more and more the hospital is asking the school to help pay for these shortfalls, even though they [the hospital] are encouraging these types of deals."

Percy's View of All Departmental Administrators

There is variation in department administrators' performance, and their bosses are the department chairs. Percy believes many of the departmental administrators lack the appropriate skills set and experience in managing clinical operations. "My office has to provide much oversight and micromanagement. Chairs should be advocates. But administrators must keep the medical center out of trouble. Maybe we should tie some of the administrators' compensation to this."

Case Study Questions

1. What can Percy do to facilitate a more meaningful relationship with both the chairs and the administrators?

2. Should faculty compensation be left to the individual departments to determine? Who else might be able to assist with this process?
3. Conceptually, is it acceptable to have faculty who do not generate a profit? If so, how are these losses typically covered?
4. Should the faculty practice be centralized or decentralized? Why?

Conversation at Tony's Coffee Shop

On December 20, 2008, three departmental administrators discussed management issues, and a summary of their discussion follows:

Sam Sabathia (cardiology administrator): Another financial crisis. The cardiology chair wants to keep recruiting, and the dean of the medical school wants us to cut costs and show a profit.

Liz Burnett (medicine administrator): Well, at least we're employed. Bruce Percy wants us to enroll in a leadership development program. That's certainly going to keep me from getting a lot of my work done.

Joe Rodriguez (orthopedics administrator): Pedro Santana has some special circumstances going for him in surgery. First of all, it's surgery, and second of all, his chair understands business and is not hesitant to push for what he wants.

Sam Sabathia: But Pedro runs a good show, too. His accounts receivable days are way down. Their overhead percentages are down. Surgery gets good ratings on quality and customer service. They make money for the hospital.

Liz Burnett: It's a lot easier for them to get what they want.

Joe Rodriguez: But what is Pedro doing right, and what can we learn from him?

Sam Sabathia: Pedro doesn't always spell out precisely what he's doing. He's got a lot of staff and good staff. Dr. Blinick has a business background, and he is focused on bringing in a lot of revenue. He's got a strategy in mind, even if it's in his head, and he acts on that strategy.

Liz Burnett: So how do we get the support to allow us to produce the numbers that Dr. Percy wants?

Joe Rodriguez: And what do we want, and how do we get the support that we need from our chairs?

Case Questions

1. What are the constraints and opportunities that the departmental administrators face in reaching their targets?
2. How do they overcome the constraints and take advantage of the opportunities?
3. What should Dr. Percy do to improve the performance of the faculty practices?
4. What should the dean of the school of medicine do to facilitate effectiveness and efficiency in combined operations of the FPA and departments of the medical school?
5. What should Santana do to build on the financial successes of the department of surgery? To what extent does he need to get involved more in issues outside of the department, such as the relationships between the FPA and clinical practice in surgery?

Short Case 16
Complaining Doctor and Ambulatory Care

Anthony R. Kovner

You are the assistant director for ambulatory services. An attending physician complains, "The clerks are no good in this clinic, and neither is the director of nursing." What do you say to him? Assume that the physician is an important customer.

Later during the week, he is still not satisfied. Now you are the problem. What do you do?

Short Case 17
Doctors and the Capital Budget

Anthony R. Kovner

You are the hospital CEO. Doctors on the capital budget committee cannot agree on which equipment to recommend for purchase and for how much. They are way over budget. What do you say to them?

Short Case 18
Doctors and a New Medical Day Care Program for the Terminally Ill

Anthony R. Kovner

You are the hospital CEO. Medical staff is opposed to the hospital's providing needed day care to the terminally ill, which is forecasted to break even financially. They say this is not what the hospital is supposed to do, and it will actually or potentially compete with their business. What do you say to them?

Short Case 19
Average Length of Stay

Anthony R. Kovner

You are the hospital CEO. Two of the doctors consistently keep too many of their patients in the hospital longer than the average length of stay for several diagnosis-related groups. They say their patients are older and sicker and that they're practicing higher-quality medicine. What do you say to them?

Short Case 20
Managing Relationships: Take Care of Your Nurses

Anthony R. Kovner

Betsy Cline, the patient care director of the 14-bed pediatric cardiac intensive care unit (PCICU) at Children's Hospital, has held this post for two years. The unit has an $8 million budget. Cline has worked at Children's Hospital for 16 years. She spends 50 percent of her time on patient safety, 20 percent on staffing and recruitment, and 20 percent with nurses in relation to their satisfaction with the work and with families in relation to their satisfaction with care. The remaining 10 percent of Cline's time is spent on administrative duties. She says, "What I like is working with exceptional nurses who are very

EXHIBIT IV.7
PCICU
Organization
Chart

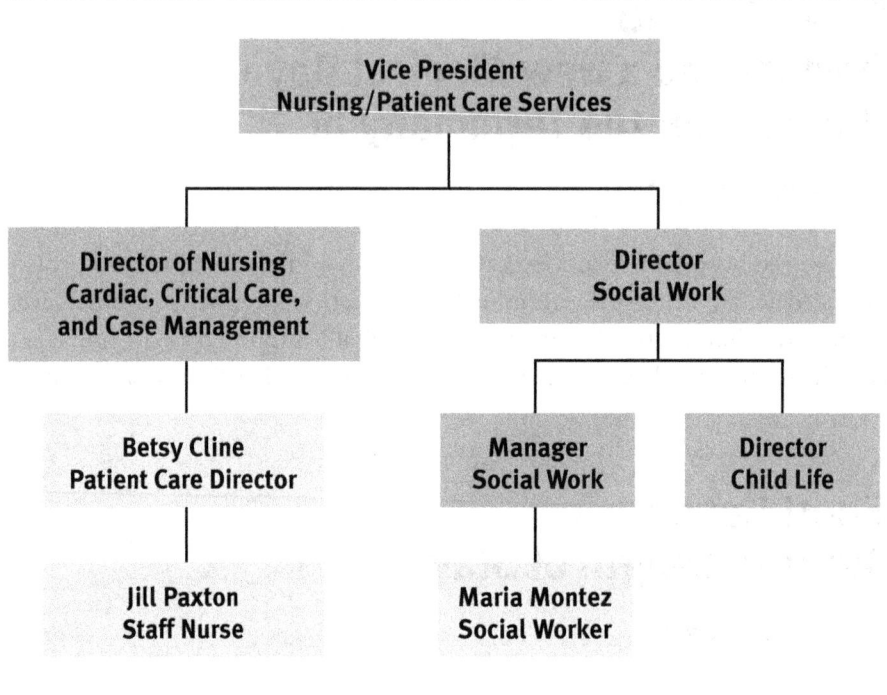

smart and do what it takes with limited resources. However, we don't always feel empowered, despite the existence of shared governance, a structure I help to coordinate." Exhibit IV.7 shows the PCICU organization chart.

Relationships with Nurses on the Unit

Nurses on the unit work three days a week, 12 hours a shift. Cline says, "My name is on the unit, not the medical director's. If anything goes wrong with the unit, they blame it on nursing. Yet I'm brushed off by people with whom I have to deal outside of the unit. For example, we have a problem with machines that analyze blood gases. I spoke with the people there about the technology. This was four weeks ago. It's a patient safety issue. I sent them e-mails. I need the work to get done. The staff don't feel empowered if I'm not empowered. This goes for other departments as well. For example, respiratory therapy starts using a new ventilator without informing us. We have never seen this machine, nor have we been in-serviced on it. They don't phone or e-mail. So I make the decision that we're not going to use the machine. With surgeons, when I tell them to wash their hands, they roll their eyes. It takes tremendous energy to deal with this."

Jill Paxton, RN, is a clinical nurse in the PCICU where she has worked for six months, having been at the hospital for nearly nine months. Paxton spends 40 percent of her time dealing with patients and families—turning, suctioning, changing dressings; 30 percent talking with physicians—negotiating plans of care and medication plans; 20 percent in medications administration and conversations with the pharmacy; and 10 percent on miscellaneous duties. She has worked on the day shift for only three weeks now, but she had also been on days for three months during orientation. Paxton says she is challenged to get the core services she needs. If she has to give a 2:00 p.m. medication, and would like the medication by 1:00 p.m., she gets it by 4:00 p.m., even if she calls. She finds it difficult to coordinate services from a child life specialist—a specialist who breaks down medical terminology to children, such as "what's about to happen to you," and who also deals with siblings. Paxton can't find the cardiac transplant consultant when she needs her and doesn't have her pager number. Paxton's main satisfactions are educating the people she's working with, repairing children and seeing them go home, and helping the family.

Relationships with Families

Cline says, "I'm clear with them in orienting families to the unit, how we do our job. We treat families with respect. Families watch me, and mentoring of nurses is important."

Paxton agrees that the unit generally does a good job supporting families. She says, "Families are kind and happy. There is a problem with turnover of doctors and residents, who aren't here two days in a row. The plan of care can get lost with attendings when they change every week. Families are told different outcomes and recovery times. Families get stressed out and are often far from home. I listen to them and ask, 'Do you have any questions?', 'What do you want to see done?', and 'Do you have any questions for the doctors?' I ask them if they want to participate in rounds. Sometimes we just listen. When families can't come in, they can call me every two hours because we have an in-house phone that accepts outside calls."

Cline and Paxton feel that families are an important part of what they do, that the unit has special structures and processes to involve families, and that what they are doing is generally working. But they lack concrete ways to measure unit performance in this regard.

Relationships with Social Work

Cline says, "The hospital has a social worker who deals with heart transplant patients. This service is fragmented, and I have difficulty getting her to come to the unit. I will go to her director or to my director if I have to. I understand she has other responsibilities, but she needs to come to rounds, to deal with issues around getting nurses for home care. Of course, social workers can't wave a magic wand."

Maria Montez, the unit social worker, has worked in the PCICU for ten years. She spends 75 percent of her time on the floors with families. She works from 9:30 a.m. to 5:30 p.m., five days a week, and there is social work coverage at other hours. The kinds of issues Montez deals with are requests for a visiting nurse; medications and associated education; ordering of oxygen; ordering a special intervention team at home if there is a need to assess; and physical, occupational, and speech therapy. If a patient is dying, Montez discusses with nursing what they can do together when crises come up.

Montez says that she has a good relationship with Cline, and that she orients the new nurses to social work. Montez respects the work that nurses do. "We're invited to each other's rounds. The work is so intense, there are so many patients. We've reached a level of understanding; if there's a problem, it's not personal. It's what we're all going through. We discuss each of the 37 patients in the three ICUs once a week at an interdisciplinary conference." Montez concludes, "If I could advise the hospital administrator, I would tell her to take care of your nurses."

Case Questions

1. What are the most important things that Betsy Cline can do to "take care of her nurses" who work in the PCICU?
2. What are the priorities for Jill Paxton?
3. How can nurses in the PCICU judge whether the unit is doing an adequate job of supporting families?
4. What advice would you give to the hospital administrator to "take better care of your nurses"?

V

ADAPTATION

A hospital is a living organism, made up of many different
parts having different functions but all these must be
in due proportion and relation to each other, and to the environment, to
produce the desired general results. The stream of life which runs through it
is incessantly changing. . . . Its work is never done;
its equipment is never complete; it is always in need of new
means of diagnosis, of new instruments and medicine; it is to
try all things and hold fast to that which is good.
—*John Shaw Billings (1889)*

COMMENTARY

Adapting to external and internal pressures for and against change is a difficult challenge for the manager of a healthcare organization (HCO). The word *adaptation* suggests a view of organizational survival and growth dependent on a specific direction of change. A closer fit between environmental demands and organizational response allows the organization to attract greater or continued resources from society.

A key paradigm here comes from marketing. In quality improvement, this is called customer-mindedness. The central idea is to find out what people want and design a product or service to meet these preferences, rather than create a product or service and convince people that they want it. Finding out what patients want and organizing to respond to those preferences is at the core of a customer-driven organization. In HCOs, the notion of patient-centered care is helping focus service delivery to meet those customer needs. Patient satisfaction surveys, focus groups, follow-up telephone calls after discharge, and community surveys are now widely used.

Organizations vary in their sensitivity to environmental pressures. HCOs function in complex environments, and failure to respond to pressures—such as competition, financing problems, and workforce issues—threatens their viability.

In all aspects of healthcare, large organizations are getting larger and capturing market share, although there is room in many markets for many smaller organizations to remain viable and grow. Competitors typically cross traditional lines. For example, large health systems may contain within them an HMO, a long-term care facility, a nursing home, home healthcare services, and neighborhood health centers. HCOs compete with each other for patients, funding, and workforce.

Medical technologies are constantly changing. Effective drugs for mental illness introduced in the 1950s led to deinstitutionalization, community-based treatment, halfway houses, and an increase in homelessness and in the jail population of the mentally ill. More than 50 percent of surgery is now done in ambulatory surgery centers and doctors' offices. Hernia surgery, which once required a 20-day hospital stay, is now routinely an ambulatory procedure. Paperless electronic health records, telemetric laboratory and radiologic testing, and computer-assisted laser surgery are already common. Digital radiology tests taken in the United States are being read by radiologists in Australia or

India. Keeping up with advances in informatics and diagnostic procedures is costly, and the benefits of those advances are difficult to accurately forecast.

HCOs are physically located in communities. But the communities they serve may be geographically local, regional, or even national, as consumers increasingly shop over the Internet and travel for services they believe to be higher in quality and less costly. Some patients have surgery in India or other countries, believing they receive adequate-quality care at a lower cost. But many organizations are locally controlled, and require strong community relations to accomplish their purpose—for example, relations with churches may be important in making sure that low-income mothers-to-be get adequate prenatal services. Some HCOs are owned by a government, with the goal of meeting the healthcare needs of nearby residents. Others serve the poor to maintain their not-for-profit tax status.

HCOs receive funding from a variety of sources, each with its own rates, regulations, and conditions. The organizations often have little influence over what they get paid by large payers and can only respond by trying to increase volume.

Payer mix is an important consideration in changing what services are started, increased, decreased, or discontinued.

HCOs are often large employers. When a healthcare facility closes, the community becomes less attractive. Conversely, opening a large new facility may be a boon to local union workers and firms.

HCOs respond to external pressures in a variety of ways, from pursuing acquisitions or mergers to selling or closing services and programs to investing (or not) in highly intensive capital technology to saturating (or not) local areas with satellite health centers. Appropriate response often requires specialized management staff in planning, marketing, community relations, data generation, and other areas. HCOs must constantly scan the environment to ensure that they can adequately respond to current developments and anticipate future trends.

THE READINGS

egun and Heatwole's cycling model of strategic planning facilitates adaptation. Traditional strategic planning does not adapt well in a dynamic environment. Begun and Heatwole emphasize continuous assessment of strategies based on feedback from benchmark analysis and dialogue with key stakeholders. They suggest using multiple scenarios and making contingency plans given the uncertainty of the future.

The supplementary readings are divided among planning and marketing articles, along with the Robinson and Dratler piece on how the Catholic Healthcare West system balances mission and margin in a capital-intensive industry. These articles focus on the organizational response rather than on the environmental pressures. Christensen, Bohmer, and Kenagy argue that the innovations that will eventually turn HCOs around are ready, in some cases—but they can't find backers. Berry and Bendapudi demonstrate the Mayo Clinic's organized, explicit approach to presenting customers with coherent, honest evidence of organizational abilities.

Griffith and White explain how planning and marketing departments of large health systems work. They review how planning departments (and internal consultants) analyze and forecast statistical data; provide expertise on complex technical problems; and maintain community values in planning decisions and capital investments. With regard to marketing and strategy, they explain how marketing is a broad approach to building exchange relationships and how to use evidence-based management to frame strategies. They also discuss segmentation of markets, listening approaches, and management of the strategic discussion.

Strategic Cycling Revisited
Note from James W. Begun,
University of Minnesota

This note updates information since this article was originally published.

The core messages of "strategic cycling" remain relevant in an environment characterized by growing pressures to improve HCOs in strategic ways. For example, to argue that HCOs can somehow deliver care that is safe, effective, equitable, efficient, patient-centered, and timely without strategic planning—by just doing more of what they currently do—is farfetched. Strategic planning allows an organization with limited resources to prioritize problems and opportunities for change, analyze and customize potential solutions, and go after them. Strategic planning is one of the most important practices healthcare administrators can bring to their organizations.

At the same time, strategic planning processes need to be more flexible and fluid than ever, to accommodate increased competition among organizations (e.g., hospitals and urgent care centers) and to be responsive to new community and personal health needs (e.g., health promotion and prevention, palliative care, behavioral and complementary health services, chronic care, and aging services). As promoted in the article, the strategic planning process, conceptually, should be "continuous"—plans are subject to revision depending on conditions that could change at any minute in significant ways. A useful piece of advice from management consultant Tom Peters (1991, 555) comes to mind: "I beg each and every one of you to develop a passionate and public hatred for bureaucracy." In the same way that bureaucracies can be mind-numbingly ineffective in changing times, so can strategic plans that rigidly prescribe activity several years into the future. (Some 30 percent of HCOs develop strategic plans with a time horizon of five years or greater [Zuckerman 2007].) Administrators should question and challenge their own plans in the interests of continuous improvement.

Three concepts would be added to the discussion of strategic cycling were it to be rewritten today. First is the concept of the learning organization. Learning has emerged as a key purpose of planning in a dynamic marketplace. Learning requires that organizations systematically collect feedback from strategic ventures. Learning has to be incorporated into the organization's mission/vision/values, and resources have to be devoted to it. Second is the concept of evidence-based management. Far too many strategies of HCOs emerge from tradition, imitation, and fad behavior (Kaissi and Begun 2008). The thoughtful consideration of evidence and customization of strategies to a local setting, coupled with a learning posture ("we will make mistakes and we will learn from them"), are part of a healthy planning process. A third concept that has emerged as useful in the planning process is the balanced scorecard. The idea that organizational performance is multidimensional, and that elements of success need to be comprehensive rather than just financial, has become widely accepted over the past decade.

Effective HCOs and their leaders will continue to plan for the future while adapting their planning processes to a dynamic environment. The strategic cycling model is a convenient and practical way to structure a flexible and fluid planning process that also promotes learning and the use of evidence in management decision making.

References

Billings, J. S. 1889. "The Plans and Purposes of the Johns Hopkins Hospital." *Boston Medical and Surgical Journal* 120 (19): 449–54.

Kaissi, A. A., and J. W. Begun. 2008. "Fads, Fashions, and Bandwagons in Healthcare Strategy." *Health Care Management Review* 33 (2): 94–102.

Peters, T. 1991. *Thriving on Chaos.* New York: HarperPerennial.

Zuckerman, A. M. 2007. *Raising the Bar: Best Practices for Healthcare Strategic Planning.* Chicago: Society for Healthcare Strategy and Market Development.

Strategic Cycling: Shaking Complacency in Healthcare Strategic Planning

Jim Begun and Kathleen B. Heatwole
From the *Journal of Healthcare Management* 44 (5), September/October 1999

Executive Summary

As the conditions affecting business and healthcare organizations in the United States have become more turbulent and uncertain, strategic planning has decreased in popularity. Strategic planning is criticized for stifling creative responses to the new marketplace and for fostering compartmentalized organizations, adherence to outmoded strategies, tunnel vision in strategy formulation, and overemphasis on planning to the detriment of implementation.

However, effective strategic planning can be a force for mobilizing all the constituents of an organization, creating discipline in pursuit of a goal, broadening an organization's perspective, improving communication among disciplines, and motivating the organization's workforce. It is worthwhile for healthcare organizations to preserve these benefits of strategic planning, at the same time recognizing the many sources of turbulence and uncertainty in the healthcare environment.

A model of "strategic cycling" is presented to address the perceived shortcomings of traditional strategic planning in a dynamic environment.

The cycling model facilitates continuous assessment of the organization's mission/values/vision and primary strategies based on feedback from benchmark analysis, shareholder impact, and progress in strategy implementation. Multiple scenarios and contingency plans are developed in recognition of the uncertain future. The model represents a compromise between abandoning strategic planning and the traditional, linear model of planning based on progress through predetermined stages to a masterpiece plan.

The popularity and significance of strategic planning reside on a pendulum in the same manner as a host of other in-favor/out-of-favor management techniques. Strategic planning is alternately hailed as the savior or denounced as the false god of organizational management. As the pendulum swings, however, much of the contemporary literature portrays planning in a negative light, as it has become fashionable to attack formal strategic planning (Gray 1986, 89; Daft and Lengel 1998, 223). Recent empirical research on the effectiveness of strategic planning is also divided; numerous studies support its efficacy, but just as many cite no relationship with organizational performance (Boyd 1991; Bruton, Oviatt, and Kallas-Bruton 1995; Powell 1992; Sinha 1990).

This article will discuss both the negative and positive features of strategic planning. The negative concerns about strategic planning are related to the dynamic environment facing organizations in general, and more recently, organizations in the healthcare industry. Discussion of the positive and negative consequences of strategic planning and the environment in which planning in healthcare organizations must take place provides a framework for the use of a strategic cycling model. This model incorporates the positive features of planning and addresses the negative consequences to guide hospitals and other complex healthcare organizations through the turbulent environment.

Potential Adverse Consequences of Strategic Planning

Many legitimate concerns about the effectiveness of strategic planning have been voiced, particularly relating to the traditional, formal, linear method. There have been situations in which formal strategic plans have been more harmful than helpful to corporate organizations, and these issues translate to the healthcare industry. Six of the major negative consequences of strategic planning follow.

1. When "planning" is initiated by an organization merely to satisfy a regulatory body's requirement for a "plan," the effort becomes

meaningless. No commitment is made on the part of key leadership, and no participation is given from those in the organization who will be responsible for implementing the plan. When the planning process becomes too bureaucratic, formalized, and irrelevant, creativity can be stifled and critical opportunities overlooked (Hax and Majluf 1991; Lenz 1985; Perry, Stott, and Smallwood 1993).

2. A bureaucratic planning process focused on top-down development may lack coordination and integration with other critical dimensions of the organization. The need for strategic integration includes not only the operational element of the organization and middle management, but other related functions such as financial resource management and information management (Hax and Majluf 1991; Henderson and Thomas 1992).

3. One of the most common complaints regarding strategic planning is the lack of flexibility and responsiveness, particularly in a dynamic and rapidly changing environment. In many organizations, strategic planning has become so much of a science, with graphs, charts, statistics, and projections, that there is no accommodation for the art, intuition, and innovation that is so necessary if planning is to be effective (Luke and Begun 1994). Plans that are too rigid and detailed can inhibit flexibility and innovation (Aaker 1992; McDaniel 1997).

4. An interesting phenomenon that can be a significant negative consequence of planning is the automatic buy-in that can occur when a "masterpiece plan" is created. After creation of the masterpiece, the tendency is to try to make the plan work. Two factors are at work: (1) a fear of loss of face if plans change fosters an adherence to the plan even in situations where a change of course is clearly indicated (Mintzberg 1994); and (2) "organizations will generally tend to make changes closely related to their current strategies . . . to stay within their strategic comfort zone beyond which the organization does not wish to venture" (Shortell, Morrison, and Friedman 1992, 35).

5. Using the past to project the future is also a potential negative consequence of a formal planning process. The often-erroneous assumption that the future will follow past trends can lead to the development of flawed strategies. This emphasis on the past can lead to "the creation of strategies that are either repetitions of a largely irrelevant past or imitations of other organizations" (Wall and Wall 1995, 49). Ohmae (1982) refers to this flaw as "strategic tunnel vision," where the greater the need to broaden the vision, the more likely the tendency to narrow the focus, eliminating potentially viable options.

6. A final and deadly complaint against strategic planning is that too much attention and effort are placed on the development of the plan and

strategies, and very little on implementation and monitoring. In many cases, the plan becomes the end of the process, not the spark to move the organization to change (Abell 1993; Curtis 1994).

The Positives of Good Strategic Planning

The listed adverse consequences are all legitimate complaints about the potential of strategic planning. Just as many positive consequences are associated with planning, and these play a part in the success of many organizations. Following are several positive elements that are important to preserve as a new planning model is developed:

1. Strategic planning can provide an overarching direction or roadmap for an organization. As the various constituencies of the organization develop their individual objectives, the strategic planning process provides a framework so that efforts are coordinated with organizational strategies. The strategic planning process can help ensure that the key managers understand and are working in support of common organizational objectives (Hax and Majluf 1991).
2. Organizational discipline and control are also identified as positive results associated with a strategic planning process. The previous section identified the potential problems inherent in a process that "controls"; however, in any organization, particularly in unstable dynamic situations, a mechanism should be in place that forces the organization to envision the future, to look long term, and to be vigilant of potential opportunities and threats. In volatile settings, it is important to "find patterns in what appears to be a chaotic and constantly changing environment. The leaders will be the ones who are able to see order within the chaos . . . and who know how to use it" (Primozic, Primozic, and Leben 1991, 5).
3. Strategic planning can also provide the basis for an organizational decision-making process. Strategic planning provides the information and analysis needed to evaluate situations, opportunities, and strategies. A strategic planning process that encourages participation broadens the organization's perspective by considering divergent viewpoints and interpretations of possible strategies. The planning process is a catalyst through which an organization can develop consensus among the leadership on major strategies (Birnbaum 1990).
4. Improving overall communication among the various disciplines of an organization is another positive benefit associated with a

strategic planning process (Langley 1989). The process educates the organizational team on the issues and choices faced by the organization, and can direct managers to think beyond their own departmental time frames and work with the organizational timelines in a focused and coordinated manner (Perry, Stott, and Smallwood 1993).

5. Another potential benefit of a strategic planning process is its motivational influence. Workers find the knowledge that their organization constantly assesses the dynamic environment and plans strategies to ensure organizational survival reassuring. The workforce is more secure in its future knowing that the organization is planning for whatever the future brings.

Planning in a Dynamic Environment

Many business organizations in the United States have discovered that the environment is changing too rapidly for a static, reactive planning process. Instead, attention has shifted to taking advantage of temporary gains, creating new products and markets, and staking out new competitive spaces (D'Aveni 1994; Hamel and Prahalad 1994; Moore 1996). The healthcare industry is following corporate America in facing a turbulent, uncertain environment. Healthcare is transitioning from a stable, comfortable, and complacent past to a confusing present and unpredictable future. All of the key aspects of the industry are experiencing dramatic shifts. A simple continuum analysis demonstrates the turbulence of the current healthcare environment. This continuum of the "Cs" (depicted in Exhibit V.1) highlights the challenges facing the healthcare industry.

EXHIBIT V.1
Healthcare Continuum Shifts

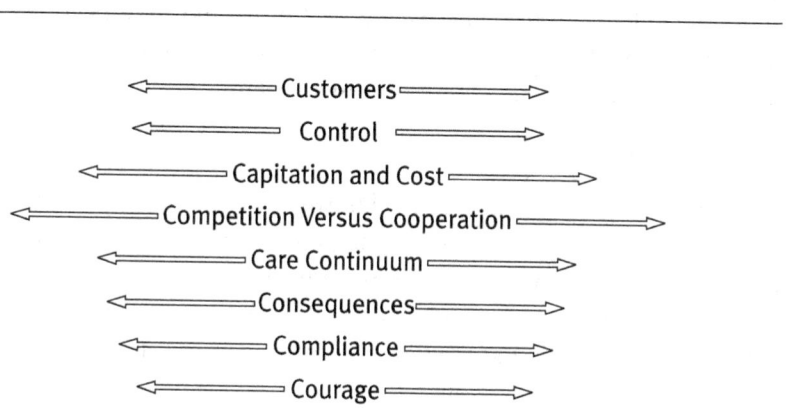

Traditionally, patients and physicians were the "customers" of most healthcare organizations. Now, business and industry and insurers are major customers. In fact, in many instances, the desires of the patient and physician are secondary and the insurers dictate the hospital provider.

Control

In the past, most healthcare organizations held independent control of their strategies and futures. Now, most are part of systems or alliances—or are considering strategies to merge or partner. The individual healthcare organization must give up some control of its destiny and focus planning efforts on the partnership in addition to each member.

Capitation and Cost

The current reimbursement environment is schizophrenic, with varying degrees of managed care penetration causing a shifting mix of payment types from capitation to cost-based to percentage of charges. The future promises even more changes in reimbursement, and planning with future revenues and financial resources unknown will be challenging at best.

Competition Versus Cooperation

Most healthcare organizations face conflicting marketing strategies. The competitive environment has grown dramatically and organizations now face predatory attacks. At the same time, however, cooperative efforts among previous rivals are becoming commonplace.

Care Continuum

The care continuum refers to the paradigm shift from treating illness to focusing on wellness and prevention. This has been a relatively new focus for the healthcare industry. However, as the healthcare industry becomes increasingly responsible for the overall health of a defined population, the emphasis on improving health will become a primary focus.

Consequences

The "consequences" continuum acknowledges the many stakeholders that are now affected by any strategy developed by a healthcare organization. An organization's planning process must consider the consequences on other related organizations and constituencies. Equally important is the evaluation of the repercussions that strategies developed by these stakeholders will have on the healthcare organization.

Compliance

The recent increase in state and federal regulatory oversight as a means of quality control has had a dramatic effect on the healthcare industry, with increased scrutiny of the operation of healthcare delivery organizations. The public's confidence in the healthcare industry has been shaken as major accusations of fraud and abuse have been leveled at the industry. Strategies will not only need to address compliance, but also prove ethics and value.

Courage

All of these changes signal a need for healthcare leaders who have the skills to make the necessary changes—who have the vision and flexibility to lead and plan in turbulent times.

In summary, the healthcare industry is facing major changes. Changing customers, a changing product and mission, changing payment mechanisms, conflicting marketing strategies, more and different stakeholders, and a need for new leadership skills are just some of the major changes in the healthcare industry. The good news is that a dynamic and uncertain environment is not all bad. The fractious nature of the environment might prove to be the catalyst to shake the complacency from the current strategic planning process found in most healthcare organizations and encourage the development of more flexible, comprehensive models. The higher levels of tension and conflict can generate new perspectives (Stacey 1992, 39).

Strategic Cycling—A Planning Model to Shake Complacency

The previous discussion reveals that the process of strategic planning must adapt and evolve to be effective in the new healthcare environment. Although much of the current literature on strategic planning focuses on the negative qualities, the need for a process for appropriate future planning remains. In fact, most of the articles condemning strategic planning have created new terms such as strategic improvising, strategic processing, strategy application, issues management, and a wealth of other descriptive labels that still identify a thoughtful, proactive method or process to evaluate and set a course of action for an organization.

Much of the current literature on improving strategic planning focuses on a particular aspect or element of planning or addresses a specific complaint regarding a formal planning process. However, the previous discussion on the potential downsides of strategic planning and description of the environment in which healthcare organizations must chart their course indicates the need for a broader perspective. What is needed is a process that preserves the positive aspects of planning that are the "baby in the bathwater," while infusing the process with the flexibility and adaptability to not only respond to the rapidly changing environment, but to anticipate and thrive on it.

The strategic cycling model presented in Exhibit V.2 is a cycle or continuous process that provides a broad focus on critical issues that a healthcare organization should consider in planning strategically. The model differs from other contemporary frameworks in its emphasis on planning as a continuous feedback process rather than a set of stages that result in a relatively permanent and institutionalized plan (Ginter, Swayne, and Duncan 1998; Zuckerman 1998).

The strategic cycling model is arranged in a circular manner to avoid the linear and proscribed formal planning processes that create rigid, inflexible masterpiece plans. However, the model does not necessarily move in a clockwise manner. The arrows located in the center indicate the flexibility and responsiveness of the model, in which the process can react and adapt quickly

EXHIBIT V.2
Strategic
Cycling Model

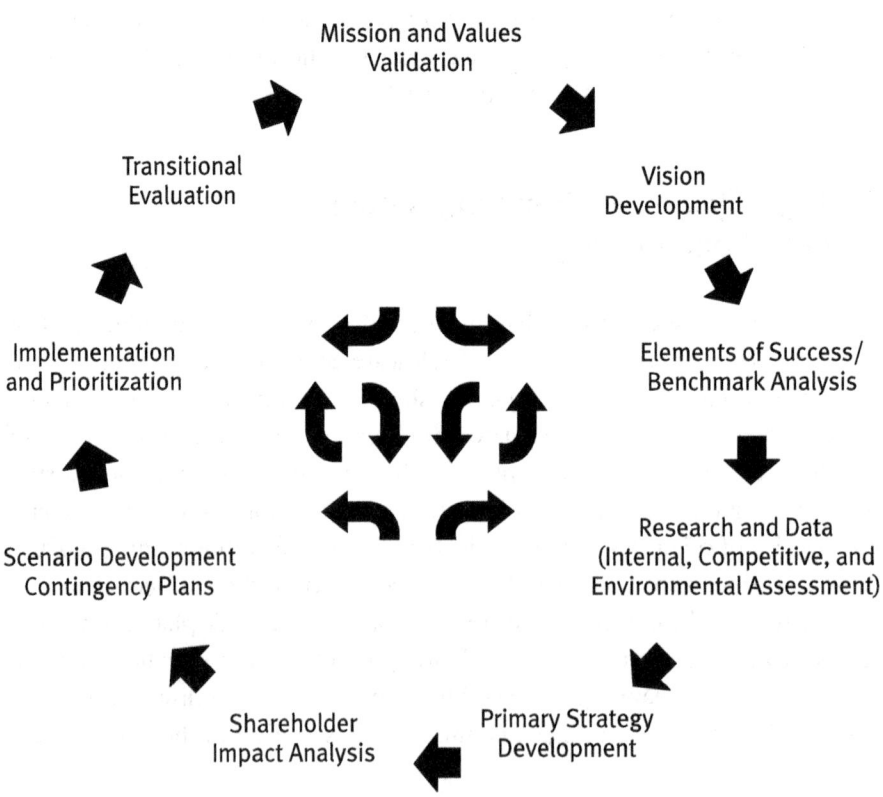

to changes in the environment. For example, an ongoing assessment of the competitive environment can detect threats that cause the leadership of the organization to develop a competitive strike contingency plan; or an analysis of the effect of certain strategies on a major stakeholder can create a need to reprioritize the strategies.

The strategic cycle is a process and not a plan. It represents a moving and flowing process of analysis and evaluation to continuously monitor the environment and adapt the organization. This cyclical or process emphasis with consideration of the relationships and contingencies must be included in a strategic planning process in these transformational times. Such a perspective facilitates systems thinking—a framework for seeing interrelationships and patterns that is often presented in terms of a continuous cycle emphasizing feedback effects (Senge 1990).

The elements of the strategic cycling process provide a broad framework to structure an approach to planning. The elements are general guidelines that should be violated to preserve innovation and creativity. Without some guidelines, however, the positive features of strategic planning dissipate. The elements of the strategic cycling model are described in more detail below.

Mission and Values Validation and Vision Development

The model uses the mission, values, and vision of the organization as the foundation for the process. However, if the mission, values, and vision become too abstract or, conversely, too specific with no room for interpretation, the planning process can become a rote confirmation of an obsolete direction. Strategic cycling calls for a revalidation of the underlying foundation of the organization. Missions are often believed to be carved in stone; however, the turbulent environment can dictate a necessary adjustment or even a major change in an organization's mission, values, and vision.

Elements of Success/Benchmark Analysis

The healthcare industry is just now beginning to catch up with its industrial and corporate counterparts in the compilation, analysis, and dissemination of comparative performance data. Most healthcare organizations track trends in their own performance for a variety of financial and clinical indicators, but those data alone lack relevance in a broader sense. Mandated reporting requirements on both state and federal levels are now providing healthcare leaders with a wealth of comparative data. In most cases, the benchmark data are adjusted for differences in populations with regard to age and severity of care for more valid comparisons. Hospital "report cards" are becoming widely published for both consumer and payer review. Decisions regarding which provider to use are made based on the comparative data.

As part of the planning process, organizations must evaluate their comparative position in the market and determine the elements of success by which they will evaluate their own performance. The analysis identifies "best practice" hospitals and the scores on particular indicators that can become benchmarks or targets for the planning organization. Organizations that want to remain competitive must engage in benchmarking; "avoiding these comparisons is like burying your head in the sand" (Cleverley 1989, 33). This step in the planning process identifies measurable goals and keeps the organization continuously looking for benchmarks to improve its performance in relation to other similar organizations. The benchmark analysis not only alerts the organization to potential problem areas; it provides an opportunity to correct indicators before they are published in public reports.

Research and Data Analysis: Internal, Competitor, and Environmental Assessment

This element of strategic cycling is the standard bearer of traditional planning. In the past, strategic plans collected data and performed the infamous Strengths/Weaknesses/Opportunities/Threats (SWOT) analysis. This element is still an important part of a planning process; however, rather than compiling a book of data, graphs, and trend lines that gathers dust on a shelf, the process of data assessment becomes an ongoing effort of monitoring and adjusting the organization in response to the analysis. A large amount of literature on environmental scanning, competitor analysis, and portfolio analytical tools suggests that these techniques continue to remain important in strategic planning (Drain and Godkin 1996; Ghoshal and Westney 1991). To avoid the negatives associated with this aspect of planning, focus should be placed on the use of the data and analysis to develop and implement strategies to prevent falling victim to the paralysis-by-analysis syndrome (Lenz 1985).

The means to create opportunities for product and service offerings that are not possible in the present environment and of "changing the environment to better suit the organization's goals" (Reeves 1993, 229) must also be considered. Possibilities for altering and creating new environments expand in uncertain times.

Primary Strategy Development

Although the term "strategy" in this element of strategic cycling is singular, the strategy development stage involves the development of multiple strategies. In this stage, the more scientific compilation of data and analysis combines with the less formal intuition and interpretation skills to develop workable strategies for the organization. An analysis of data and trends alone can lead to the development of erroneous strategies. The planning team must evaluate and interpret the data using experience and intuitive logic (Thomas, McDaniel, and Anderson 1991).

The coordination of the strategies among the various disciplines of the organization is a critical step in the process. This important activity solicits input and participation to avoid the problems discussed earlier in this article, where those responsible for implementation of the strategies had not been involved in nor did they believe in the validity of the strategies. Numerous anecdotal stories in the literature describe strategies that have been developed in direct conflict with other organizational directives. Clearly, one of the more important efforts involves integrating strategic development through the management team to all parts of the organization.

Shareholder Impact Analysis

Shareholders or stakeholders are "individuals, groups, or organizations who have a stake in the decisions and actions of an organization and who attempt to influence those decisions and actions" (Blair and Fottler 1998, 2). In the changing healthcare environment, shareholder impact analysis has become an even more critical aspect of strategic planning. Most healthcare organizations are now part of a system or alliance with other providers such as hospitals, physicians in PPO arrangements, and often with insurers to create a total product. Because of these vital relationships, planning becomes more complicated and the stakeholders must be considered in the planning process. In addition, the inter-relatedness among the stakeholders requires that the plans of these other individuals, groups, and organizations be considered as well. The concept of shareholder impact analysis is becoming a major focus in the planning literature. Whether called "linkage analysis" (Primozic, Primozic, and Leben 1991), "fostering generative relationships" (Lane and Maxfield 1996), or other creative terminology, the key is to evaluate relationships that can add value to the organization and to consider these potentially beneficial (or competitive) relationships in the development of organizational strategies.

Scenario Development/Contingency Plans

Scenario development and contingency planning are techniques that acknowledge that planning does not come with a crystal ball and that major assumptions can change with dramatic implications for the organization. Scenarios are "vehicles for helping people learn" (Schwartz 1991, 6). Obviously, an organization cannot anticipate all possible scenarios, nor do organizations have the time and financial resources to develop plans for all contingencies. The process of thinking about and planning for the unanticipated has the beneficial effect of moving leaders beyond their strategic comfort zone. The effort of scenario development and contingency planning leaves the organization better prepared for the unexpected. Scenario-based planning addresses one of the more serious negatives of strategic planning where only one possible "future" is considered.

Scenario-based planning can be very sophisticated, with computer models to run "what ifs," and the resulting analysis can be used to evaluate and develop possible actions in response to alternative situations that could arise (Georgantzas and Acar 1995). However, even if an organization does not have the computer or financial resources to simulate complex scenarios, a beneficial effect can be found in continuously evaluating and considering possible environmental changes or adverse conditions and thinking about the organization's options in response to these changes. This element of strategic cycling makes an organization more proactive and responsive, which will be a key factor of success in the turbulent healthcare environment.

Implementation and Prioritization

An often-cited negative consequence of strategic planning is that more effort goes into the development of a plan than into implementing it. One of the most important elements—it could be argued to be the most important element—of the strategic cycling process is the execution. Too often, the organization congratulates itself on the analysis, decisions, and creation of the plan, but rather than providing direction to a dynamic process of implementation, the "plan" is put on a shelf and forgotten. Implementation is one of the most critical aspects of the strategic planning process, but is often given little attention, which basically renders the plan useless.

Another important consideration in the implementation stage is the assignment of priorities. As resources are allocated to implementation of defined strategies, the allocation should be based on the strategies that have the most effect or are most critical—the top priorities for the organization. All of the key players in the organization must be committed and dedicated to the implementation of the strategies.

Transitional Evaluation

In the strategic cycling model, a continual evaluation of the implementation of the strategies completes the feedback loop. If strategies are not effective, the evaluation redirects the implementation process or redefines the strategy. Monitoring and evaluation provide for corrective action and put some control into the process. Evaluation and monitoring "make the planning effort a tangible reality rather than an academic exercise" (Birnbaum 1990, 221). In the model, the evaluation step can link back to any stage in the cycle to correct the implementation. If more data are needed, the process is flexible. If changes have taken place in the environment, then the scenario-development stage could provide possible alternative implementation efforts. Without an evaluation step, the planning process would be in serious contention to attain all of the negative results identified earlier in this article.

Conclusions

In the dynamic healthcare environment, strategic planning can be a vital and useful process to provide direction and guidance to a healthcare organization. But the possible negatives that can be associated with an ill-conceived process must be carefully considered. This article offers a strategic cycling model to broaden the planning perspective and address the potential drawbacks. The model takes into consideration the beneficial aspects of planning and focuses on a flexible, responsive, and proactive method of surviving the turbulent times. Although the current literature seems to focus on the downsides to strategic planning, a broader conceptualization of the strategic planning process provides real opportunities for healthcare organizations to face the uncertain future with confidence.

References

Aaker, D. 1992. *Developing Business Strategies.* New York: John Wiley & Sons.

Abell, D. 1993. *Managing with Dual Strategies: Mastering the Present, Preempting the Future.* New York: Free Press.

Birnbaum, W. 1990. *If Your Strategy Is So Terrific, How Come It Doesn't Work?* New York: American Management Association.

Blair, J. D., and M. D. Fottler. 1998. *Strategic Leadership for Medical Groups.* San Francisco: Jossey-Bass.

Boyd, B. 1991. "Strategic Planning and Financial Performance: A Meta-analytic Review." *Journal of Management Studies* 28 (4): 353–74.

Bruton, G., B. Oviatt, and L. Kallas-Bruton. 1995. "Strategic Planning in Hospitals: A Review and Proposal." *Health Care Management Review* 20 (3): 16–25.

Cleverley, W. 1989. "How Boards Can Use Comparative Data in Strategic Planning." *Healthcare Executive* 4 (3): 32–33.

Curtis, K. 1994. *From Management Goal Setting to Organizational Results.* Westport, CT: Quorum.

Daft, R. L., and R. H. Lengel. 1998. *Fusion Leadership.* San Francisco: Berrett-Koehler.

D'Aveni, R. A. 1994. *Hypercompetition.* New York: Free Press.

Drain, M., and L. Godkin. 1996. "A Portfolio Approach to Strategic Hospital Analysis: Exposition and Explanation." *Health Care Management Review* 21 (4): 68–74.

Georgantzas, N., and W. Acar. 1995. *Scenario-Driven Planning: Learning to Manage Strategic Uncertainty.* Westport, CT: Quorum.

Ghoshal, S., and D. Westney. 1991. "Organizing Competitor Analysis Systems." *Strategic Management Journal* 12: 17–31.

Ginter, P. M., L. E. Swayne, and W. J. Duncan. 1998. *Strategic Management of Health Care Organizations*, 3rd ed. Malden, MA: Blackwell.

Gray, D. 1986. "Uses and Misuses of Strategic Planning." *Harvard Business Review* 64: 89–97.

Hamel, G., and C. K. Prahalad. 1994. *Competing for the Future.* Boston: Harvard Business School Press.

Hax, A., and N. Majluf. 1991. *The Strategy Concept and Process.* Englewood Cliffs, NJ: Prentice Hall.

Henderson, J., and J. Thomas. 1992. "Aligning Business and Information Technology Domains: Strategic Planning in Hospitals." *Hospital & Health Services Administration* 37 (1): 71–87.

Lane, D., and R. Maxfield. 1996. "Strategy Under Complexity: Fostering Generative Relationships." *Long Range Planning* 29 (2): 215–31.

Langley, A. 1989. "In Search of Rationality: The Purposes Behind the Use of Formal Analysis in Organizations." *Administrative Science Quarterly* 34: 598–631.

Lenz, R. T. 1985. "Paralysis by Analysis: Is Your Planning System Becoming Too Rational?" *Long Range Planning* 18 (4): 64–72.

Luke, R., and J. Begun. 1994. "Strategy Making in Health Care Organizations." In *Health Care Management*, 3rd ed., ed. by S. M. Shortell and A. D. Kaluzny, 355–91. Albany, NY: Delmar.

McDaniel, R. R., Jr. 1997. "Strategic Leadership: A View from Quantum and Chaos Theories." In *Handbook of Health Care Management*, ed. by W. J. Duncan, P. M. Ginter, and L. E. Swayne, 339–67. Malden, MA: Blackwell.

Mintzberg, H. 1994. *The Rise and Fall of Strategic Planning.* New York: Free Press.

Moore, J. F. 1996. *The Death of Competition.* New York: HarperCollins.

Ohmae, K. 1982. *The Mind of the Strategist.* New York: McGraw-Hill.

Perry, T., R. Stott, and W. N. Smallwood. 1993. *Real-Time Strategy.* New York: John Wiley & Sons.

Powell, T. 1992. "Research Notes and Communications—Strategic Planning as Competitive Advantage." *Strategic Management Journal* 13: 551–58.

Primozic, K., E. Primozic, and J. Leben. 1991. *Strategic Choices: Supremacy, Survival, or Sayonara.* New York: McGraw-Hill.

Reeves, P. 1993. "Issues Management: The Other Side of Strategic Planning." *Hospital & Health Services Administration* 38 (2): 229–41.

Schwartz, P. 1991. *The Art of the Long View.* New York: Currency Doubleday.

Senge, P. 1990. *The Fifth Discipline.* New York: Currency Doubleday.

Shortell, S., E. Morrison, and B. Friedman. 1992. *Strategic Choices for America's Hospitals.* San Francisco: Jossey-Bass.

Sinha, D. 1990. "The Contribution of Formal Planning to Decisions." *Strategic Management Journal* 11: 479–92.

Stacey, R. 1992. *Managing the Unknowable.* San Francisco: Jossey-Bass.

Thomas, J., R. McDaniel, and R. Anderson. 1991. "Hospitals as Interpretation Systems." *Health Services Research* 25 (6): 859–80.

Wall, S., and S. Wall. 1995. *The New Strategists.* New York: Free Press.

Zuckerman, A. M. 1998. *Healthcare Strategic Planning.* Chicago: Health Administration Press.

Discussion Questions for the Required Reading

1. What is strategic planning?
2. Begun and Heatwole emphasize continuous assessment of strategies based on feedback from benchmark analysis and stakeholder impact. Why don't most HCOs use this model? What would it take for these organizations to adopt the Begun and Heatwole model?
3. Who is responsible for carrying out adaptive activities for the small, midsized, and large nonprofit HCO?
4. Where does marketing fit into an organization's plans for adapting to changes in its environment?

Required Supplementary Readings

Berry, L. L., and N. Bendapudi. 2003. "Clueing in Customers." *Harvard Business Review* (February): 100–106.

Christensen, C. M., R. Bohmer, and J. Kenagy. 2000. "Will Disruptive Innovations Cure Healthcare?" *Harvard Business Review* (September–October): 102–12.

Foreman, S. 2004. "Montefiore Medical Center in the Bronx, New York: Improving Health in an Urban Community." *Academic Medicine* 79 (12): 1154–61.

Griffith, J. R., and K. White. 2010. "Knowledge Management," "Human Resources Management," and "Marketing and Strategy." In *Reaching Excellence in Healthcare Management.* Chicago: Health Administration Press.

Robinson, J. C., and S. Dratler. 2006. "Corporate Structure and Capital Strategy at Catholic Healthcare West." *Health Affairs* 25 (1): 134–47.

Steiger, N., and A. Balog. 2010. "Realizing Patient-Centered Care: Putting Patients in the Center, Not the Middle." *Frontiers of Health Services Management* 26 (4): 15–25.

Discussion Questions for Required Supplementary Readings

1. What is distinctive about the marketing approaches carried out at the Mayo Clinic?

2. The authors suggest that healthcare may be the most entrenched, change-averse industry in the United States. Why is this so? How is performance-based reimbursement changing the situation, if at all?

3. What can academic medical centers do to extend the reach of their mission and serve surrounding communities? Are they obligated to do this?

4. Give an example of an environmental pressure affecting large group practices, and suggest alternative ways in which the group practices can adapt to these pressures.

5. How do large hospitals raise the capital they need to adapt to change? How does Catholic Healthcare West balance mission and margin in the capital-intensive hospital industry?

6. What is involved if an HCO commits to realizing patient-centered care?

Recommended Supplementary Readings

Arndt, M., and B. Bigelow. 2000. "The More Things Change, the More They Stay the Same." *Health Care Management Review* 25 (1): 65–72.

Berkowitz, E. N. 2006. *Essentials of Healthcare Marketing*, 2nd ed. Boston: Jones and Bartlett.

Bigelow, B., and M. Arndt. 1994. "Great Expectations: An Analysis of Four Strategies." *Medical Care Review* 51 (2): 205–33.

Collins, J. C., and J. I. Porras. 1996. "Building Your Company's Vision." *Harvard Business Review* (September–October): 65–77.

Davenport, T. H., and J. G. Harris. 2007. *Competing on Analytics.* Boston: Harvard Business School Press.

Garvin, D. A., and M. A. Roberto. 2001. "What You Don't Know About Making Decisions." *Harvard Business Review* (September): 108–16.

Griffith, J. R., and K. White. 2006. "Planning and Internal Consulting" and "Marketing and Strategy." In *The Well-Managed Healthcare Organization*, 6th ed. Chicago: Health Administration Press.

Griffith, J. R., and K. R. White, with P. Cahill. 2003. *Thinking Forward: Six Strategies for Highly Successful Organizations.* Chicago: Health Administration Press.

Kizer, K. W. 1998. "Healthcare, Not Hospitals: Transforming the Veterans Health Administration." In *Straight from the CEO.* New York: Simon and Schuster.

Kotter, J. P. 1995. "Leading Change: Why Transformation Efforts Fail." *Harvard Business Review* (March–April): 2–10.

Mintzberg, H. 1994. "The Fall and Rise of Strategic Planning." *Harvard Business Review* 72 (1): 107–14.

Porter, M. E., and E. O. Teisberg. 2006. *Redefining Healthcare.* Boston: Harvard Business School Press.

Reichheld, F. F. 2001. "Lead for Loyalty." *Harvard Business Review* (July–August): 76–84.

Rindler, M. E. 2007. *Strategic Cost Reduction.* Chicago: Health Administration Press.

Senge, P. M. 1990. *The Fifth Discipline: The Art and Practice of the Learning Organization.* New York: Doubleday Currency.

Zuckerman, A. M. 2006. "Advancing the State of the Art in Healthcare Strategic Planning." *Frontiers of Health Services Management* 23 (2): 3–15.

THE CASES

Adaptive capability involves organizational responses to new conditions. Organizations must be innovative or proactive in responding to the pressures of competitors and regulators and to the expectations of various stakeholder groups—from customers to physicians. One indicator of adaptive capability is the presence of specialized units to carry out certain functions, such as strategic planning and marketing, that are concerned specifically with adapting rather than with operations.

Strategic planning is an important managerial function. It can be conducted through a special unit, through some part of a special unit, directly by management, or by some combination of the above. Top management sees to it that information about the organization's business is gathered. Questions about the organization's mission, services, customers, competition, and strategies are addressed.

Milio (1983) reminds us that organizations have limited problem-solving capacities; they avoid uncertainty, engage in biased searches for ways of adapting, act on the basis of limited knowledge, and select alternatives on the basis of past successes.

Decisions to adapt can run counter to organizational goals and system maintenance. Even if the decisions can be shown, in hindsight, to have been technically appropriate, they may have been politically inappropriate. Managers may fail to consider the values of important stakeholders when they plan how to attain their mission and strategy. We are assuming, of course, that the HCO already has a carefully worked out mission and strategy, which it constantly reassesses in terms of competitive and regulatory pressures and in terms of the preferences and expectations of stakeholders, such as physicians and nurses.

The three long case studies in this section deal with questions of adapting the organization to meet the needs of employees and patients. How these questions are answered and what strategies are selected may have consequences that are different for specific organizations and for specific managers. In the case "Challenges for Mammoth Health System," the CEO, Barb Northrop, is faced with a set of choices involving setting priorities for her organization, given the health system's desire to become an employer of choice. In "An Investment Decision at Central Med Health System," an investment decision will impact product focus and delivery for the health system, and have broad

323

implications for a variety of stakeholders. In "Cultural Competency at Marion County Health Center," Patricia Cole must address problems associated with racial and ethnic health disparities, perceptions of discrimination, and issues associated with cultural diversity, considering both the perspectives of multiple stakeholders and implications for the future of the health center.

The five short cases examine different issues around adaptation from multiple perspectives. The first short case study raises the basic issues from a management perspective—that of a new chief of ob-gyn—and tests your skills at developing an organized, coherent response. In the second short case, hospital board members provide their perspectives about a CEO's decision to sell an HMO. A physician perspective is examined when increasing competition forces a private physician to consider a new strategic direction for her practice in the third short case. The fourth short case explores the issue of disparities in care from the perspective of a hospital CEO faced with evidence that his hospital is providing disparate care. In the final short case, both clinical and management perspectives must be considered in the context of an opportunity for a health clinic to become a patient-centered medical home.

Reference

Milio, N. 1983. "Health Care Organizations and Innovation." In *Health Services Management: Readings and Commentary,* 2nd ed., ed. by A. R. Kovner and D. Neuhauser, 448–64. Chicago: Health Administration Press.

Case M
Challenges for Mammoth Health System: Becoming the Best Around

Ann Scheck McAlearney

Mammoth Health System

The six hospitals that made up Mammoth Health System (MHS) enjoyed some of the best weather the United States had to offer. Nonetheless, Barb Northrop, the chief executive officer (CEO) of MHS, had the same view as her employees—four walls of a relatively large cubicle. Her cube was one among many located on the second floor of the system's corporate office building. She had insisted on this arrangement when corporate services had moved to the new site. Senior executives, directors, managers, and staff analysts all had cubes, leaving window views for the meeting rooms and conference rooms located along the building's exterior walls.

Northrop had assumed the CEO role six months ago, and she was still trying to digest all the issues and opportunities confronting the health system. Currently, MHS was struggling to compete with the region's other major health system, and MHS had not been winning the battle. Aurora Health System, capitalizing on its reputation as an academic specialty referral center, had spent the previous five years gradually expanding its market share and luring away capable employees from MHS. Northrop's recent promotion to CEO from chief nursing officer (CNO) presented her with the new opportunity to assess reality for MHS and to make decisions that could set MHS on a better path.

Taking Stock of MHS

When Northrop had taken the helm at MHS, her first step had been to assemble her executive team and get a sense of the extent of MHS's problems and opportunities. Her chief quality officer, Rebecca Robinson, was particularly helpful, especially given Robinson's access to data and expertise with data analysis.

Robinson pointed out that MHS patient satisfaction scores were very positive, and she showed Northrop how these scores had been above 90 percent for the past three years. Northrop, however, was not convinced. She knew that patient satisfaction scores tended to be high and suspected that these scores did not tell the whole story—after all, patients were selecting Aurora hospitals over MHS hospitals. Northrop decided she needed to learn more, so she enlisted the help of her new management fellow, Kevin Pickett, to investigate the topic of patient satisfaction measurement at MHS and elsewhere.

Patient Satisfaction Measurement

Pickett was excited about his first big project working for Northrop, and began to learn everything he could about patient satisfaction. Reviewing MHS's patient satisfaction survey data, he saw that satisfaction was high and had been high for several years, just as Robinson had noted. However, he was also skeptical. What did 90 percent mean at MHS? What could this be compared to?

After doing a little digging, Pickett found that many hospitals' individually reported patient satisfaction scores were above 90 percent. In fact, high levels of patient satisfaction were touted on most hospitals' websites, but again he wondered, what did 90 percent mean?

Examining the Evidence for Patient Satisfaction Measurement

Pickett decided to investigate the evidence further and logged into the hospital's library website, where he had access to a variety of searchable databases. Beginning a rudimentary search, he selected the PubMed database first; he then added the Academic Source Complete, Health and Consumer Information, and Business Source Complete databases so he could conduct a search for evidence both within and outside the healthcare literature.

Knowing that the broad term "patient satisfaction" would return too many articles for him to review, Pickett combined search terms such as "patient satisfaction rates" with "comparison." Nonetheless, he was still overwhelmed by the number of articles his search uncovered, so he decided to narrow his findings by refining his search to retrieve only review articles. Pickett knew that review articles were often helpful because they reviewed and summarized a number of different articles on a given topic. Using this focused search strategy, he was able to cull through the refined search results to uncover a few key papers, and began to scan the articles so he could start to make sense of the evidence.

Patient satisfaction scores, Pickett learned, were less informative when surveys were conducted internally and not benchmarked against other institutions. However, national firms conducted patient satisfaction surveys for their clients, and these firms could aggregate their data and compare individual hospitals' and health systems' scores with those of hospitals with similar characteristics. A benchmarked comparison such as this could provide individual hospitals with more specific information about their patient satisfaction levels because these levels had been measured in the same way as levels had been measured in other hospitals, thus enabling across-hospital comparisons.

With a few more clicks, Pickett soon found the website for Press Ganey, a firm known for survey-based measurement of patient satisfaction in healthcare, and began to explore the information it provided. He noted that Press Ganey did indeed provide the comparative benchmark information that MHS might find helpful, and it also offered clients an opportunity to drill down into their patient satisfaction data by providing reports by unit, by department, and so forth.

Pickett reported back to Northrop with a major recommendation—MHS should consider revising its patient satisfaction measurement program and begin to benchmark itself against other hospitals using a survey and measurement process that enabled across-site comparisons as well as unit-level information on satisfaction levels.

Getting a New Baseline

Northrop was not particularly surprised by Pickett's recommendation—she suspected there were opportunities to learn more from patient-based surveys—so she set about the task of obtaining board-level support for the new expense of using a national firm to perform patient satisfaction surveys. She made the compelling case that this investment could provide information about how MHS could better compete against Aurora and other regional hospitals, as well as highlighting how benchmarked data could be used to guide other efforts to improve quality of care and patient service within MHS.

The board agreed to Northrop's proposal, and the stage was set for MHS to get new patient satisfaction data. Robinson was happy to lead the process, and all was moving along nicely—until the new numbers came out.

When compared to similar hospitals and health systems across the country, MHS's patient satisfaction rates were abysmal—only 11 percent of patients were reportedly satisfied with the care and service they received at MHS. According to the new benchmarked data, MHS was among the worst in patient satisfaction nationwide. What was going on?

Looking Further

Northrop was surprised at the poor showing for MHS, but also secretly pleased. She knew that this new information could provide the motivation for MHS to embark on what she perceived as needed organizational changes—and she knew that organizational change was never easy. The shockingly low patient satisfaction scores might well provide a "burning platform" that could promote a sense of urgency to change things around a bit at MHS.

However, Northrop also knew that these poor numbers would not be accepted blindly by either the physicians or board members who monitored these metrics. She enlisted Pickett's help once again to examine the unit-level patient satisfaction rates to learn more from the new satisfaction surveys.

Looking further at the satisfaction data, Pickett noted that one area in particular stood out—MHS employee attitudes were rated very poorly, and this had clearly translated to low levels of patient satisfaction. Pickett took this detailed information to Northrop and was curious about how she would react.

Examining Employee Satisfaction Data

Northrop considered herself a data person and was delighted that the new satisfaction survey data had sufficient detail to enable MHS to investigate issues that might be contributing to poor patient satisfaction. The detailed information about poor employee attitudes suggested there were problems throughout MHS that were contributing to negative attitudes, and, in Northrop's eyes, these problems presented opportunities.

Because she had been an employee at MHS, Northrop knew the organization regularly collected information about employee attitudes and their satisfaction as part of its annual employee survey. She asked Pickett to investigate further and provide her with a summary of employee satisfaction survey data from the past five years.

This request took a little time to complete, but within the week Pickett was able to show Northrop results of the MHS employee satisfaction survey that appeared consistent with the negative employee attitudes recently found in the patient surveys. What surprised Northrop, though, was that despite fairly low turnover rates at MHS, employees, on average, were not particularly pleased with MHS as a place to work—and this had not changed much over the past five years.

Employees Were Not Satisfied

The overall sense Northrop gleaned from these survey scores was that employees perceived that MHS was a "good" place to work because of factors such as the location, the benefits, and the fact that employees felt fairly secure about not losing their jobs because of layoffs. However, the scores indicated that MHS was far from "great," and, in fact, showed consistently low marks in "focus on people," "caring about employee development," or "likelihood to recommend MHS as a place to work." Further, while the results showed some variation by department, they had also been relatively stable over the past five years the survey had been performed.

Northrop was convinced. As she reflected to Pickett, "MHS certainly seems to have some work to do to improve employee satisfaction—and this has been the case for some time. It's time for us to start paying attention."

Considering How to Improve

Northrop asked Pickett to get Robinson and bring their computers and their data to the second-floor conference room. She also wanted them to bring along full cups of coffee so they would be ready to tackle the problems they now saw MHS faced.

When Pickett returned with Robinson, Northrop welcomed them both and immediately turned to the conference room's whiteboard to write one word: "Baldrige."

Northrop went on to explain that the Baldrige program had been established as a public–private partnership focused on quality improvement and performance excellence in US organizations. As she noted, the Baldrige Performance Excellence Program (2012a) tries to help organizations across industries improve, highlighting three focus areas:

1. Help organizations achieve best-in-class levels of performance.
2. Identify and recognize role-model organizations.
3. Identify and share best management practices, principles, and strategies.

Not surprisingly, Robinson was familiar with the Baldrige program, and quickly found the program websites listing the Baldrige Criteria and providing information about previous winners of the Baldrige Award in the various categories (e.g., small business, education, manufacturing) (Baldrige 2012b). She discovered that while the Baldrige Award had been presented to outstanding organizations since 1988, the first award in the healthcare sector had not been given until 2002. Since then, a handful of HCOs had been recognized with the award, but none in MHS's local area.

Northrop was excited. Looking over Robinson's shoulder, she pointed to the information on the website about the Baldrige Criteria for Performance Excellence. As described on the website, "The Criteria work as an integrated framework for managing an organization. They are simply a set of questions focusing on critical aspects of management that contribute to performance excellence" (Baldrige 2012c). The seven listed criteria were as follows:

1. Leadership
2. Strategic planning
3. Customer focus
4. Measurement, analysis, and knowledge management
5. Workforce focus
6. Operations focus
7. Results

In addition, the website contained "Health Care Criteria for Performance Excellence," a PDF version of the workbook that helps organizations guide their Baldrige performance improvement efforts (Baldrige 2011).

While Northrop knew that MHS had a long way to go, she suspected that the Baldrige Criteria could provide an evidence-based framework to guide MHS's efforts to improve in patient satisfaction and other performance areas. She was particularly concerned about the workforce focus area, given the data MHS had gathered about employee attitudes.

Reviewing the workforce focus section of the guidebook, Northrop was particularly struck by their use of the term "high performance." As she read in the booklet, "The Workforce Focus category examines your ability to assess workforce capability and capacity needs and build a workforce environment conducive to high performance" (Baldrige 2011). Turning to Pickett, she asked him to investigate the notion of high-performance work practices in HCOs to see what that meant and to find additional information that could focus MHS's efforts to improve.

Use of High-Performance Work Practices in Healthcare Organizations

Pickett's review of both the peer-reviewed and "gray" literature (i.e., reports, articles, and information available in non-peer-reviewed sources such as trade journals, the Internet, and through consultants and other organizations) showed that the topic of high-performance work practices (HPWPs) had been of interest for some time, and that several recent research studies had emphasized the topic over the past year. Digging more deeply, Pickett found that in the past year alone, a conceptual model had been proposed to examine HPWPs in HCOs (Garman et al. 2011), and the applicability of this model had then been investigated through a series of case studies of HCOs that were considered good places to work (McAlearney et al. 2011). Also related to this evidence was a third article in the series exploring the issue of how HCOs might create a business case for investment in HPWPs (Song et al. 2012), but as Song and her colleagues explained, a business case was, in practice, difficult to quantitatively establish.

As Garman and colleagues (2011, 202) state, "HPWPs can be defined as a set of practices within organizations that enhance organizational outcomes by improving the quality and effectiveness of employee performance." Their examples of such work practices include involving employees in organizational decision making, applying selective hiring practices, and using rigorous recruiting practices. Various work practices can be considered HPWP "subsystems," thus providing an organizing framework for how to think about four main areas of HPWPs: (1) staff engagement, (2) leadership alignment and development, (3) staff acquisition and development, and (4) frontline empowerment (Garman et al. 2011; McAlearney et al. 2011).

While Pickett's own introduction to MHS had been through the highly selective fellowship application process, he was unsure about how other employees were recruited and selected for the various jobs spread across the many MHS entities. Further, he knew from his review of the most recent MHS employee survey that the vast majority of employees did not feel included in MHS decisions—at their individual job level, at their unit level, or at the broader organization level. Instead, Pickett sensed—as he reviewed the practices and subsystems proposed as a model of HPWPs in HCOs (see sidebar)—that MHS had a long way to go.

Moving Ahead

Northrop knew that focusing on people was the right thing to do, but she also knew she could not change the organization on her own. Given MHS's poor

---

High-Performance Work Practices (HPWPs) Proposed to Influence Employee and Organizational Outcomes in HCOs

HPWP Subsystem 1: Staff Engagement
  Communicating mission and vision
  Information sharing
  Employee involvement in decision making
  Performance-driven rewards/recognition
HPWP Subsystem 2: Leadership Alignment/Development
  Leadership training linked to organizational goals
  Succession planning
  Performance-contingent rewards
HPWP Subsystem 3: Staff Acquisition/Development
  Rigorous recruiting
  Selective hiring
  Career development
  Extensive training
HPWP Subsystem 4: Frontline Empowerment
  Employment security
  Employment safety
  Reduced status distinctions
  Teams/decentralized decision making

Source: McAlearney et al. (2011).

marks in both patient and employee satisfaction, she suspected that the HPWP model might provide a framework for examining MHS's "people practices," and for uncovering specific areas for improvement. They already had compelling baseline data in both areas that suggested MHS was far from perfect; thus the case could be made that the status quo was no longer acceptable.

Yet, as the literature was starting to show (e.g., Song et al. 2012), investing in HPWPs was still being pursued as a "leap of faith" rather than because it could demonstrate a proven return on investment. In addition, Northrop knew that the broader Baldrige application process itself was expensive, to say nothing of the investments that would be required in MHS to support needed changes throughout the health system if MHS had any hope of making a case for performance excellence in their Baldrige application.

As Northrop reviewed the evidence that Robinson and Pickett had presented, she wondered what she should do next. She knew that she needed the support of her executive leadership team and solid commitment from the health system's board if she was going to make progress and transform MHS. However, she also knew that she had to proceed carefully if she was going to propose substantial changes for the organization—especially as she had only been leading MHS for a short time.

Case Questions

1. What are Northrop's current options for MHS? What are the pros and cons of the different options she might recommend?
2. What option do you recommend that Northrop propose for MHS? Why?
3. Given the option you select, outline a proposal that Northrop could use to make her case to the board. What do you need to include in your proposal to make this case as strong as possible? What additional information would you need to support this proposal?
4. Outline a communications plan that Northrop can use to present the outline of this proposal to MHS employees. Again, what should be included in this plan? Is there anything that should be left out?

References

Baldrige Performance Excellence Program. 2012a. "About Us." *National Institute of Standards and Technology.* Accessed August 3. www.nist.gov/baldrige/about/what_we_do.cfm.

———. 2012b. "Baldrige Award Recipients' Contacts and Profiles." *National Institute of Standards and Technology.* Accessed August 3. www.baldrige.nist.gov/Contacts_Profiles.htm.

———. 2012c. "Criteria for Performance Excellence." *National Institute of Standards and Technology.* Accessed August 3. www.nist.gov/baldrige/publications/criteria .cfm.

———. 2011. "2011–2012 Health Care Criteria for Performance Excellence." *National Institute of Standards and Technology.* Accessed August 3. www.nist .gov/baldrige/publications/upload/2011_2012_Health_Care_Criteria.pdf.

Garman, A., A. S. McAlearney, M. Harrison, P. Song, and M. McHugh. 2011. "High-Performance Work Systems in Health Care Management, Part 1: Development of an Evidence-Informed Model." *Health Care Management Review* 36 (3): 201–13.

McAlearney, A. S., A. Garman, P. Song, M. McHugh, J. Robbins, and M. Harrison. 2011. "High-Performance Work Systems in Health Care Management, Part 2: Qualitative Evidence from Five Case Studies." *Health Care Management Review* 36 (3): 214–26.

Song, P., J. Robbins, A. Garman, and A. S. McAlearney. 2012. "High-Performance Work Systems in Health Care, Part 3: The Role of the Business Case." *Health Care Management Review* 37 (2): 110–21.

Case N
An Investment Decision at
Central Med Health System

Emily Allinder, Jason Dopoulos, Breanne Pfotenhauer, David Reisman, Erick Vidmar, Jason Waibel, and Ann Scheck McAlearney

Background

Central Med Health System (CMHS) was created on January 1, 1996, with the mission of "providing expert healthcare to the people of North Central Iowa." The nonprofit organization is composed of two general, acute care hospitals, Central Med Hospital and Shelty Hospital, with a combined total of 395 beds. The service area consists of a six-county region in North Central Iowa: Rich, Crawford, Ashville, Morris, Huron, and Knowell counties. Central Med is the largest provider of healthcare services between the cities of Cletan and Flagship. The health system provides a complete range of primary care and specialty practices. Central Med Hospital offers a Level II trauma center and a Level II perinatal department. Other featured services include cardiac care, comprehensive neurological services, cancer care, behavioral health, maternity services, sports medicine, surgical services, pediatric therapy services, speech therapy services, industrial health and safety services, home care, and hospice care.

All services and business units are driven by the mission, vision, and values of Central Med. Central Med's vision is to provide "expert care close to home." The organization seeks to be the provider of choice for residents of North Central Iowa and strives to dissuade residents from traveling to Cletan or Flagship for care. The core values as stated by Central Med include:

- *Quality*: We will be known for excellence in all that we do.
- *Customer service*: We will work to fulfill the individual needs of every patient, family member, and visitor.
- *Innovation*: We will continually strive to develop and work with the latest processes available in every department.
- *Teamwork*: Our staff will work together to provide our patients with the best care possible.

Financial Status

CMHS is a financially stable organization. Operating margins have been consistent with similar BBB bond-rated organizations over the past three years and currently stand at 3 percent. A $12 million endowment provides consistent investment returns, which contributed to a total margin of 8 percent last fiscal year. CMHS maintains a prudent balance sheet with a debt-to-capitalization ratio of 25 percent. Days cash on hand has averaged 225 over the last three years, and the current ratio was 2.5 last year, demonstrating the facility's ability to cover its operating expenses. CMHS has historically used debt to finance capital projects, but due to evaporation of liquidity in the municipal bond markets, the system decided to fund certain projects with cash from operations.

The Problem

Like other nonprofit healthcare providers, CMHS struggles to enhance patient care with limited financial and capital resources. Investments in new clinical programs are evaluated carefully to ensure that patients have access to the appropriate new programs and services. CMHS strives to balance the need to invest in the clinical programs that are most important to its patient population with the need to remain financially viable.

CMHS leadership is currently faced with a difficult decision. The system has $13 million to invest in a clinical expansion project, and stakeholders throughout the organization have varying ideas about which program is most deserving of the new capital investment. While certain members of the leadership team want to invest in an expanded radiation oncology program, others are interested in bolstering heart services by enhancing the interventional cardiology program.

Option 1: Radiation Oncology

The American Cancer Society, the *Journal of Oncology Management*, the Health Care Advisory Board, and other expert sources project a 20 to 25 percent increase in the number of newly diagnosed cancer cases in the next ten years. In addition to newly diagnosed cases, the five-year relative survival rate has increased significantly as a result of newer technologies and treatments. As people live longer, the demand for cancer services will grow. Exhibit V.3 provides additional information about projected demand for radiation oncology services, and the sidebar describes the perspective of a nurse executive interested in expanding this program at CMHS.

Dr. Moh, the only radiation oncologist at CMHS, sees up to 70 patients a day, which is 40 percent more patients than the average radiation oncologist. The facilities are cramped and the schedule is tight, but somehow he is able to complete the day's work. Perhaps the friendly culture of CMHS

EXHIBIT V.3
Current Market Share—Radiation Oncology

	Total 2007 Radiation Oncology Pts.	Central Med 2007 Radiation Oncology Pts.	Central Med 2007 Radiation Oncology Market Share
Ashville	138	50	36.2%
Crawford	135	61	45.2%
Huron	189	15	7.9%
Knowell	163	24	14.7%
Morris	68	3	4.4%
Rich	419	327	78.0%
Total	1,112	480	43.2%

Projected Market Share—Radiation Oncology

	2007	Year 1	Year 2	Year 3	Year 4	Year 5
Conservative (43%–51%)	43.2%	43.3%	45.2%	47.2%	49.2%	51.1%

A Nurse Executive's Argument for Building a New Radiation Oncology Facility

Isabelle Gonzalez had served as the chief nursing officer at CMHS for 20 years. She had worked in several different departments, and was well respected and admired by her colleagues and superiors. She was known for her solid work ethic and unwavering dedication to the success of CMHS and to the provision of excellent patient care services.

Isabelle felt that building a new facility to house the radiation oncology department and its equipment was the best option. She noted that the existing facilities were "old, inefficient, cramped, and not patient friendly." She was concerned that Central Med could lose a considerable amount of market share if the health system did not remain on the leading edge of cancer care. "Cancer patients are very sick and require a high intensity and frequency of care," Isabelle stated. "We have a duty to our patients to provide comprehensive cancer services close to their homes. Besides, radiation oncology is a growing service line that contributes significantly to our operating margin."

---

keeps the staff content with current operations, but Dr. Moh believes something needs to be done differently to continue to provide high-quality care.

Every radiation oncology department in the country needs two components: a board-certified radiation oncologist and the essential equipment to create a treatment plan. CMHS has both of these components, but there is growing concern regarding the need for additional equipment to accommodate treatment plans. Linear accelerators are traditionally used to program a patient's treatment plan and can be accessed for each appointment. CMHS currently has two machines and averages between 40 and 50 patients per day.

The literature recommends that one machine treat 30 to 35 patients per day; therefore, it is important that CMHS has two machines running. Technical difficulties are a problem because CMHS's linear accelerators are unmatched. This means that if one machine goes down, the patient plan for that machine cannot be transferred to the other machine. This results in wasted time and resources.

In addition to these operational challenges, Dr. Moh is concerned that CMHS is vulnerable to competitors who might want to enter the radiation oncology market in CMHS's primary service areas. Such competition would be difficult to withstand with CMHS's current facilities. Dr. Moh knows he needs to act quickly to secure the future success of the program.

Option 2: Interventional Cardiology

Although the cardiology program has been quite successful for CMHS, further investment in the interventional cardiology segment of the department is desperately needed. Current industry trends favor interventional cardiology procedures over traditional open-heart operations. Expert industry organizations predict that this trend will continue. CMHS needs to make a significant investment in its interventional cardiology program if it wants to retain and expand market share in this specialty. Additional data about interventional cardiology are provided in Exhibit V.4, and the perspective of a board member interested in expanding the program is provided in the sidebar.

As the number of patients requiring specialized cardiology care continues to increase throughout the service area, CMHS has been struggling to expand its service offerings to this patient population. New cholesterol-lowering and antihypertensive medications introduced over the past ten years have resulted in significantly extended life spans for cardiology patients. However, Americans leading more sedentary lifestyles and eating high-fat diets have contributed to a larger number of patients requiring specialized cardiac care. At the same time, a large competing health system in the area has recently invested in a significant expansion of its cardiovascular service line. Dr. Peak, an interventional cardiologist and CMHS's director of cardiology, knows that

	Total 2007 Interventional Cardiology Pts.	Central Med 2007 Interventional Cardiology Pts.	Central Med 2007 Interventional Cardiology Market Share
Ashville	276	75	27.2%
Crawford	270	92	34.1%
Huron	378	23	6.1%
Knowell	326	36	11.0%
Morris	136	5	3.7%
Rich	838	491	58.6%
Total	2,224	722	32.5%

EXHIBIT V.4
Current Market Share—
Interventional Cardiology

Projected Market Share—Interventional Cardiology

	2007	Year 1	Year 2	Year 3	Year 4	Year 5
Conservative (32%–52%)	32.5%	39.7%	43.2%	46.8%	49.9%	52.3%

A Board Member's Argument for Expanding the Interventional Cardiology Program

An influential hospital board member, Brandon Gerner, argued that CMHS should invest the $13 million in an expanded interventional cardiology program. Gerner felt the radiation oncology program was not headed in a positive direction. In his opinion, the program should be discontinued and the money should be allocated to the interventional cardiology program, which would produce higher margins for the institution. "Let's beef up our interventional cardiology program," stated Gerner. "The future impact of radiation oncology has been drastically overestimated, and the need for interventional cardiology will continue to grow as the population continues to age. Furthermore, favorable reimbursement for interventional cardiology procedures is likely to continue in the future, making this a sound financial decision for the organization."

---

to ensure the future success of the cardiology division, he needs to secure additional financial support from hospital leadership.

The cardiology program at CMHS has overcome significant challenges in the past. Several years ago the division faced a need for more cardiac surgeons and operating rooms to handle the increased number of coronary artery bypass graft procedures. The solution to the problem was to remodel the cardiac operating rooms and recruit several highly qualified physicians. The program has since become one of the more profitable units at CMHS and a model that other divisions within the hospital hope to emulate.

Advances in treatment options for cardiology patients have focused on minimally invasive interventional procedures that are more comfortable for patients and have significantly reduced recovery times. In fact, the number of minimally invasive interventional cardiology procedures performed at CMHS has nearly doubled in the past few years. These procedures are completed in specially designed treatment areas where sophisticated imaging equipment is used to guide small catheters and instruments through patients' cardiovascular systems. The single interventional cardiology suite at CMHS is no longer adequate to serve this expanding clinical need. Dr. Peak knows that to retain market share in this competitive environment, CMHS needs to invest significant capital in the creation of additional interventional cardiology treatment areas.

Implications of the Investment Decision

Given CMHS's location, the health system is continually concerned about its ability to retain market share and avoid losing patients to hospitals in Cletan or Flagship. While the financial stability and reputation of CMHS are enviable, the hospital has been unwilling to expand beyond the North Central Iowa region. Further, CMHS's clear mission and strong organizational culture have made affiliation options such as alliances or other cooperative arrangements with competitors virtually impossible to consider. As a result, any CMHS investment will be pursued on its own.

In previous discussions about investment options, hospital leadership has raised alternative uses for the $13 million at CMHS. However, the board has rejected other alternatives and has narrowed the options to the two currently on the table. They are unwilling to further explore avenues that might make the two options jointly possible. Even though an exclusive investment in radiation oncology will threaten the success of the interventional cardiology program, and vice versa, the board wants to force a decision between the two, and it wants the decision made now.

Case Questions

1. What are the pros and cons of each alternative investment? Does the radiation oncology project or the enhanced interventional cardiology program better align with CMHS's mission and vision? Why?
2. Whom does CMHS serve? At what cost?
3. Which stakeholders at CMHS will be affected by this decision? Which stakeholders should be included in discussions leading to a decision about which alternative investment to pursue?
4. What time sequence would you propose for the planning process around this investment?
5. What additional information would you need to make a solid business decision? Are there nonfinancial data you should consider?
6. What implications would exist for the alternative service that is not selected for investment? What might happen to volume and market share for that service?
7. If the two alternatives were not mutually exclusive, what types of financing strategies would you propose to permit investment in both options?

Case O
Cultural Competency at Marion County Health Center

Maria Jorina and Ann Scheck McAlearney

Marion County Health Center (MCHC), a not-for-profit community health center, is located in Indianapolis, Indiana. Within its women's clinic, MCHC runs a breast cancer screening program intended to provide preventive services and educational programs to women residing in the county. The clinic offers screening mammograms, clinical breast exams, STD testing, pregnancy counseling, and a variety of instructive materials on cancer and health promotion for women. The clinic's patient population reflects the racial makeup of the county: 60 percent of its patients are white, 30 percent are African American, and the remaining 10 percent represent a mix of Native American, Asian, and other racial groups. About 65 percent of the clinic's patients are over the age of 40, and many are poor and unemployed.

When Patricia Cole, the new administrator of MCHC, reviewed the most recent health center statistics reporting breast cancer screening rates, she was concerned to see not only that MCHC rates were below the state and national averages, but, most disconcertingly, that white women had consistently higher rates of initial and repeated screening visits than their African-American counterparts. Annual mammogram screenings are currently recommended for women over the age of 40, when self and clinical breast exams are considered less effective at detecting cancer. Because many of the center's patients are older than age 40, low breast cancer screening rates were troubling, to say the least. In addition, Cole was well aware of the continual emphasis of the Indiana Office of Minority Health on reducing healthcare disparities among racial and ethnic minorities in the state. Given that MCHC's mission pledged to "provide access to care regardless of race, ethnicity, or country of origin," Cole wondered what factors might be contributing to this difference, and what she as the health center's administrator could do about it. She decided to ask Emily Parsons, the director of all MCHC screening programs, to investigate.

A Review of Breast Cancer Screening Services at MCHC

After receiving her assignment from Cole, Parsons went directly to the MCHC women's clinic so that she could see, firsthand, how care was being provided. Upon entering the clinic, she first noticed that most of the women in the waiting room were white. She also saw a number of brochures placed on the counters and coffee tables situated in the waiting room. These brochures covered subjects ranging from STD prevention and pregnancy to cervical and breast cancer screening.

Parsons wanted to speak with some of the physicians working at the clinic to see if she could learn about how the physicians interacted with their patients. She was particularly interested in learning under what circumstances and how often the topic of breast cancer screening was brought up during patient visits. Fortunately, all four clinic physicians agreed to brief meetings, so Parsons cleared her schedule.

The Physicians' Perspectives

Parsons' meetings with the four clinic physicians were strikingly similar. MCHC physicians appeared to believe that the benefits of breast cancer screening were already well known. Further, several physicians noted that because MCHC's breast cancer screening program had been extensively advertised in the local media, they did not feel obligated to emphasize the benefits of screening to the patients they saw in the clinic. As all four physicians noted, MCHC provided educational materials at the clinic that were widely available for patients to read while they waited for their appointments; thus, the physicians did not feel the need to specifically discuss screening during the short periods of time they had with their patients. The physicians' collective sentiment appeared to be that if a patient had questions, she could raise those questions during the visit. Parsons was surprised by such conviction, especially given that three of the four physicians were women.

Parsons also got the impression that the physicians did not believe that early breast cancer screening was equally beneficial for all patients. Several of the physicians made comments to the effect that "most African-American women did not see their providers regularly anyway," so telling them about the screening program was suggested to be a waste of these physicians' time. Another physician explained that because African-American women were statistically less likely to get breast cancer, he believed these women did not need the same amount of health education on this topic. When Parsons brought up MCHC's mission, all four physicians expressed sincere belief that they were providing care equally.

A final impression from her meetings was that the clinic physicians did not seem to feel comfortable discussing the importance of breast cancer screening with their patients because they had not received any specific training about how to introduce and discuss this subject. Several physicians noted that they found it especially difficult to communicate with nonwhite patients because they believed that some of these patients did not have sufficient knowledge of medical terminology to fully understand what the physicians were telling them. All four physicians expressed a sentiment that relating to nonwhite patients was generally impaired by racial and cultural differences.

Some Patients' Perspectives

Parsons was quite startled by the physicians' comments and felt that she needed to learn even more about what was going on in the clinic. She decided to ask patients what they thought about the benefits of screening, see if they had any questions, and see if they would share their thoughts with her about the need to perform breast self-exams.

After obtaining permission from the MCHC's institutional review board to speak with patients about their perspectives and experiences, Parsons interviewed a number of both white and African-American women at the end of their clinic visits to learn about their views of breast cancer screening.

Among the women who agreed to be interviewed, the majority of white patients expressed general satisfaction with MCHC's breast cancer screening program and noted that it had indeed been well publicized in the local media. With few exceptions, this group believed that breast cancer screening was beneficial to all women, and that screening should be a part of health promotion programs throughout the county. A majority of women in this group also commented that they did not feel the clinic's physicians brought up cancer screening first, and patients often had to ask about it themselves.

The African-American women's responses painted quite a different picture for Parsons. A great majority of these women noted they believed breast cancer screening was only necessary when recommended by the physician and reported that they did not feel comfortable asking about screening if the doctor did not introduce the topic. When asked whether they had seen advertisements promoting MCHC's screening program on TV or in local newspapers, the majority of African-American women said they had not. Many of these women did not have cable television, and most did not regularly read a newspaper. Further, most of the African-American women Parsons interviewed were not aware of the benefits of breast self-examinations and reported not knowing how to do them.

Many of the African-American women reported having difficulty seeing a physician on a regular basis. Some women noted that doctor visits were inconvenient, with several expressing frustration that to visit the clinic, they had to ask for time off work. A couple of women also commented that the clinic's location was an issue because they had to take two buses to get there. Several other women complained that going to the clinic involved paying for daycare for their children, and this was an expense they could not always afford.

Additional Issues Surface

After hearing from both the physicians and a number of patients, Parsons presented her findings to Cole. Parsons' view was the MCHC physicians were not culturally competent, and they seemed unable to relate to their nonwhite patients. Cole could not disagree.

To make matters worse, Cole then told Parsons she had recently received a letter of complaint from one of the MCHC employees in the clinical quality department. In this letter the employee expressed her dissatisfaction with the MCHC work environment and provided several examples of insensitivity on the part of MCHC staff, who were reportedly ignorant about cultural differences and intolerant of this employee's religious practices.

Cultural Differences Among Employees

Because of an ongoing shortage of domestically trained medical staff, a problem common across the country, MCHC had begun hiring foreign-trained candidates to fill vacant patient coordinator positions. Most recently, the department of clinical quality had hired a new patient coordinator, a Pakistani female, whose duties included greeting and assisting patients and visitors, helping patients with scheduling tests and procedures, obtaining test results, maintaining the accuracy of patient information in the health center database, and resolving issues related to insurance claims and referrals.

This newly hired patient coordinator, Ms. Neely, had come to the United States ten years previously and had worked in healthcare for that entire time. Neely had received nursing training in Pakistan, and she had worked there as a registered nurse for five years. Since coming to the United States, Neely had taken and passed the National Council Licensure Examination for Registered Nurses (NCLEX-RN) and obtained a license from the state of Illinois, where she initially resided. Neely had recently moved to Indiana, where MCHC was located. While she applied initially for an RN position posted on the MCHC website, she was instead offered a patient coordinator job. Even though Neely felt she was overqualified for the patient coordinator position and deserved the RN position instead, she felt obligated to accept the position to support herself and her teenage daughter. In addition, Neely had been assured by the human resources manager during the job interview process that her position could been seen as a stepping stone, and with more experience and an Indiana state license, she would be given additional challenges and responsibilities.

A Complaint About Cultural Competency

In her letter to the MCHC administrator, Neely complained that after having worked at MCHC for nine months and having obtained an Indiana RN license, she still had not been given an opportunity to take on more challenging tasks. She noted that she felt that her work was being micromanaged by the nurse supervisor, and she perceived that she was given too many "boring" tasks such as resolving patient insurance claims and scheduling tests. Further, she noted that there had not been any discussion about a promotion any time soon. Neely also commented that she felt that her colleagues and supervisors looked down on her because of her nationality and her accent. She stated that these work colleagues made it obvious that her accent was difficult to understand, and they spoke noticeably louder when addressing her. She further commented that these colleagues always appeared uninterested when she talked about her culture and traditions. Finally, Neely stated, on several occasions her supervisor had expressed discontent when she requested time off for her religious holidays.

Incorporating Additional Evidence

Upon receiving this letter, Cole recalled having overheard one of Neely's colleagues, Ms. Gilbert, complaining to another staff member in the clinical quality department about some of her reservations. Cole decided to see if Parsons could learn more about what was going on in the department, so she suggested that Parsons talk to Gilbert and continue her investigation.

Parsons found Gilbert in her office and also found her more than willing to talk about what was going on in the department. As Parsons soon learned, Gilbert had apparently been surprised and disappointed when a college friend who had been a Marion County resident all her life had applied for the patient coordinator position at the same time as Neely, but did not get the job. Gilbert stated that she believed that all jobs should be offered first to domestically trained professionals who have the skills and competencies to provide adequate services to the MCHC population. Next, Gilbert described how she and her colleagues felt that it was culturally insensitive of Neely to bring her traditional Pakistani dishes to office potlucks and American holidays parties because most people working at MCHC were not used to the spices in these dishes. Gilbert noted that she and her colleagues had discussed how Neely should have learned how to make traditional American dishes by now since she had lived in the United States for at least ten years. Third, Gilbert noted that she and her colleagues found it unprofessional that several times a day, Neely left her workplace to perform her prayers. Gilbert complained that during Neely's absences, important calls could be missed, and the continuity of patient care could be disrupted. Finally, Gilbert commented that because Neely's faith required her to always wear *shalwar kameez*, a traditional Pakistani garment of pants and a tunic, Gilbert and her colleagues felt that Neely bent the office rules by getting to wear "relaxed" clothing every day of the week instead of only on Fridays, as allowed of the other staff. Even though Neely wore a white medical coat on top of her shalwar kameez, everyone felt she was not following the rules. In summary, Gilbert's account indicated the department felt a general distrust toward Neely, regardless of her performance as a patient coordinator.

Now What?

Parsons scheduled an appointment to meet with Cole and discuss the additional information she had learned from her meeting with Gilbert. While they both realized that Gilbert's comments could be interpreted as just one person's opinion, they also sensed that there must be elements of truth in her words given the letter Neely had sent to Cole.

Cole was both unhappy and perplexed with the situation she now knew she faced at MCHC. While in college and graduate school, she had learned about the existence of racial and ethnic health disparities, discrimination, biases, and the importance of cultural diversity, but she had never personally dealt with these issues before. Nor had she ever expected to find them in her workplace. It was clear to Cole that MCHC had some issues to resolve around both discrimination and cultural competency, and she had to take the lead to develop a strategy to address and resolve these problems.

Case Questions

1. What are the cultural competency problems MCHC faces? What makes these problems similar, and what makes them different?
2. What organizational and cultural barriers can be identified in this case?
3. What strategies should be developed to overcome these barriers?
4. What kind of priority should these problems have for Cole, the MCHC administrator? Does Cole have to act as the sole decision maker in this situation? Who else could be involved in developing strategies to address these problems?
5. Whose interests should be considered in this situation and at what cost?

Short Case 21
New Chief of Ob-Gyn: The Next Three Years

Anthony R. Kovner

Since Dr. Mikhail has taken over as chief of ob-gyn at North Heights Medical Center in New York City, the following have occurred: a slight increase in deliveries; a significant expansion of primary care centers and number of visits; a large increase in the number of abortions done; a large increase in research grants received; improvement in facilities; and an improvement in patient service. However, patient revenues have decreased slightly because of improvements in health for premature births (preemies), and use of the preemie nursery has decreased significantly. North Heights serves a low-income, diverse population and is a large hospital and health system with a $200 million budget.

The following discussion has occurred among a group of consultants brought together by Dr. Bright, the medical director:

Dr. Strong: The service needs to increase its share of the market. St. Brennan's Hospital represents a threat in this regard and Washington Hospital represents an opportunity.

Dr. Light: There is a leakage in primary care away from North Heights. Hire an outreach worker to find out the reasons for the leakage and do something about it.

Dr. Bright: Dr. Mikhail should increase marketing efforts, including advertising.

Dr. Quick: Dr. Mikhail should continue with the present strategy. Deliveries are down in the Bronx, and market share is slowly increasing.

Dr. Rough: Dr. Mikhail should reduce the number of full-time staff and produce the same number of deliveries with a smaller budget.

Dr. Clever: Dr. Mikhail should alter his research strategy and seek grants aimed at interventions that will increase the number of deliveries.

Case Questions

1. What are the key facts in the situation?
2. What are the problems and issues?
3. What should Dr. Mikhail do, and why?

Short Case 22
To Sell or Not to Sell

Anthony R. Kovner

Clark Medical Center in New York City is losing $2 million a year on sales of $750 million. Clark Hospital serves a low-income, diverse population and is located in an old facility. Besides owning a hospital, the Medical Center owns HelpYou, a Medicaid HMO with more than 250,000 patients. HelpYou contributes its surplus of $2 million per year to Clark Medical Center, which meets the medical center's deficit.

Sam Hayes, Clark's CEO, has determined that the best way to save the hospital is to sell the HMO and believes that Clark can get up to $200 million for it. Sam has convinced all but two members of the executive committee that "this is the way to go." The two unconvinced board members are Luke Reacher and Harry Smith, who have the following conversation about the prospective sale at Joe's Pub:

Luke: I'm not against selling, but the HMO is worth $300 million, and I would only sell if Sam told us in advance how much of the money is "net" and what he would use it for.
Harry: I think we should sell the hospital and invest in the HMO. The hospital continues to lose money. Why do we pay Sam $1 million a year anyway?
Luke: Shouldn't we at least review the experience of other hospitals that have sold their HMOs?
Harry: Sam says we're unique.
Luke: The next question is, what should we and what can we do about the situation as board members? The hospital board has already agreed to sell the HMO if we can get $200 million.
Harry: No one will offer us that. What if they offer us $100 million?
Luke: What worries me is that Sam will take the $100 million to pay off underfunded reserves for malpractice and the nurses' pension plan. This may be up to half of the $100 million.

Case Questions

1. If selling the HMO is such a bad idea, why are the hospital CEO and the board in favor of the sale?
2. What is the hospital likely to do with the proceeds of the sale?

3. What are the choices available to Luke and Harry?

4. What do you recommend that Luke and Harry do now, and why?

5. List barriers to implementing your recommendations and how Clark Medical Center and its board can overcome them.

Short Case 23
A New Look?

Ann Scheck McAlearney and Sarah M. Roesch

Dr. Elinor Cooke is a renowned cosmetic surgeon, highly dedicated to healing and restoring well-being for those affected by aesthetic issues. She believes that her line of work builds the confidence and self-esteem of those who seek her services. Dr. Cooke received her medical degree from Case Western Reserve University and then completed four years of residency and two additional years of residency in plastic surgery at the Ohio State University Hospitals. Dr. Cooke's current practice, North City Aesthetic and Plastic Surgery, Inc., affiliated with Northside Community Hospital, is located in a suburb of Cleveland on a beautiful wooded lot next to Lake Erie. In addition to Dr. Cooke, there is one other doctor affiliated with North City, Dr. Ryan Thomas, who specializes in men's reconstructive surgery. The practice also employs two nurses and an office manager. The practice enjoys an excellent reputation and is known for its compassionate approach to care.

While North City Aesthetic and Plastic Surgery is considered one of the premier practices in the Midwest market area, Dr. Cooke is concerned about some of the changes she has observed in the field of plastic surgery. When she started her practice in the early 1980s, cosmetic surgery was a relatively new field. Plastic surgery was available for those affected by disfigurement, but not readily available for those who wanted to fix something just because they didn't like their appearance. Over the years, Hollywood, new techniques, and new trends sparked tremendous growth in the cosmetic surgery industry, and with this growth, the profile of a typical cosmetic surgery practice changed. Whereas patients used to be amazed that a tummy tuck, breast augmentation, facelift, or rhinoplasty was possible, now the average patient tends to want more than surgery alone.

Another trend Dr. Cooke has observed is the increasing level of competition for aesthetic surgery services. She is aware of the expanding availability of surgical procedures through ambulatory surgery centers, but a recent invitation to a Botox party event provided evidence of a new competitive threat—even if the quality of care provided might be suspect. Dr. Cooke's

North City practice has managed to grow based on patients' word-of-mouth recommendations and other physicians' referrals rather than through advertising. Yet given local and regional competition for well-paying patients, Dr. Cooke knows that she must develop her own strategy to ensure that her practice can survive and thrive into the future. The practice's prosperity is important to Dr. Cooke, and she is continually looking for ways to grow her practice's business.

Dr. Cooke, who also has a bachelor's degree in business, is a problem solver by nature. In considering the new trends in the aesthetic surgery area, Dr. Cooke senses that she has a choice to make. Abdominoplasty (tummy tuck) is the most popular form of surgery that she performs. After surgery, the patient often has trouble with activities such as moving from a sitting to a standing position, walking, and caring for the postoperative drains. Dr. Cooke has often thought it would be nice to have a 24-hour care alternative for postoperative patients.

One particularly intriguing option is to develop a "hideaway" for her aesthetic surgery clients where they can relax and recover after their procedures. She knows that her patients desire complete confidentiality at all times, and that they also want a high degree of professional and personal attention—before, during, and after the procedures. Creating a hideaway would allow Dr. Cooke to provide top-notch medical care in a spalike atmosphere, and enable her staff to offer professional and personal attention to the healing patients during the days following surgery. Further, given her knowledge of the important connections between individuals' minds and their bodies, she is certain that a relaxing atmosphere would enhance the healing process while offering a safe place for her demanding clientele to recover. Moreover, there is no such facility in the Cleveland area, and she feels that this would definitely give her practice an edge over other practices. She also feels that her building's scenic locale would be perfect for this type of postoperative hideaway.

While Dr. Cooke suspects that this hideaway concept would have considerable appeal to her well-heeled patients, she knows that potential patients are not the only individuals she would need to consider in developing a new approach for her North City practice. When she shared her idea with Dr. Thomas, he was less than enthusiastic. Dr. Thomas reminded her that they were surgeons, not innkeepers. He noted that the overhead costs associated with such a practice change would be high, and he was particularly worried about management of the facility. Dr. Thomas also brought up the issue of insurance liability. Then he mentioned that he had heard that St. Clare's, another community hospital, was also looking into opening a similar type of facility not too far away.

Dr. Cooke, discouraged, yet not defeated, understands Dr. Thomas's concerns. As the lease is soon up on the building for her current practice, Dr.

Cooke knows she will need to make any decision about changing the direction of her practice quickly so that she can take action. The possibility of a facility opening at St. Clare's motivates Dr. Cooke to further investigate her idea. She believes the wooded lot with lake views that her practice occupies would be an ideal location for a recovery retreat. And she feels that Dr. Thomas's male patients would also benefit from a discreet hideaway to recover.

Case Questions

1. What are the pros and cons of changing the focus of Dr. Cooke's practice?
2. What would you predict would be the reactions of the various stakeholders to Dr. Cooke's new business concept (e.g., patients, referring physicians, Northside Community Hospital, her professional colleagues)?
3. What would you recommend for Dr. Cooke?

Short Case 24
Disparities in Care at Southern Regional Health System

Ann Scheck McAlearney

Tim Hank leaned back in his chair and closed his eyes. While he had been afraid the reports might have bad news, he now had to figure out what to do with this new information. Flipping through the first binder on his desk, reporting results of the recent Robert Wood Johnson Foundation–sponsored assessment of the cardiovascular care provided by his organization, he was increasingly concerned. Southern Regional Health System was based in Jackson, Mississippi, an area known for a highly diverse population and high poverty rates. Black and Hispanic residents in the area were about three times more likely to live in poverty than were whites. Unemployment was also a big problem that affected whites and nonwhites differently—in the Jackson area, black residents were two and a half times more likely to be unemployed and Hispanics over twice as likely to be unemployed as white residents. Beyond poverty and employment differences, though, was the issue of different care given to different patients. This issue of disparities in care was receiving increasing national attention, but Hank had thought the care they provided at Southern Regional was "color blind." Given the health system's mission of providing "excellent quality of care for all," he assumed that the care was equitably delivered across patients and patient populations.

Apparently, this was not the case. This first report showed that there were indeed disparities in the care provided by Southern Regional. Data on heart care had been collected by race and ethnicity for the past year, and these baseline data showed differences. For instance, using the four core measures for heart failure that the Centers for Medicare & Medicaid Services currently collects and reports, only 41 percent of patients were receiving all recommended heart failure care, and the numbers were worse based on race and ethnicity. The analysis showed that while 68 percent of whites received all recommended care, the comparable number among nonwhites was 27 percent. For one measure—the percentage of heart failure patients receiving discharge instructions—only 65 percent of Hispanic patients received the information, compared to 85 percent of non-Hispanic patients. Also troubling Hank was the fact that none of these measures was close to 100 percent—this certainly wasn't the type of care he'd want offered to his own family. Yet he truly didn't understand how his hospital could be providing such disparate care.

The second binder on his desk offered little information to ease his concern. This report, the "Assessment of Organizational Readiness to Change" for Southern Regional Health System, showed that few individuals in his hospital were aware of the nationwide problem of disparities in care, and even fewer were aware that such an issue might be problematic within their own hospital. Now he had the data for Southern Regional that showed significant gaps in care provided to African American and Hispanic patients relative to white patients, but the accompanying readiness-to-change evaluation showed a strong tendency among hospital employees and physicians to resist any proposed changes and instead "go with the flow." Hank knew that his ability to bring the issue of disparate care to the forefront of hospital concerns and successfully make strides to reduce these disparities would be a legacy he would love to leave. Yet he didn't know how he could possibly begin to address this issue at Southern Regional Health System.

Case Questions

1. What should Hank do with the information contained in these reports?
2. What reactions would you predict he might receive from various hospital stakeholders, such as other executives, physicians, board members, or the community?
3. What can Hank do to raise the level of urgency at Southern Regional Health System to address the issue of disparities in care?
4. What are the constraints he will face?

Short Case 25
A Patient-Centered Medical Home at Twin Rivers?

David Muhlestein and Ann Scheck McAlearney

The Twin Rivers Family Medicine Clinic

The three years since you became office manager at Twin Rivers Family Medicine Clinic could be described as relatively stable. The four physicians who jointly own and provide services for the clinic have been working together for nearly a decade, are on good terms with each other, work hard, and provide excellent medical care. The clinic is favorably located in the moderately affluent suburb of a midsized city where it leases space in a medical office building. Clinic patients range in age from newborns to the elderly.

Two of the three nurses who assist the physicians have been here for more than five years and the third, a recent nursing graduate who replaced a retiring nurse, has been in the office for six months. The office staff, consisting of you and two clerical workers, has been able to stay on top of billing and successfully oversaw the transition one year ago from an outdated electronic health record (EHR) system to an integrated EHR. This new EHR is used by the hospital system the clinic is affiliated with and allows patient records to be seen instantly when patients present at most of the area hospitals. In addition, the EHR includes a secure online patient portal where patients can schedule appointments, view test results, and e-mail their physicians.

Financially, the past two years have been relatively good for the clinic. While payment rates have not increased as much as they have in previous years, you have found several ways to lower overhead costs (including automating some billing) and slightly increase volume without increasing the time your physicians spend in the clinic (approximately 55 hours a week). The result has been consistent operating margins for the clinic over the past five years; on revenues of nearly $2 million, the clinic spends approximately 65 percent on overhead and staff salaries, with the remainder paid evenly to the physicians. Currently, all of the physicians respect your judgment in managing the clinic, and they trust your business acumen. Their preference is to focus on patient care as much as possible, and they are not interested in adding a new physician to the practice. Meanwhile, the rest of the staff, while not strongly resistant to change, is comfortable with the present state of the clinic. Requiring additional work hours from the staff without an accompanying increase in salary, however, would be met with resistance.

Of the 9,000 patients currently in the clinic's panel, approximately half are seen one time or less per year. The physicians cumulatively see an average of 400 patients per week. Approximately half of the physicians' appointments are brief follow-up visits that require about at most 10 minutes of physician time. The other appointments usually last from 15 to 20 minutes and then require additional time for charting and documentation. The physicians begin seeing patients at 7:00 a.m., and the last appointment is generally scheduled for 4:30 p.m., but given unforeseen delays and accommodation for same-day appointments, generally at least one of the physicians is in the office until at least 6:30 p.m.

In addition to seeing patients and charting, physicians also are required to sign billing forms, write doctors' notes and call in prescriptions to local pharmacies. The physicians currently are not regularly on call, though they occasionally take call for specific patients. Some of the follow-up appointments and prescription writing could be performed by a nurse practitioner or physician assistant, which the clinic has considered hiring for $100,000 a year (salary and benefits).

The Opportunity

Recently, a national insurance company that covers 40 percent of the clinic's patient panel has come to you and offered Twin Rivers the chance to take part in a patient-centered medical home (PCMH) pilot program it is introducing throughout the country. The PCMH model attempts to focus more on providing well care rather than sick care by incenting medical practices to actively monitor patients, provide preventive care, use evidence-based best practices, and deliver team-based care centered around an individual patient's needs. The primary care focus of PCMHs aims to prevent illness and provide an opportunity for patients to interact more holistically with their primary care physicians. While there is no formal requirement to become a PCMH other than attempting to follow these tenets, the opportunity to become accredited as a PCMH by organizations such as the National Committee for Quality Assurance (NCQA) exists. Becoming accredited formalizes the steps a primary care practice has made to become a PCMH and facilitates contracting as a PCMH with insurers.

For each of the covered lives that a physician provides services for, the insurance company is offering to pay Twin Rivers up to $10 a month initially to act as a PCMH. Then, after a first-year baseline is set, the company will introduce the possibility of bonus payments to the clinic, based on calculated savings resulting from improved care coordination and lower utilization rates. In conjunction with the potential for bonuses, if the clinic has above-expected costs, then some of the "excess" costs will be passed on to the clinic in the form of decreased reimbursements.

To take part in this PCMH pilot program, Twin Rivers will be required to extend clinic office hours, offer 24/7 primary care access, explicitly coordinate the care of individuals with chronic illnesses, and ensure that preventive care is provided for all patients in its panel. The insurance company will then guarantee half of the monthly payment and will pay the additional half on the basis of Twin Rivers' ability to deliver appropriate, patient-centered care to its patient panel. This determination will be made on the basis of quality metrics, such as the proportion of diabetics who are given regular eye exams, the proportion of women who receive regular Pap smears, and the proportion of children who receive appropriate immunizations on schedule. A quick analysis assures you that Twin Rivers would already qualify for nearly 75 percent of the quality measurement–dependent funds, and that achieving 95 percent of quality requirements would be possible within two years. You feel that care coordination is the direction your market is headed, and whether or not you agree to participate in this pilot program, you will eventually need to move to a PCMH-type model and accept some amount of financial risk.

Considering the Changes Required

If you agree to enter into a contract with the insurance company to participate in the PCMH program, the first change you must make is to extend clinic office hours. Currently, nurses are salaried, arriving shortly before 7:00 a.m. and leaving at 4:00 p.m., though one may stay later if patients come in late. In contrast, clerical staff are hourly employees and work 40 hours per week. Their schedules are staggered so that one starts at 6:30 a.m. and the other at 10:30 a.m. to provide full coverage for the clinic. For the physicians, their current schedule for morning hours would be adequate under the new contract, but evening hours would need to be expanded. In addition, there might be a need to provide extended clinic hours on weekends so that patients' schedules and care needs could be fully met.

For off-hours emergencies under the PCMH model, patients will need access to primary care through the clinic. Two options to ensure constant primary care access are (1) for your physicians and nurses to rotate being on-call, or (2) to contract with a third-party nurse hotline that will answer calls whenever the physicians do not want to be on call. Nurses on the hotline would then screen calls and either refer the calling patient to the emergency room or tell the patient to contact their clinic physician the next day. You have learned that the hotline costs $40 per call, payable by the clinic, but you have no indication how much this service, once implemented, will be used.

Under the new PCMH model, care coordination will be critical. The new contract will make the clinic responsible for overseeing the care of its patients through all levels of care (not just care provided at the clinic) and ensure that appropriate preventive care is delivered to all patients. You have determined that to manage the care of and follow-up with the clinic patient panel, you will need to hire at least one new employee. This new employee will be responsible for scheduling preventive care screenings and visits, following up regularly with patients, confirming that patients understand and are taking their medications, and coordinating with providers to ensure that care is documented when it is provided by clinicians who are not connected to the clinic's EHR system. For this care coordination role you have calculated that hiring a nurse would cost around $70,000 a year (salary and benefits), and that this additional nurse would be able to provide basic clinical support and help out in the clinic during busy periods, in addition to providing care coordination services. You have also calculated that if the decision were made to hire a nonclinical coordinator, the cost would be less ($45,000 a year for salary and benefits), but the focus of this individual's position would be exclusively on care coordination and would not allow the flexibility to provide additional clinical support.

Concerns

You have discussed this opportunity individually with each member of the present staff and each of the practicing physicians. You sense that the general mood is cautious optimism that the plan will lead to better patient care, but this is coupled with reluctance to drastically change work flow or work responsibilities. One physician has specifically voiced concerns that she wonders whether quality will be affected if patients turn to nurses for advice after hours. In addition, she noted she would prefer to keep the practice the same size it is now. A second physician is strongly in favor of increasing the size of the practice by hiring physician assistants. The remaining physicians did not state a preference for expanding the practice, but you suspect they lean toward keeping the status quo. One concern among the staff is a desire to avoid entering more information into computers that will add to their present responsibilities.

Looking Ahead

Currently, only this single insurer has proposed a PCMH-type payment arrangement. Other insurers, though, have explored such arrangements, and if you adopt the PCMH model now, the clinic likely could qualify for at least one more similar contract over the next few years. While the current insurer has not mandated this PCMH arrangement, you are somewhat concerned that if you do not agree to this model, they may exclude you from their network sometime in the future. Looking into the future, you have made some rough estimates about the effect of adopting the PCMH model. You predict that overall patient visits will increase by approximately 10 percent the first year, primarily because of shorter, preventive care visits that could be performed by a nurse practitioner or physician assistant. Average time that physicians spend with patients during non-follow-up visits may also increase as physicians seek to address more preventive care issues during visits, though by how much is certainly unknown. Total revenue is expected to grow by approximately 15 percent because many of the preventive services are favorably reimbursed. You expect that 50 percent of the monthly PCMH payments and the growth in clinic revenue will go toward general overhead (including billing, supplies, and leasing more exam rooms), with the remainder available to hire additional staff and increase net profits. Finally, you have no projections about whether the clinic would qualify for any bonus payments in future years, though you are relatively confident that you will avoid any penalties in the first year.

Case Questions

1. Will you accept the insurance company's offer to become a PCMH? Why or why not? What are the largest drawbacks of adopting the PCMH model? What are the potential benefits? How does the added risk factor into your decision?
2. Assuming you choose to adopt the PCMH model, how will you get buy-in from the physicians and from the staff? How will your approach differ between the parties?
3. What new employee(s) will you hire, and what will their roles be?

ACCOUNTABILITY

Let's not be too hasty; haste is a dangerous thing.
Untimely measures bring repentance.
Certainly, and unhappily, many things in the Colony are absurd.
But is there anything human without some fault?
And after all, you see, we do go forward.
—C. P. Cavafy (1992)

COMMENTARY

Society gives resources to organizations that add value to the inputs and provide society with goods and services. The owners or governing bodies of these organizations have five functions, according to Pointer and Orlikoff (2002): formulating the organization's vision and key goals and ensuring that strategy is aligned with vision and goals; ensuring high levels of management performance; ensuring high-quality care; ensuring financial health; and ensuring the board's effectiveness and efficiency. The CEO is the board's agent on-site.

Two factors are vital for aligning organizations for accountability: (1) a specification of organizational performance that is mutually agreed on in advance by stakeholders, and (2) the capability of managers to control the resources and behaviors necessary to achieve the specified performance objectives.

Expectations of Organizational Performance

Stakeholders assess levels of organizational performance in a variety of ways. Some organizations use "balanced scorecards" as strategic management tools. As posited by Kaplan and Norton (1996), the measures come from four perspectives: (1) financial, such as return on investment or market share; (2) customer service; (3) internal business processes, such as hospital readmission rate for the same illness; and (4) learning and growth, keyed to employee morale and suggestions.

Management accountability ranges accordingly across the four functions. For example, to improve customer service, managers can conduct marketing studies to learn what patients like and dislike about the organization's services. Managers can reorganize work so that fewer people provide more services for each patient or physician. Managers can reevaluate organizational routines regularly, especially in terms of impact on patient outcomes and on physician convenience.

Managers can tour the facility regularly. Managers can let patients and clinicians know what service levels they should expect and what behavior is expected from them. Managers can also report regularly to other stakeholders—such as purchaser and employee representatives—on performance, plans, and issues. These stakeholders can be included on policymaking and advisory committees. Management information systems can be developed for planning and evaluating services. Information should include the population served and the use of various services; the quantity, cost, and quality of services provided; and patient and provider satisfaction. Summarized reports of regulators and accrediting bodies can be shared with stakeholder groups. Organizational goals and performance can be analyzed, as can information about trends in turnover, use of overtime, and absenteeism, and in fundraising, profitability, and purchases of new capital equipment.

The process of decision making can be examined and improved. By making itself more formally accountable, the leadership incurs substantial costs in management time spent on the process, dollars spent on information system upgrades, and conflicts raised by discussions about present and future direction. But the leadership may also reap substantial benefits: plans and initiatives that are more acceptable to stakeholders, and therefore more feasible to implement; greater commitment from key clinicians to organizational goals; and a sharper focus on the organization's mission so that goal attainment is more easily achieved and justified to employees and customers.

Stakeholder Claims on the Organization

Organizational performance can be improved (or negatively affected) by legislation, regulation, and the media. For example, if Medicare payments are reduced, this may shift costs to other payers and reduce well-being and access for beneficiaries, especially when certain physicians no longer participate in the Medicare program.

Managers generally have less control over external stakeholders. And healthcare is particularly challenging because of the difficulties in specifying measureable outcomes and in gaining agreement among stakeholders with different ideas about goals, strategies of the organization, and the appropriate role for not-for-profit governing boards. Some organizations have made great advances in the area of accountability. According to Berry and Bendapudi (2003), the Mayo Clinic manages a set of visual and experiential clues so patients recognize that care is organized around their needs rather than around doctors' schedules or hospital processes. Mayo employees are hired because they embrace the organization's values. These values are emphasized through training and are reinforced in the workplace.

To encourage collaboration among professionals, physicians at Mayo are paid salaries; sophisticated internal paging, telephone, and videoconferencing are used; and electronic medical records have been fully implemented. The facilities are designed to relieve stress, offer a place of refuge, create positive distractions, convey caring and respect, symbolize competence, minimize crowding, facilitate way finding, and accommodate families.

Managers can ensure that key stakeholders are identified and that their expectations and satisfaction levels are regularly measured. For objectivity in this regard, measurements can be made by external organizations explicitly structured for this purpose, such as Consumers Union, which publishes *Consumer Reports* magazine.

References

Berry, L. L., and N. Bendapudi. 2003. "Clueing in Customers." *Harvard Business Review* 81 (2): 100–104.

Cavafy, C. P. 1992. "In a Large Greek Colony, 200 BC." *C. P. Cavafy: Collected Poems.* Princeton, NJ: Princeton University Press.

Kaplan, R. S., and D. P. Norton. 1996. "Using the Balanced Scorecard as a Strategic Management System." *Harvard Business Review* 74 (1): 75–85.

Pointer, D. D., and J. E. Orlikoff. 2002. *Getting to Great: Principles of Health Care Organization Governance.* San Francisco: Jossey-Bass.

THE READINGS

Patrick Charmel is president and CEO of Griffin Hospital and also CEO of Planetree, Inc., a not-for-profit association of more than 150 US and international hospitals dedicated to patient empowerment and patient-centered care. His aims are similar to those of "The Triple Aim," an initiative of the Institute for Healthcare Improvement (IHI): (1) improve the health of the population; (2) enhance the patient experience of care (including quality, access, and reliability); and (3) reduce, or at least control, the per capita cost of care.

As Charmel explains in his interview, "We set out to be a great place to provide an exceptional patient experience, to deliver great care, and to be a great place for caregivers." Charmel's sense of accountability led to inviting Planetree to become a part of the Griffin Health Service Corporation in Derby, Connecticut. As he explains, Griffin Hospital provides a great showplace for people interested in learning about the model. Griffin was the first hospital in the country to build a completely new facility based on Planetree's patient-centered care principles.

Charmel stresses the importance of understanding the patient experience from the patient's point of view. This includes focus groups, telephone and mail surveys, community image surveys, rounding, and the establishment of a patient and family advisory council. Executives spend one hour per month observing patients' experiences. Their personal stories convey the persistent challenges of navigating a complex healthcare system. The experts on what constitutes a satisfying patient experience are the patients themselves.

The required supplementary readings pursue similar themes. The Commonwealth Fund posits an ambitious agenda for high-performance health systems in the United States. McCarthy sketches attributes of high-performing health systems now in the United States. Griffith and White develop ways for hospitals to move from acute care to community health. Finally, Porter and Teisberg sketch out how healthcare organizations (HCOs) could become more accountable by facilitating a more competitive, market-oriented economy in healthcare.

Defining and Evaluating Excellence in Patient-Centered Care

Patrick A. Charmel
From *Frontiers of Health Services Management*, 26 (4): 27–34.

Introduction

Griffin Hospital is a 160-bed acute care hospital located in the highly competitive healthcare market of the northeastern United States. Despite the number of larger and better-known healthcare institutions in adjacent communities, Griffin has gained a reputation as a hospital of choice through a focused effort to satisfy the full range of patient and family needs. Griffin's approach to patient-centered care is guided by the Planetree philosophy, which promotes patient–provider partnerships through access to information and family involvement and emphasizes caring for and supporting staff so that they can better care for and support patients. At the core of this model is the patient and responsiveness to the patient's needs, expectations, and preferences.

A Multipronged Approach to Understanding the Patient Experience

As illustrated in the articles by Taylor and Rutherford and Steiger and Balog, any undertaking to be responsive to patient needs must be founded on an effort to understand the patient experience—not from the vantage point of a CEO, physician, or nurse, but from the patient's perspective. For those of us who work in hospitals, the language and processes of healthcare are familiar and routine. For patients and their families, they are anything but. Engaging patients to share their experiences and communicate what is most important to them ensures that, despite our fluency in hospital operations, day-to-day routines and improvement efforts are grounded in the revealing perspectives of those who come to us for care.

While much of my discussion with patients and family members was distinctly positive, their personal stories also powerfully convey the persistent challenges of navigating a complex healthcare system.

Griffin Hospital's approach to this work is multipronged. It includes focus groups, telephone and mail surveys, community image surveys, rounding, and the establishment of a patient and family advisory council.

Collectively, these methods have amplified the voice of patients and family members and have recast the traditionally passive recipients of care as agents of organizational change. These processes have illuminated opportunities for improvement and have resulted in the implementation of varied strategies to enhance the patient experience. Changes to discharge teaching and billing communications, patient education about the hospitalist program, efforts to reduce noise levels, and the design and services of the recently opened Center for Cancer Care are just a few of the improvements and enhancements driven by patient feedback.

Though multifaceted, Griffin's approach to engaging patients and family members is hardly all-inclusive. Inspired by Rutherford and Taylor's recommendation that executives spend one hour per month observing patients' experiences, I carved out some time during a recent week to do just that. Admittedly, it was not easy to find the time with so many competing demands jockeying for the top priority. Nonetheless, the true priority was indisputable, and my time connecting with patients and family members proved to be well spent.

It was gratifying to hear patients and their loved ones commend the kindness, friendliness, and responsiveness of staff. While much of my discussion with patients and family members was distinctly positive, their personal stories also powerfully convey the persistent challenges of navigating a complex healthcare system even in an organization like Griffin Hospital with a 20-year history of working to demystify the healthcare experience. The son of an 86-year-old patient with emphysema struggled to make sense of the case management process, wanting to do what would be best and safest for his father but unsure of how to maneuver through the logistical and emotional maze of placing his father in a nursing home. Another patient awaiting the results of a biopsy casually mentioned the she has never met her primary care physician, but hoped to, "one day." And another family who took turns at the bedside of their loved one with a broken knee and wrist from two falls in two days wrestled with her helplessness and with how to make sure all of her needs were met when they couldn't be there.

Patients are human beings struggling with real issues. They are not room numbers, diagnoses, or numbers on a page. The personal experiences these patients and families shared with me underscore that we must be vigilant in our efforts to personalize and demystify the patient experience, but they also accentuate the challenges facing staff. In my casual conversations with them, patients with hearing impairments struggled to hear me and more than once responded to questions I hadn't asked, seemingly to spare me the inconvenience of repeating myself. Others were medicated, and family members noted with amusement that the patient would likely not remember our conversation in a few hours. The implications of such communication barriers take on much greater significance when it comes to caregivers imparting important clinical information to patients. It is one thing for a patient not to remember a conversation with a visitor because she is medicated; it is quite another for her not to remember instructions on how to take a new medication, or for a patient with hearing loss to feign comprehension of important discharge information because she feels uncomfortable asking a caregiver to repeat it. As a patient-centered hospital, we are obliged to tackle these communication issues. This is not news. Communication challenges are pervasive in any hospital. However, experiencing the barriers firsthand shed a new light on the day-to-day experiences of staff and make clear that there is no magic bullet for effective communication. Instead, these efforts must be persistent, comprehensive, and versatile to meet the individual needs of patients.

Broadening the Definition of the Patient Experience

More than anything, these interactions with patients and family members validated that from the standpoint of patients, the healthcare experience encompasses much more than clinical capabilities, medical science, technology, and the other important details that occupy healthcare executives. Instead, patients spoke to me about the kindness and smiles of the staff, the happy-go-lucky housekeeper, reaching out to the hospital chaplain for support, the delicious soup they were served, and how much they appreciated having family around. Their comments stress that if we are to organize the way care is delivered around the priorities of patients, we are obliged to look beyond the narrow definition of the patient experience that until recently has dominated the healthcare executive's perspective.

Naturally, the experts on what constitutes a satisfying patient experience are patients themselves. More than 30 years ago, a patient's experiences at a California hospital left her feeling detached, ill-informed, and insignificant to her own healing process. She conceived a new model for healthcare in which providers partner with patients and families and patient education, dignity, and well-being are prioritized with providing top-quality clinical care. Named after the tree in Ancient Greece where Hippocrates taught the first medical students, the Planetree model she founded has weathered the test of time. In fact, it is more relevant than ever. The growing membership of Planetree affiliates includes a global community of 250 hospitals, medical centers, and continuing care communities in the United States, Quebec, the Netherlands, Brazil, and Japan. Members include a varied range of healthcare organizations, from 25-bed rural community hospitals to large academic medical centers and integrated healthcare systems (Planetree, Inc. 2010).

As Steiger and Balog point out, patient-centered care is not a new idea. The early patient-centered pioneers of Planetree began their work to transform healthcare by exploring with patients, families, and professional caregivers their thoughts and ideas for creating a better patient care experience in the hospital environment. By identifying diverse aspects of the hospital experience specified by patients as important to them, this feedback shaped the core components of the Planetree model (Frampton, Gilpin, and Charmel 2008). Caring interactions with providers, access to meaningful information, involvement of family, a healing physical environment, and the recognition of the role of spirituality, the arts, and food in healing mirror the important aspects of the hospital experience prioritized by the patients I spoke with during my recent rounds.

Considered collectively, these components go beyond the isolated cosmetic improvements, scripting, or customer service initiatives that Steiger and Balog and Taylor and Rutherford caution against. Rather, they provide a comprehensive framework for cultural, operational, and environmental transformation that cultivates healing environments in which patients can be active participants and caregivers are positioned to thrive.

Patient-Centered Care as a Concrete Aim Versus an Ambiguous Aspiration

Few leaders would dispute the merit of any endeavor whose stated goals are actively participating patients and thriving caregivers. However, unless progress toward such goals can be measured, patient-centered care will remain an ambiguous aspiration rather than a concrete aim. The question remains, then—how do we, as leaders, define, evaluate, and measure patients' active participation and caregivers' ability to thrive? Personal interactions and letters of compliment and complaint surely identify isolated instances of excellence or need for improvement, but anecdotal evidence is insufficient as a meaningful metric of progress toward a tangible vision of how care will be delivered.

Hospital Consumer Assessment of Healthcare Providers and Systems (HCAHPS) patient perception of care survey data can provide a more global evaluation of the patient experience, but it, too, has its limitations. At Griffin Hospital, this data has been used to inform deliberate and focused improvement initiatives. The scores capture patients' perspectives, but the numbers do not speak for themselves. Administering the survey by phone has provided opportunities to capture patients—in their own words and in their own voices—articulating what went well about recent hospital stays and what could have been improved. These telephone calls are recorded, compiled into audio files, and shared with staff to reinforce that the stories and the people behind the HCAHPS data are what motivate ongoing improvement efforts in such important aspects of the patient experience as communication, responsiveness, discharge, cleanliness, and noise.

However, while patient responses to HCAHPS survey questions ranging from "always happens" to "never happens" have provided useful information, these responses alone do not address the full range of patients' and families' desires from their hospital experiences. The HCAHPS survey is made up of 27 questions. Interactions with patients accentuate that survey questions alone could not possibly capture the totality and complexity of the patient experience.

For example, during a recent telephone survey, a discharged patient was asked the 27 HCAHPS questions. Then the caller asked, "Is there a specific employee whom you would like to see congratulated or thanked for the care he or she provided during the visit?" The patient's response speaks volumes about the seemingly simple gestures and accommodations that combine to leave lasting positive impressions on patients, and notably many of them are absent in responses to the standard HCAHPS questions:

> The nurses I would like to thank at Griffin Hospital would be Kristen for helping me, checking in on me, printing up crossword puzzles for me when I was there for so long and I was bored out of my mind and for her genuine personality and treating me more like family than a patient. I'd like to thank Mikey for staying with me and helping me and talking with me even though it was after her shift had ended. I'd like to thank Mimi for letting me drink out of a real person's cup instead of a plastic cup since I was there for a whole week and for treating me like a real person. I would like to thank Reggie for telling me that she offered me in her prayers... I'd like to thank Michele, Kate and Claire for also helping me a lot and being there and again treating me more like family than as a patient and going above and beyond what was expected as part of their daily routine.

Defining Excellence in Patient-Centered Care: The Patient-Centered Hospital Designation Program

A more meaningful measure of Griffin Hospital's effectiveness in delivering patient-centered care was its recognition in 2008 as a Designated Patient-Centered Hospital. Developed by Planetree, the Patient-Centered Hospital Designation Program is the only program to formally recognize hospitals that have comprehensively embraced and implemented patient-centered care. Designed to provide consistency in how we define excellence in patient-centered care, the program was developed with extensive input from hospital executives and staff and overseen by a designation advisory committee made up of hospitals, Planetree staff, and outside experts. The criteria are designed to be applicable to all acute care hospitals, irrespective of size, location, or formal affiliation with Planetree, and designation is one of the awards recognized by The Joint Commission on its Quality Check website, www.qualitycheck.org (Planetree, Inc. 2010).

To achieve recognition as a Designated Patient-Centered Hospital, a hospital must satisfy 50 criteria. The criteria are wide-ranging, reflecting key attitudes, behaviors, and policies one would expect to find in a patient-centered healthcare setting. These include a number of the practices identified by Taylor and Rutherford, including shared access to medical records, open visitation, and family members' participation in care, opportunities for patient and family input into hospital operations, patient choice in meal selection, and patient and family involvement in change-of-shift report. In addition, the criteria challenge hospitals to consider how best to balance patient empowerment with important safety considerations, to ensure that transparency and partnership remain priorities even when the unexpected occurs, and to apply patient-centered approaches to billing processes and community education and outreach initiatives.

Recognizing that the patient experience ultimately originates with those providing their care, several other criteria focus on nurturing a work environment that is professionally and personally supportive of staff. Of course, patient-centered care must not come at the expense of excellent medicine. On the contrary, it complements clinical excellence and contributes to it through the cultivation of mutually beneficial partnerships and enhanced communication between patients and caregivers. Accordingly, an evaluation of quality outcomes is also part of the designation program.

Consistent with the theme of the two feature articles—that partnerships with patients and families are the foundation of patient-centered care—the crux of the decision to award a hospital the Patient-Centered Hospital Designation is the feedback gleaned from patients and family members during focus groups. It is not enough for leaders to profess that a patient-centered culture is in place; this must be validated by patients, family members, and staff. To date, ten hospitals in North America have been recognized as Designated Patient-Centered Hospitals.

Given the depth and scope of the designation criteria, perhaps it is not surprising that Designated Patient-Centered Hospitals are doing better than most in satisfying a wide range of patients' needs, as reflected in their HCAHPS scores (see Exhibit VI.1). As a group, the nine Designated Patient-Centered Hospitals in the United States perform above the CMS national average in nine of the ten publicly-reported HCAHPS categories and at the national average in the tenth category. The most significant differences appear in the overall rating and willingness to recommend questions.

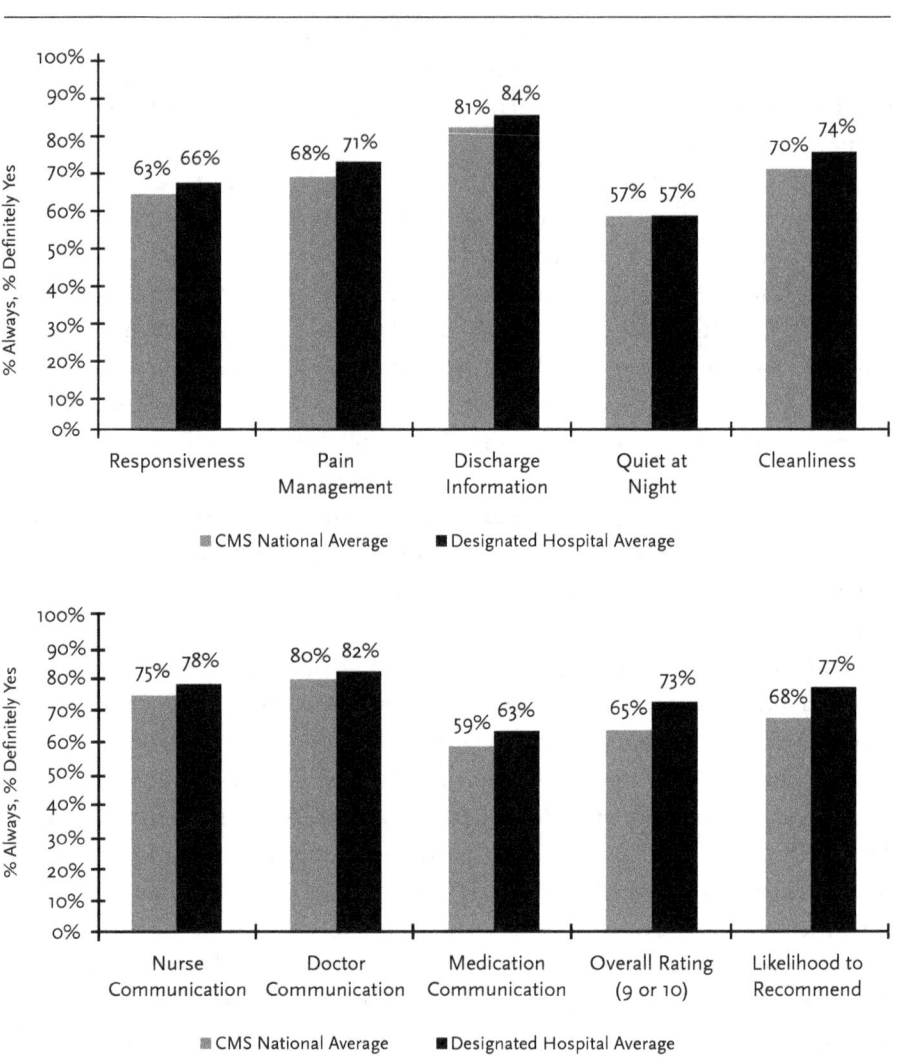

EXHIBIT VI.1

HCAHPS Comparison of US Planetree Designated Hospital Average and CMS National Average

Source: Adapted from CMS (2010).

New Incentives Strengthen the Business Case for Patient-Centered Care

Steiger and Balog write that "operationalizing patient-centered care requires investment." The experiences of the Designated Patient-Centered Hospitals, though, suggest the potential for a considerable return on investment, especially given the events of the last few months. When President Barack Obama signed into law the healthcare reform legislation in March, the long-anticipated proposal for financial incentives for hospitals that meet certain quality performance standards—including measures that focus on patient perceptions of care—became a reality, effectively solidifying the economic significance of providing patient-centered care (US Congress 2010).

These new incentives will undoubtedly compel more healthcare leaders to champion the importance of providing patient-centered care. Declarations of a philosophical commitment to partnering with patients and families, though, must be married with tangible changes in practice. Leaders must guide their organizations in translating concepts into action. This is not easy. Espousing the importance of open communication is simple; the challenge lies in operationalizing an approach to make sure that transparent, respectful, and reciprocal communication is the expectation and not the exception. Abandoning the tendency toward proprietorship and competition to share concrete practices like PeaceHealth St. Joseph Medical Center's "Safe to Speak Up" campaign is what will ultimately drive more widespread implementation of patient-centered care.

To this end, in 2008 Planetree developed the *Patient-Centered Care Improvement Guide* (Planetree, Inc., and Picker Institute 2008). Funded by the Picker Institute, the guide captures the collective wisdom of organizations implementing patient-centered care at an advanced level and the experiences of those who have encountered and overcome barriers. It focuses on the specifics of implementation and guides organizations through incorporating the concept of patient-centered care into the day-to-day business of caring for patients, families, and staff.

Conclusion

Of course, though, the most powerful resources available to those of us on a journey of patient-centered care culture change are not manuals or a series of articles; they are the people who make up our organizations: patients, families, staff, medical staff, volunteers, board members, and patient and family advisory council members. As leaders, our most important responsibility in providing patient-centered care is being receptive and responsive to their stories, their frustrations, and their ideas. These moments of listening and engaging in meaningful dialogue are the building blocks for partnerships and for providing patient-centered care.

References

Centers for Medicare & Medicaid Services (CMS). 2010. "CMS Hospital Compare Database." [Online information; retrieved 5/1/10.] www.hospitalcompare .hhs.gov.

Frampton, S. B., L. Gilpin, and P. Charmel (eds.). 2008. *Putting Patients First: De-signing and Practicing Patient-Centered Care*, 2nd ed. San Francisco: Jossey-Bass.

Planetree, Inc. 2010. "About Planetree." [Online information; retrieved 4/13/10.] www.planetree.org/about.html.

Planetree, Inc., and Picker Institute. 2008. *Patient-Centered Care Improvement Guide*. Derby, CT: Picker Institute.

U.S. Congress. Senate. 2010. *Patient Protection and Affordable Care Act*. 111th Cong., 1st Sess. [Online document; retrieved 4/13/10.] http://democrats .senate.gov/reform/patient-protection-affordable-care-act.pdf.

Interview with Patrick A. Charmel, FACHE, President and Chief Executive Officer of Griffin Hospital

Stephen O'Connor

Patrick A. Charmel, FACHE, is president and CEO of Griffin Hospital and its parent, Griffin Health Services Corporation, in Derby, Connecticut. As CEO of the corporation, he is also CEO of Planetree, Inc. Planetree is a not-for-profit organization supporting an association of more than 150 US and international hospitals dedicated to patient empowerment and patient-centered care.

Griffin has been the recipient of numerous awards and recognitions, including *Fortune's* 100 Best Companies to Work For, the Health Leaders Media 2008 Top Leadership Team in Healthcare, the Premier Healthcare Alliance 2010 Premier Award for Quality, and HealthGrades 2009, 2010, and 2011 Distinguished Hospital for Clinical Excellence and The Health Grades Outstanding Patient Experience awards.

Mr. Charmel served on the National Advisory Council for Healthcare Research and Quality. He is a board member, and past chair, of the Connecticut Hospital Association and has received the John D. Thompson Distinguished Visiting Fellow Award from Yale University, an honorary doctorate degree and the Distinguished Alumni Award from Quinnipiac University (where he is also a university trustee), and the Deane C. Avery Award from the New London *Day* newspaper in recognition of commitment to the public's right to know.

Mr. Charmel is a co-editor of *Putting Patients First: Best Practices in Patient-Centered Care*, which received ACHE's James A. Hamilton Award in 2004. He earned an undergraduate degree from Quinnipiac University and a master's degree in public health from Yale University.

Dr. O'Connor: Tell us about Griffin Hospital and Griffin Health Services Corporation and your position as president and chief executive officer.

Mr. Charmel: Griffin is a 160-bed community teaching hospital and is the largest entity within the Griffin Health Services corporate family. We are involved in some unique activities, such as our work with Planetree.

We are the only hospital in the country that houses a federally funded Prevention Research Center, and among our areas of expertise are obesity prevention, nutrition, and physical activity. Working with the top nutrition scientists in North America, we developed a comprehensive food scoring system that assists consumers in making healthy choices when buying food. The scoring system, which has been commercialized under the name NuVal™, is being licensed to supermarkets and disseminated to hospitals and managed care companies who do nutrition counseling and disease management. Over 90,000 foods have been scored, and these scores are influencing people's decisions, moving them to more healthy choices. In participating supermarkets, every food item on the shelf has a NuVal score next to the price and weight on the shelf tag, making it easier for consumers to figure out which food has higher nutritional value.

We pursued development of the scoring system because of our commitments to Planetree and to preventive healthcare. Planetree's foundation is in patient empowerment through access to information. Planetree tries to engage patients and to provide the information they need to make decisions about their health and well-being. This aim is part of Griffin's broader commitment to community health, health promotion, and wellness, a somewhat uncommon commitment for an acute care hospital.

Dr. O'Connor: What is it about your leadership style that has allowed the hospital to acquire so much positive recognition and national attention over the years?

Mr. Charmel: Griffin has always fancied itself an innovator, and we like to challenge the status quo. This is not a stated goal of the organization, but something that has evolved over time. We like to be entrepreneurial and look at new ways of doing things. Initially, this focus on innovation came from a need to differentiate Griffin in the marketplace. Twenty years ago the hospital was not differentiated. It had a poor reputation and suffered a long period of decline. If allowed to continue along that trajectory, the hospital would not have survived. We went through a process in which we engaged the community and sought their input. We did not get a lot of specifics, so we began to talk to employees as a proxy for the community. We talked to some of the approximately 1,000 employees who live in the surrounding area, asking them what an ideal hospital experience would look like for them and their families. Once we understood, we contrasted ourselves with the stated ideal. There was a gap between what we said we wanted to be and what we acknowledged we were; it created a lot of dynamic tension in the organization. It was the first time we were really honest with ourselves. We made a firm commitment to our staff and our community that we would get to that ideal state. A strong sense of ownership on the part of everyone associated with the organization has been instrumental in getting to that ideal. The staff and community felt proud when we began to make strides and show improvement. Our efforts led us to being considered a great place to work. We are visited all the time by companies inside and outside of healthcare who ask about our strategic plan for becoming an employer of choice. We tell them that we never had one. We never set out to be an employer of choice, but we did set out to be a great place to provide an exceptional patient experience, to deliver great care, and to be a great place for caregivers. We realized that we could never be a great place to be cared for unless we really took care of our caregivers and engaged them in the process of organizational transformation.

Dr. O'Connor: Employee pride appears to be an essential ingredient for Griffin.

Mr. Charmel: A few years back when we were ranked fourth in the country on the *Fortune* 100 Best Companies to Work For list, we had the highest pride rating of any one of the Best Places to Work companies. We came to realize that pride is absolutely fundamental. It is not about employee satisfaction, but employee pride. How do you create that sense of pride in the organization? By having credible management, delivering on promises, walking the talk, setting high standards and meeting them, and being sure to reward and recognize employees in the process. Initially, Griffin set out to create programs and services that were responsive to consumers, by emphasizing customer service and by creating a great service experience. The discipline we developed has served to improve clinical performance as well. We went from being a laggard in service and clinical quality to being a leader in our state, in terms of objective measures of quality, and one of the leaders in the country. Again, this has resulted in a strong sense of employee pride, which facilitates continued improvement. Griffin is a small hospital that became an influential leader, and we try to remain an organization that others seek to emulate. We have helped many organizations, directly and through Planetree, and we are committed to continuing to help others.

Dr. O'Connor: What is Planetree and why has Griffin Hospital been so deeply involved in following its tenets and approaches?

Mr. Charmel: When Griffin was struggling we engaged our employees in the community to define an ideal hospital. Initially, we experimented, focusing on one service at a time, beginning with our then-failing maternity service. We turned it around by talking to women of childbearing age and to women who'd had babies here and elsewhere, and by creating a new patient-centered model of maternity care, which became the first hospital-based birthing center in New England. We went from a service in decline to one that was rapidly growing with very high patient satisfaction. It was a good first step, but the hospital's overall reputation did not improve. We were not so presumptuous to think that because we improved one service line we could apply that same approach hospitalwide. We needed to find other models of patient-centered care.

That led us to Planetree, which at the time was a single, 13-bed unit in the 500-bed Pacific Presbyterian Medical Center that is now California Pacific Medical Center. That model Planetree unit came about through the initiative of a patient, Angie Thieriot. As Angie battled a rare viral infection, she was disheartened by the lack of personalized care at the hospital. Her response was to start Planetree, which began as a consumer health library in downtown San Francisco. Angie believed that hospitals could become more responsive to consumers by empowering them through access to information so they could be actively involved in decisions affecting their care and well-being. This was pre-Internet late 1970s. Back then healthcare consumers, at least when they were hospitalized, certainly were not engaged. "Ideal" patients were compliant and passive and let providers do things without questioning them or complaining. That "ideal" did not serve patients' interests.

Thieriot and her team started a consumer health library and created a ground-swell of informed consumers. The hospital where she had the bad experience invited her to work with them to create a prototype unit. The unit revolutionized the physical environment of inpatient care delivery by involving family members and removing typical barriers and restrictions between caregivers and patients. Griffin discovered Planetree when it was in its infancy. Planetree had several model units, mostly on the West Coast, with one in New York City. We discussed a relationship but did not want to be a model unit—the model unit approach was very prescriptive. We sought a looser relationship so that we could experiment. Griffin was the first affiliate of Planetree, and really the first hospital in the country, to build a completely new facility from the ground up based on Planetree's patient-centered care principles. We had the freedom to design a hospital around these principles, and we won many industry design awards. The hospital's image and reputation improved dramatically. There was a lot of industry attention and recognition, which we deflected to Planetree in California, and that attention was a challenge for them. They were a small, socially minded organization trying to change the world but did not have a strong infrastructure to field those inquiries and help organizations who wanted assistance. In 1998, after Planetree began to show signs of stress, we offered them the opportunity to become part of our corporate family. They were an independent, not-for-profit organization and were not based within a provider organization, so becoming part of the Griffin organization provided a great showplace for people interested to learn about the model. People could see Planetree in practice, kick the tires, and talk to caregivers, and we could keep Planetree's operating costs down because of our shared resources and infrastructure. Planetree came to Connecticut and has since grown dramatically, to 150 organizations with about 500 care sites across the United States and a number of foreign countries. Our work with Planetree maintains our commitment to the model that led to our success as a hospital and allows us to spread the philosophy to others as well. The work has been very rewarding. Within the last six months, the Veterans Health Administration has contracted with Planetree to facilitate the implementation of patient-centered care across the VA healthcare system.

Although I'm the CEO of the hospital and its subsidiaries, Susan Frampton, PhD, the president of Planetree, has led its expansion and is responsible for Planetree's tremendous success. She is a very skilled and passionate executive. Planetree is the leader of the patient-centered movement in this country. Planetree shares its best practices through patient-centered care improvement guides available free of charge online at the Picker Institute and the Planetree websites. These guides allow those who don't want to become Planetree alliance members to access the best practices of the world's premier patient-centered hospitals. Organizations are realizing that they need to become more patient focused to meet the expectations of more demanding consumers (especially those paying more out of pocket) and to succeed and thrive in the coming era of pay for performance and value-based purchasing.

Dr. O'Connor: Your approach to leadership has been distinguished by frequent, open, and honest communication with employees. What role has communication played in developing credibility, trust, and enhanced relationships with your employees?

Mr. Charmel: Because our organization struggled early on, we felt the only way we could survive and be successful was to engage our staff in meaningful ways. My leadership style is honest and very open to sharing information. We are strong proponents of transparency—it's what we believe in, and it prompts us to perform at a higher level. Being open and transparent about our performance puts pressure on the organization to continually improve. Employees know that transparency, openness, and engagement is the expectation. We have a strong culture and philosophy that keeps us in line as leaders. If we are not being true to our values, employees will tell us, which can be challenging at times. A common phrase here is "That is not Planetree." When we hear that, it may be because we did not explain things clearly and the employee misunderstood, or it may be because the employee is right and we compromised when we should not have.

Dr. O'Connor: Tell us about the role of leadership communication during the anthrax inhalation death at Griffin in 2001.

Mr. Charmel: That was a pretty remarkable experience. The patient presented to the emergency department and was found to have inhalation anthrax. This occurred during the national anthrax scare, but there had been no anthrax in our area. The state health department did not believe the test results. They were very skeptical, and we had to convince them to be persistent because we thought we were right. When it became apparent that the patient did have anthrax, there was a strong effort to restrict information flow. This restriction was inconsistent with our culture and it caused tensions between us and various authorities, including the FBI. When the information was still fresh, the FBI did not want me to share it with staff. By that time, staff were aware of the possibility of an anthrax case. I was concerned for their safety, the safety of our community, and our families. While still protecting the patient's privacy, we told employees what we had found, what we were going to do about it, and what the risks were. We wanted to talk to the community, too. When law enforcement told us not to, I said, "You can't stop me." I only realized later that they were carrying guns and certainly could have stopped me. But we did share the information, and I think we did the right thing. We understood that there were some law enforcement benefits of not sharing the information, but they were exaggerated. Disclosing the information reinforced our culture during a very stressful time. Our patient-centered principles guided us. Unfortunately, the patient died. The patient's death was unavoidable. The experience cemented for us that even in the face of strong opposition and adversity, we tried to do the right thing.

Dr. O'Connor: The career of a healthcare executive often involves numerous moves for developmentally progressive career opportunities in different geographic locations and different organizations. However, you have spent your entire career, from undergraduate intern to president/ CEO, at Griffin Hospital and have stated that "Often it is better to bloom where you are planted rather than seek a bigger pot." Please expand on and illustrate what you mean by this statement.

Mr. Charmel: I was told repeatedly by recruiters, my colleagues, and my professors that I was limiting my career opportunities by staying at Griffin. Frankly, they have stopped telling me that, but they tried for a long time. The conventional wisdom is that you start at a small hospital, develop a good track record, then use that as an opportunity to step up to a larger, more complex, prestigious organization with greater compensation. I am a firm believer in continuity of senior leadership. High-performing organizations are usually characterized by stable, credible, competent leadership. I feel some obligation to this organization because I have asked the staff and board to make many sacrifices and commit to excellence. They have met every challenge and fulfilled every commitment. Griffin has given me tremendous opportunities. I don't know too many organizations, large or small, that have had the kind of impact this organization has had. The career development advice I suggest is to not necessarily buy the conventional wisdom. I've spoken to a lot of people who have gotten to where they want to be career-wise but have jumped around a lot and don't have the same sense of fulfillment or accomplishment I have. They have sacrificed in the process. I don't think moving between organizations is necessary, and there are other examples like me. Employees in organizations that have a lot of senior management turnover spend too much time figuring out who has the power, how things are going to change, and either keeping their heads down or figuring out who they're going to align with. We haven't seen a lot of that here.

Discussion Questions on Required Readings

1. Why do most HCOs fail to meet Griffin Hospital's practice in improving the patient experience?
2. What are the barriers for other HCOs that attempt to adopt these best practices?
3. How do you respond to naysayers who argue that this kind of approach leads to higher cost of care and complaining patients getting luxury services they are not willing to pay for?
4. Why don't more hospitals adopt Planetree practices, including shared access to medical records, open visitation, family members' participation in care, opportunities for patient and family input into hospital

operations, patients' choice in meal selection, and patient and family involvement in change-of-shift report?

Required Supplementary Readings

Commonwealth Fund Commission on a High Performance Health System. 2007. *A High Performance Health System for the United States: An Ambitious Agenda for the Next President.* New York: The Commonwealth Fund.

Griffith, J. R., and K. R. White. 2011. "Beyond Acute Care to Community Health." In *The Well-Managed Healthcare Organization,* 7th ed. Chicago: Health Administration Press.

McCarthy, D. 2011. "Integrative Health Care Delivery Models and Performance." In *Health Care Delivery in the United States,* 10th ed., edited by A. R. Kovner, J. R. Knickman, and V. D. Weisfeld. New York: Springer Publishing Company.

Porter, M. E. and E. O. Teisberg. 2004. "Redefining Competition in Health Care." *Harvard Business Review* 82 (6): 65–76.

Discussion Questions for Required Supplementary Readings

1. What are the barriers and opportunities to implementing medical homes and accountable care organizations as of 2011?
2. How can acute community hospitals improve their community benefit programs now?
3. Why have successful integrated health system models—such as Mayo, Geisinger, Kaiser-Permanente, and the VA—not spread more widely?
4. What are the pros and cons of the Porter/Teisberg model for achieving the goals of healthcare reform?

Recommended Additional Readings

Dentzer, S. 2010. "Geisinger Chief Glen Steele: Seizing Health Reform's Potential to Build a Superior System." *Health Affairs* 29: 1200–1207.

Institute of Medicine. 2001. *Crossing the Quality Chasm: A New Health System for the 21st Century.* Washington, DC: National Academies Press.

Lutz, S. 2007. "Transparency—'Deal or No Deal?'" *Frontiers of Health Services Management* 23 (3): 13–23.

McAlearney, A. S. 2003. *Population Health Management: Strategies to Improve Outcomes.* Chicago: Health Administration Press.

Medicare Payment Advisory Commission. 2009. "Accountable Care Organizations." In *Report to the Congress: Improving Incentives in the Medicare Program.* Washington, DC: MedPAC.

Oliver, A. 2007. "The Veterans Health Administration: An American Success Story." *The Milbank Quarterly* 85 (1): 5–35.

Reid, R. J., K. Coleman, R. A. Johnson, P. A. Fishman, C. Hsu, M. P. Soman, and E. B. Larson. 2010. "The Group Health Medical Home at Year Two: Cost Savings, Higher Patient Satisfaction and Less Burnout for Providers." *Health Affairs* 29: 835–43.

Reid, T. R. 2009. *The Healing of America.* New York: Penguin Press.

Schroeder, S. A. 2005. "What to Do with the Patient Who Smokes?" *Journal of the American Medical Association* 294 (4): 482–87.

Shortell, S. 2010. "The Role of Accountable Care Organizations in Health Care Reform." Health Policy Brief, no. 3, Carey School of Business, Arizona State University.

THE CASES

Accumulating evidence indicates that a significant amount of medical care resources are misallocated relative to the health needs of Americans. At a time when nutrition, health education, and even literacy among low-income groups are neglected, hospitals have too many hospital beds, physicians perform too much surgery, and too few family practitioners and general physicians are available to low-income patients. Who is accountable? What are the risks to the manager of pursuing organizational accountability?

When a patient reports his experience, such as in Case P, "Letter to the CEO," what can the manager do to resolve these issues satisfactorily, especially now that the patient has left the facility? Patients are often hesitant to complain because they fear or respect the authority of caregivers or because they fear retaliation in levels of service provided to them.

As a rule, patients (and providers) do not wish to get involved in organizational functioning. They want things to run smoothly. Patients expect to be treated equitably compared to other patients. They expect not to be harmed by clinicians and others. For many patients, time is valuable, and they expect it not to be wasted. Patients want to be relieved of pain. They expect appropriate access to care, and some want explanations of their problems and their treatment options with probable related costs and benefits. Patients wish to be treated with dignity and with respect for their privacy. They wish to pay a fair price. How patients feel about their care varies by factors such as demographic and provider characteristics, patient condition, and services offered.

Managers expect patients to return to the facility for additional care, to complain if they feel they are not being properly treated, to make decisions about their own care, to expect only what is possible from caregivers (e.g., certain illnesses are not curable, sufficient staff are not always available), to respect the rights of other patients and providers, and to respect the facility's equipment and supplies. These expectations seem reasonable. Why then do some caregivers not behave as patients expect and vice versa?

First, effective mechanisms of accountability are frequently lacking. A culture that puts the patient first is not always present. Also, consumers may lack price or consumer information to make informed choices, and insurance companies may limit their choice of providers. When providers are paid primarily based on their costs, they may lack an incentive to be efficient. When physicians are paid fee-for-service, there may be an incentive to provide extra services rather than spend extra time talking with patients. On the other hand, when physicians are paid on salary or based on capitation, they may see fewer patients in the office.

When patients (or clinicians) are dissatisfied, they may take or threaten to take their business elsewhere. This becomes problematic in areas with few providers relative to the size of the population. Or they may complain. However, letters such as the "Letter to the CEO" may be few and far between, especially with that level of detail. Instead, patients may form organizations (as in chronic care homes or in the community) to advocate for their rights. Or patients can sue to recover costs, including pain and suffering, from a provider's malpractice insurer. Patients can lead healthier lives, so they are less dependent on the healthcare system, or they can raise their threshold of tolerance for pain or discomfort. Consumers can influence organizational performance by obtaining positions on governing boards or talking to the media. Government regulatory agencies, national accrediting agencies, and large purchasers can represent consumers and patients in holding providers accountable for meeting minimally adequate standards of care, and they can reward providers for outstanding performance, financial or otherwise.

Managers are paid to help the organization attain goals and to obtain a level of resources and productivity necessary for system maintenance (as Don Wherry, CEO, attempts to do in Case Q, "Whose Hospital?"). We believe that accountability is blurred unless some mutual agreement is specified among key stakeholders about mission, goals, satisfactory ways of measuring goal attainment, and ways to change organizational goals. Some of the consequences when such specification does not occur are shown in "Whose Hospital?"

The case study "What More Evidence Do You Need?" focuses on a different kind of accountability—to whom and for what is CEO Mark Wiley accountable? On one hand, Wiley is accountable to patients and the community for the Triple Aim goals of improving community health, enhancing the patient experience, and reducing per capita costs. On the other hand, he says what governing boards are primarily concerned with is "profits, profits, and profits." Such goals conflict, and Wiley's challenge is how to manage and communicate about necessary trade-offs to achieve compromises he can justify to staff, community, and his own conscience.

The short cases in this part of the book deal with the concept of accountability from different perspectives. "The Conflicted HMO Manager" describes the conflicts of interest between the manager and the organization. "What Benefits the Community?" and "CEO Compensation: How Much Is Too Much?" describe the conflicts for the hospital between acute care and community benefits provision and the difficulties in deciding and being accountable for decisions about executive compensation in not-for-profit organizations. "A Real Story of a Patient's Experience in Vancouver" shows that problems of organizational accountability to patients may be similar even under a single-payer system in Canada. "What's in a Name?" presents the conflict in values between a corporate philanthropic provider and the hospital that is its intended beneficiary. Finally, "Patient Satisfaction in an Inner-City Hospital" describes issues associated with patient satisfaction from the perspective of both physicians and managers.

Case P
Letter to the CEO

Anonymous
From *Quality Management in Health Care* 14 (4): 219–33, 2005

Dear Chief Executive Officer: The Perceptions of a Recently Discharged Patient

Editor's Note: *The following material represents a report based on the actual hospital experience of a health professional and his wife, who also is a health professional. They are well qualified to make the assessments set forth in this report.* Quality Management in Health Care *is treating this as a quality management case study, and, to preserve the authors' confidentiality, is omitting their names and that of the hospital.*

Foreword

Dear CEO,

Attached is a description of my recent experience at your hospital. I and my wife share this with you because we are committed to improving the delivery of health care services in hospitals. We believe that our perceptions reflect problems in the system of care and are in no way meant to reflect upon individuals.

We hope you will find the perceptions useful.

We have many professional colleagues and many friends who work at your hospital. We plan to continue to get our health care there. In fact, I expect to have another operation there 3 months from now.

We shall be happy to discuss any aspect of care with you or your staff, and do whatever we can to improve care. We plan to share this document with my physicians and with your Director of Nursing.

Sincerely,
Patient and Spouse

Perceptions of a Hospital Experience

Operation: Cardiac Arterial Bypass Graft (CABG) October 2004
Operative Report:

 I. Semi-urgent coronary bypass grafting employing aortosaphenous bypass grafts to the first and second circumflex marginal coronary artery.
 II. Anastomosis of the right internal mammary artery (skeletonized) to the right coronary artery.
 III. Anastomosis of the left internal mammary artery (as a pedicule) to the left anterior descending coronary artery (2 venous and 2 arterial grafts).
 The heart was returned to the pericardial cavity.
 The heart spontaneously defibrillated in a few minutes.
 The procedure was tolerated well and the patient was discharged from the operating room in good general condition.

This is our story of a common surgical procedure that saves lives every day, but is painful and stressful for patients and their families. The heart has spiritual meaning—our "heartfelt" thanks; "I love you with all my heart." We also know that we cannot live without our hearts. Knowing that my heart would stop beating for a large part of the surgery brought with it the special fear of truly being on the brink of death or of coming back (or not coming back from the dead). My wife and I were both terrified.

I underwent cardiac catheterization at an urban medical center in the Fall. The surgical plan at that time included insertion of a stent. However, the physician found a 70% blockage of the main anterior artery and similar damage to the posterior vessel. He said, "In 2004, in this city, a stent is not an option." The bypass graft had to wait until Plavix, the drug I took in anticipation of the stent, had passed out of my system. This circumstance was similar to that experienced by former President Clinton earlier in the year. The cardiologist required that I be given heparin, and kept under continuous hospital monitoring until a quadruple bypass could be performed 6 days later.

The quadruple bypass graft was performed by an outstanding surgeon, who typically performs more than 300 each year. Four days later I was sent home with plans for rehabilitation therapy to begin in 3 weeks. As I write this account 5 weeks after surgery, I am up and about and feeling much healthier, with more energy than before the surgery. So we could conclude that nothing went wrong. But, can we be so sure? True enough, the attending physicians provided excellent technical care and were also admirably comforting. The nurses were extremely pleasant and, for the most part, efficient. Nevertheless, we observed numerous errors or potential errors (near misses) in the way that ancillary staff, nurses, and even some physicians failed in or neglected their responsibilities, both medical and humane. There were system failures, largely in the provision of nonclinical, so-called hotel services. Opportunities were lost for staff to teach and provide emotional support, and that seriously marred the entire hospital experience. We have organized this narrative on the following themes.

Errors and Potential Errors

1. *Potential infections:* I never observed any physician, nurse, or staff member wash hands before approaching us, nor were we told that they had washed elsewhere.

2. *Fire hazards:* At least 8 gurneys, in addition to wheelchairs and linen carts, clogged the hallway outside my room, in violation of state regulations and JCAHO standards.

3. *Medication error:* Late one afternoon, a physician prescribed Cipro to be administered twice daily. A nurse gave me the first dose that evening. The next day she brought only 1 dose.

    Only on the third day she did follow orders and deliver morning and evening doses.

4. *Potential medication error:* The evening nurse came to say goodnight on one of the presurgery nights because she said she had nothing else to do for me. Only after my spouse asked about prescribed bedtime medications did the nurse leave to check, and returned to say, "Oh, I see he does have medications and I didn't see that in the computer." My spouse asked why these medications were not found in the computer.

    The nurse replied, "Oh, I guess they *are* listed for 10:00 PM. I'll get them for you." That same night, Proscar, one of my drugs, was missing from the medication drawer. The same nurse finally had to get Proscar from the pharmacy and brought it to me at 11:30 PM.

5. *Potential unnoticed cardiac event:* Another nurse left my heart monitor disconnected for 40 minutes prior to my transfer to another unit, explaining that he needed to have me ready for the transport crew. (Disconnecting a monitor takes about 3 seconds.)

6. *Potential blood clot:* At one point, the registered nurse failed to notice that the heparin intravenous bag was empty. My wife had to call him, and it took him more than 15 minutes to replace the fluid.

7. *Allergic reaction to tape:* I broke out in a skin rash from tape used during the cardiac catheterization. My wife told a physician resident, who ordered silver nitrate. On the evening before surgery, my wife told the surgical resident about the tape allergy, recommending that he not use the same tape during surgery. The resident said that the allergy was not

recorded in the chart and asked us to find out from the catheterization laboratory what kind of tape they had used.

But that was an impossible assignment for a patient or spouse. My wife asked that at least a yellow self-stick be put on the chart to note the tape problem. The resident told us to remember to tell the surgeons about it in the morning.

As our anxiety about the surgery mounted, my wife called a nurse acquaintance on the hospital staff. She finally was able to learn the name of the offending tape (Dermaclear) and placed a large warning on the chart.

8. *Informed consent:* The same surgical resident asked me to sign a consent form that did not specify any surgical procedure. He said that he would fill it in afterwards.

9. *Potential delayed recovery.* Three days after surgery, I was too tired to speak to the physical therapist (PT) who visited with instructions. The PT called my wife at home and asked her to be available the next day to help persuade me to participate in therapy. They set a time for the meeting; my wife arrived on time, but the PT failed to appear at all that day.

10. *Potential dental problems:* I occupied 2 private rooms in sequence during my stay. Neither had a toothbrush, floss, or toothpaste. There was a mouthwash of some sort—but not the kind that studies have shown works as well as dental floss in preventing gum problems.

System Failures
Absence of follow-up

1. A cardiology fellow, who worked me up in preadmission testing, promised to attend the cardiac catheterization but never showed up.

2. The evening before surgery, the anesthesia resident was unable to confirm that the attending anesthesiologist would be present throughout the cardiac surgery and would be handling only 1 patient. The resident's reaction to my inquiries suggested that she considered them bizarre. She said she would find out, but never returned with an answer. Once again, my wife called someone she knew, who verified that the anesthesiologist would be handling only my case.

Poor Communication

1. Immediately after the catheterization and prior to surgery, the cardiologist called my wife to report that I would have to be monitored and remain in the hospital until surgery. He had already told me the same thing. But when I arrived in the postcatheterization unit, a nurse congratulated me on going home that day. Similarly, a patient facilitator

for the catheterization service left a message for my wife that she could take me home in a few hours.

2. I and the entire unit had no phone service for several hours one day. On another day, my extension number, untypically, did not match the room number. So my callers ended up disturbing another patient.

3. No one explained how to get a newspaper. My wife or a physician friend brought one each morning by 8:00 AM. Only days later did we learn that a newspaper deliverer came to the floor each morning.

4. We could not get TV service for several hours in one of the rooms. The TV service's phone was continually busy.

5. No one told us what personal clothing and supplies to bring to the hospital either for the catheterization or for the surgery.

6. No one informed us how we could make use of helpful volunteers, social services, or pastoral counseling. We never saw a nutritionist, who could have explained the presurgery diet, which seemed low on salt, or the desirable posthospital diet.

7. No one explained how to work the electric bed. It may surprise readers, but my wife, a nurse, did not know either (but being a public health nurse she soon figured it out).

8. When my wife was asked to leave the recovery room following her brief visit with me, the nurse offered a phone number for checking on my condition during the night. Confident that she had a contact with a registered nurse (RN), my wife left the hospital. But when she called the number a few hours later she got the main switchboard operator who reported on my condition, secondhand.

Insensitivity to Patients

1. At 10:30 PM, the night before the surgery, several nurses were laughing and talking outside of my room for one half hour, until I requested quiet.

2. On at least 2 occasions, nurses spoke loudly over the speaker in my room, in search of a nurse who was not there.

3. The waiting area of the cardiac catheterization laboratory was in the corner of a crowded, cold hallway, with only 1 chair for me. My wife had to stand. There was no privacy for me in a patient gown. Hospital staff passed regularly through this hallway, threading between us and the laboratory equipment that cluttered the hall.

Environment and Housekeeping

1. My private room featured a broken chair, dirty windows, and inadequate light for reading. The nurse sent for a reading lamp, which arrived the next day, broken. The lamp was never fixed or replaced. On several

occasions, full waste baskets were not emptied. The bathroom towels were thin and worn.

2. Environment: The room temperature in one of my rooms was consistently either too hot or too cold.

3. Unnecessary moves: The postangiogram unit was closed from Saturday noon to Monday morning, forcing my transfer to another floor—up one crowded elevator, down another.

4. When I arrived in the new unit, there was no holder for my cardiac monitor, and I had to carry it in my hand for several hours.

5. Missing belongings: When transferred from one unit to another, my belongings were not transferred with me. It took several requests and phone calls to retrieve them.

Food Service

The food was consistently tasteless, sometimes delivered late (after 10:00 AM one morning) and, one evening, to the wrong room. We were never told that we could bring in take-out food (at least prior to surgery, we did anyway). On one occasion, my wife saw a dietary manager in the visitor cafeteria and told him that my food had been found in another unit and that it was cold. He advised her to call the dietary department and ask the nutritionist to provide a new meal. When my wife called, the woman who answered the phone said rudely, "We don't have a nutritionist here. He should never have told you that." She finally agreed to send up a new meal.

Lost Opportunities (to Provide Comfort, Improve Health, and/or Improve Safety)

1. No one gave us information or any educational materials about cardiac disease, risks affecting the course of disease after discharge, or behavior that might keep me healthy. By flipping the TV channels, we saw that the hospital has some educational videos on various topics, including meditation.

2. The cardiac surgery house staff (which sometimes included a nurse practitioner) usually visited in groups of 5 or more, but never introduced themselves by name or professional title. They spoke in murmurs, mainly to each other. They actually stood away from me, as if I had a communicable disease. They never provided emotional support or taught us anything about my illness or approaches to preventing future cardiac problems.

3. Only nurse friends, who visited me, offered emotional support or asked about our feelings and fears. Only 1 hospital aide offered hope, a hug, and kind words before surgery. My wife asked for a visiting nurse

following discharge. The hospital nurse declined. She then asked for physical therapy at home and one of the nurses said that a PT would be arranged, but it never was.

Discussion

According to a physician friend, I am incredibly lucky that I was diagnosed and treated as quickly as I was. Another physician told us "of people with my problem 10% die each year." For probably saving my life we are grateful to talented and caring physicians and nurses. Our internist is the real hero for following up on my vague and not very serious symptoms. We are grateful that we have adequate insurance and live in the United States, where I had to wait only 1 week to get the echocardiogram that began my course of care. We were fully paid by our employer during my recovery and my wife's care for me in the hospital.

Fortunately for us, we had the financial resources to go back and forth to the hospital, fly in our children, and buy whatever I wanted, from take-out food to TV and phone. We worry about people who do not have our resources, notably health insurance, or who do not speak English, have no primary care physicians who care about them, and whose spouses cannot manage to arrange good patient care.

There were many wonderful RNs and aides who cared for me. One of the RNs got me up to the chair, got me to use the nebulizer, and arranged for me to have a bed bath. That is ordinary nursing care in some hospitals, but we saw it as especially kind.

Nothing we encountered resulted in poor outcomes, but there were too many near misses, and we suspect similar mishaps occur at almost all hospitals.

The near misses usually are not reported and therefore do not inspire changes in hospital routines. Hospital managers and others can claim that our negative experiences were minor (some would say petty—like the non-functioning TV) and blame a lack of adequate funding. The managers might make a similar claim about the "lost" opportunities we noted, saying "There is a nursing shortage." This is not the place to discuss revenues and expenses, except to note that the hospital charged more than $68,000 for this 11-day stay, not including physician fees.

We believe that many of the problems we have identified result not from inadequate resources, but rather from insufficient focus on patients and a lack of accountability for performance at the patient level of care. If our experience is typical, it has important implications for hospital administrators and for the training of patient care managers.

Case Questions

1. How do you feel about the level of patient care given in this medical center? How do you think other patients feel? The doctors? The managers?
2. What are some of the problems with patient care in this hospital? What are the most important problems that the manager can do something about?
3. What are the causes of these problems?
4. As the hospital CEO, what would you do, if you had received this memorandum?
5. How would you have solved the problems to which the memorandum refers?
6. What organizational factors would constrain implementation of your recommended solutions?
7. How would you, as the CEO, overcome these constraints?

Case Q
Whose Hospital?

Anthony R. Kovner

Tony DeFalco, a 42-year-old electrical engineer, and president of the board of trustees of Brendan Hospital in Lockhart, East State, wondered what he had done wrong. Why had this happened to him again? What should he do now? The trustees had voted, at first 10 to 6 and then unanimously, to fire Don Wherry, the new chief executive officer. Brendan Hospital had hired Wherry, who had been DeFalco's personal choice from more than 200 candidates, just 18 months before. DeFalco had told the trustees that he shared the burdens of managing Brendan Hospital with Wherry, that there was no way of dissociating Wherry's decisions from his own decisions. So in a way, DeFalco pondered, the board should have fired him, too.

DeFalco had lived in Lockhart all his life, and he loved the town, commuting one-and-a-half hours each day to his office at National Electric. Lockhart was one of the poorest towns in the poorest county in central East State, with a population of about 50,000, of which 30 percent were Italian, 25 percent Puerto Rican, and 10 percent Jewish. The leading industries in town were lumber, auto parts manufacturing, and agriculture.

On June 7, 1979, Joe Black, president of the Brendan Hospital medical staff, had called DeFalco, telling him that some doctors and nurses had met over the weekend and that they were going to hold a mass meeting at the hospital to discuss charges against CEO Wherry. DeFalco had called Wherry immediately in Montreal, Canada, where Wherry was giving a lecture to healthcare administration faculty about the relationship between the chief executive officer and the board of trustees. Wherry was as shocked as DeFalco had been and returned immediately to Lockhart. That night DeFalco and Wherry went to a hospital foundation meeting near where the mass meeting was being held in the hospital cafeteria.

DeFalco and Wherry had been planning the foundation meeting for several months. It had been scheduled and rescheduled so that all eight of the prominent townspeople could attend. The key reasons behind forming the foundation were to enlist the energies of community leaders in hospital fund-raising, thereby freeing the hospital board for more effective policymaking, and to shield hospital donations from the state rate-setting authority. Brendan Hospital had held a successful first annual horse show the previous fall, netting $10,000 and creating goodwill for the hospital, largely through the efforts of DeFalco and two dedicated physicians who owned the stable and dedicated the show and all proceeds to the hospital. Because this was an important meeting, and because they had not been invited to attend the mass meeting, DeFalco and Wherry decided to attend the foundation meeting. There, they elicited a great deal of verbal support for the foundation, and for DeFalco's leadership. The community leaders were familiar with the problems of employee discontent in their own businesses and with the political maneuverings of former Brendan medical staff. It would all calm down, no doubt. The wife of the town's leading industrialist said she appreciated DeFalco's frankness in sharing the hospital's problems with them.

But, of course, everything was not yet calm. The mass meeting was held and a petition signed to get rid of Wherry. The petition was signed by half the medical staff and by half the employees as well. A leadership committee of four doctors and nurses demanded Wherry's immediate resignation, and it was rumored that if the board didn't vote Wherry out, the committee wanted the board's resignation as well. Brendan Hospital was being site-visited for Joint Commission accreditation that Thursday and Friday. A board meeting was held on Wednesday afternoon, before the site visit. After much discussion, a decision emerged to meet with the staff and employee representatives on the following Monday. The accreditation site visit somehow went smoothly.

The four doctor and nurse representatives met with the board on Monday afternoon, stating that they could not speak for the others. They delivered the petition to DeFalco, who read it to the trustees. The petition stated that the undersigned demanded Wherry's resignation because he was "incompetent, devious, lacked leadership, had shown unprofessional conduct, and had

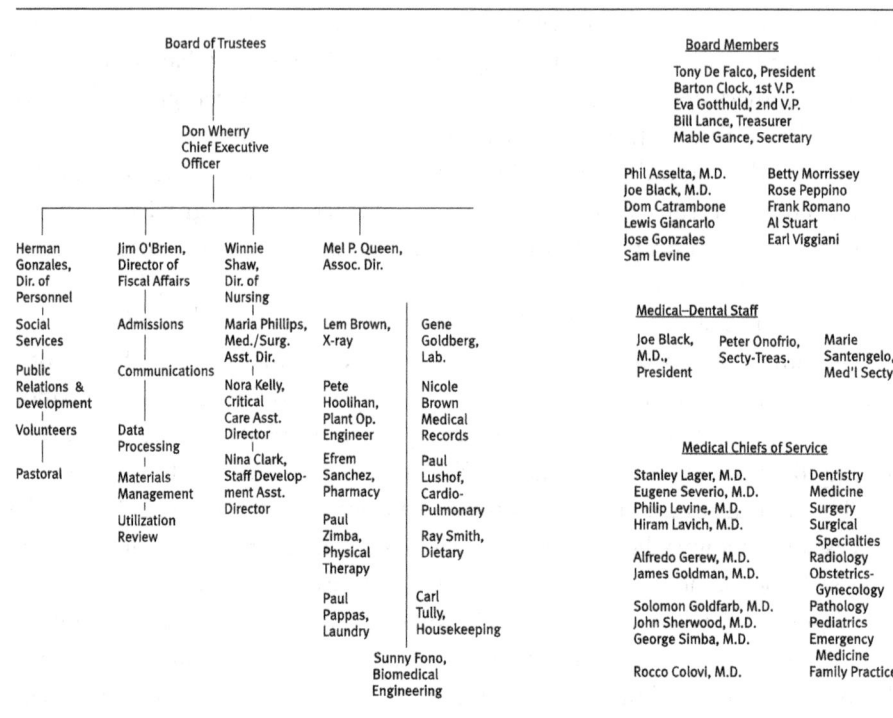

committed negligent acts." The representatives would not discuss the matter at that time. They had been delegated only to deliver the petition. Thus, DeFalco scheduled another board meeting for the following Wednesday afternoon to hear all the charges by all the accusers and to allow Wherry to confront his accusers, 13 days after the mass meeting of June 8.

The meeting of June 22 was attended by eight physicians, 18 registered nurses, five department heads, a laboratory supervisor, one dietary aide, and the medical staff secretary. (For an organization chart of Brendan Hospital see Exhibit VI.2.) All but one of the 18 hospital trustees were in attendance, including Wherry, who was a member of the board. The meeting was held in the tasteful new boardroom of Brendan Hospital, complete with oak tables and plush burgundy carpeting. The committee's presentation is summarized as follows.

The Accusers' Charges

Perrocchio: The most important thing we have to discuss today is patient care. That's why all of us are here. Many of us are here not because we have a personal gripe, but because we want to do what's best for the patient.

Tully (department head): Mr. Wherry humiliated and intimidated three department heads: Mr. O'Brien, Mrs. Williamson, and Mr. Queen.

Pappas (department head): There is a bad morale problem in the laundry.

Patrocelli (supervisor): Laboratory morale is low. There are too many people in other departments and not enough personnel in our department. Companies who deliver to us have put us on COD.

Fong (department head): Mr. Wherry humiliated Mr. Queen.

Frew: There has been a problem in staffing new areas of the hospital. We were told that these would be adequately staffed. I realize they haven't opened yet.

Tontellino: Several months ago a nursing survey was sent around by Mr. Wherry, and we all sent in our responses. We have received no response from Mr. Wherry about the survey.

Carter (RN): We need more help on the floors.

Greenberg: Insensitivity is the problem. The administrator, as you can see from all the comments made so far, is insensitive to the people who work in the hospital.

Santengelo (medical staff secretary): The director of volunteers' salary should have been explained to the rest of us. Employees should continue to get the Christmas bonuses. It means a lot to many of them. Mr. Wherry has created a whole lot of unnecessary paperwork. I don't feel he heard what we were telling him.

Lafrance (RN): There has been a lack of communication between administration and employees. Mr. Wherry actually has asked people to give him the solution to a problem they presented to him.

Shaw (RN and former director of nursing): Mr. Wherry used four-letter words in his office with me. He called one of our attending physicians a . . .

Levari (RN): When there was a bomb scare, Mr. Wherry came to the hospital and stayed for 20 minutes. Then he left before the police came, which I definitely think was wrong.

Leon (RN): It took Mr. Wherry ten months to call a meeting with the head nurses. Problems in nursing have to be solved around here by the nursing department.

Kelly (RN and assistant director): The problem has been lack of communication. I was humiliated when I presented a memo to Mr. Wherry about increases in operating room expenses. He said he couldn't understand what was in the memo, although it was right in front of him. His whole manner was rude.

Phillips (RN and assistant director): When the state inspector came on one of her inspections, she said that Mr. Wherry should be dumped.

Santengelo: He told Dr. Burns one thing and me another when we needed extra help in my office.

Bernstein (RN): Mr. Wherry was evasive and showed a lack of concern. He asked me for my suggestions. I told him to put an ad in the paper to get more help, and it was in the next day. Nurses were not present at administrative meetings.

Brown (department head): Mr. Wherry said Dr. Black would also have to sign an X-ray equipment request for $100,000. That is poor leadership.

Ferrari (RN): I didn't like the tone of his response when I called him at home to ask about treating a Jehovah's Witness in the emergency room. When we call Mr. Queen, the associate administrator, we nurses never experience that kind of problem.

Lashof (department head): I felt intimidated by Mr. Wherry. The hospital has a morale problem that interferes with patient care.

Brown (department head): He said to me, "If you can't handle the problem [we were having in X-ray], I'll find someone who can."

Charlotte (RN): I've had a problem with my insurance and the personnel department still hasn't gotten back to me for three weeks now. I am divorced and I have a little girl, and it's really creating a hardship for me. I don't understand why Mr. Gonzales, the personnel director, hasn't gotten back to me. I've called him about it many times.

Lafrance: Mr. Wherry sounded upset and annoyed when I called him at home about the electrical fire in maternity.

Gerew: The problem is communication. Mr. Wherry promised something and he didn't deliver. I have been working here for three years trying to develop a first-class radiology department. How can we cut costs and improve service in the outpatient department? I asked for help from fiscal affairs and I didn't get any.

Lavich: The family no longer has any confidence in its father. There was a unanimous vote of no confidence for Mr. Wherry in my department.

Greenberg: Mr. Wherry has a repressive style. There has been a tremendous turnover of personnel in the nursing department since he became the administrator.

Mendez: There is poor morale at the hospital. The nurses are upset. Mr. Wherry used derogatory language concerning foreign medical graduates. This was in the student administrative resident's report on what to do about the emergency room. Let's remove what is causing the problem.

Black (president of the medical staff): Department heads should be on board committees. No one came around and told department heads that they were appreciated. People at Shop-N-Bag make more money than nurses. Our medical people want to be appreciated, too.

Frew: Tony DeFalco, the board president, is seen as being in Mr. Wherry's pocket. There must be accountability for the situation that arose. I have no personal grievance. Accountability starts at the top.

Black: Dr. Fanchini was behind a good deal of what I was doing. A lot of critical things have happened, making for a crisis situation. Dr. Simba was hired to head up the emergency room, without adequate participation of the medical staff. Dr. Fanchini resigned as a board member. Dr. Burns resigned as president of the medical staff because of his personal problems. Mr. Wherry said that Dr. Severio was not really a cardiologist. The radiologists at Clarksville Hospital asked for emergency privileges. What made the medical staff unhappy was when Mr. Wherry said we weren't going to get a CT scanner and when he said that there were no problems in nursing morale. At the meeting of the medical executive committee held this Monday night, June 20, the committee reaffirmed our lack of support for Mr. Wherry, giving him a vote of no confidence by a vote of 10 for the motion, 1 against, and 1 abstaining.

Listening to the doctors and nurses, DeFalco felt as if he was a spectator watching a Greek tragedy. The committee representatives left the boardroom. DeFalco remembered when the board had met in the old private dining room only two years before, voting to dismiss the previous administrator of 22 years, Phil Drew, because Drew allegedly hadn't kept up with the times, some doctors said he had sexually harassed several of the nurses, and the hospital wasn't doing well financially. Drew had been a good man, and Tony DeFalco had promised himself that he would do everything in his power to prevent this from happening again.

Wherry's Defense

"First, I'd like to go through the state of the hospital, as it was when I got here," Wherry began nervously. And yet DeFalco thought Wherry seemed perfectly assured of himself, confident in the rightness of his cause. That was probably one of the things the doctors held against him. Wherry had attended Princeton undergraduate and Harvard Business School and had worked for a government regulatory agency in hospital cost containment before taking the Brendan job.

Wherry: There was bad leadership in the nursing department and in several other departments, a lack of medical staff leadership, and few competent department heads. Nursing is a difficult occupation. Morale is always a problem in this department. These are young people with children; they are working evenings, nights, and weekends; and the work is physically, emotionally, and administratively demanding. The doctors at this hospital are like doctors in other hospitals like Brendan, fearful of anything that threatens to affect their livelihood or freedom. I can understand that. But there is a small, embittered group with axes to grind against me. [For a list of 1978 Brendan Hospital goals and accomplishments, see Exhibit VI.3. For 1979 Brendan Hospital goals, see Exhibit VI.4.]

I have been busy with the finances of the hospital and in improving external relationships with the Latinos, state officials, and other groups. Mel Queen, the associate administrator, has been busy with the new construction and the move into our new $5 million wing.

We've had a new director of nursing on board for five weeks now, and I wish that everyone would have just given her a chance. Dr. Burns's resignation as president of the medical staff didn't help me any, and I have had a director of personnel, Gonzales, with acute personal problems, which has been a problem for me, too. Next, it's quite unusual for someone to have to defend himself on the spot to a list of specific charges that I have been waiting for these past 13 days and just now have been made aware of. I think the way this whole thing has been handled by the doctor and nurse ringleaders is disgraceful. The charges they have made are largely not true and could not be proven even if they were true. Even if the charges are true to a substantial extent, there is still not sufficient reason for your discharging me, certainly not suddenly, as they are demanding you to.

The doctors are out to get me because I'm doing the job you've been paying me to do, what I'm evaluated on, and for which I received a very good evaluation and a big raise at the end of last year, presumably because I was doing a good job. [For Wherry's evaluation, see Appendix VI.1; for DeFalco's raise letter, see Appendix VI.2.] Certainly none of you have told me to stop doing what I have been doing to ensure quality, contain costs, and improve service. During the past year I gathered information for the medical staff on a new reappointment worksheet so that reappointments aren't made on a rubber stamp process every two years. I pointed out the problems that the low inpatient census in pediatrics would create in retaining the beds in the years to come. I obtained model rules and regulations for the medical staff and shared these with the president, Dr. Black. I questioned the effectiveness of the tissue committee, which hasn't been meeting, and when it has met, whose minutes are perfunctory. I questioned the performance of the audit committee after our delegated status under PSRO was placed in question by a visiting physician, Dr. Lordi. I suggested we explore mandated physician donations to the hospital, as was passed and implemented two years ago by another East State hospital. When

EXHIBIT VI.3
Brendan
Hospital 1978
Goals and
Accomplish-
ments (from
1978 Annual
Report)

1978 Goals	1978 Accomplishments
1. Stabilize hospital finances	• $75,000 surplus • Improved Medicaid and Blue Cross reimbursement • Expenditures reduced in line with lower than expected occupancy
2. Increase fund-raising	• Modernization fund pledges on target • Successful first annual horse show
3. Improve hospital morale	• Regular employee-administration meetings • Regular publication of *Brendan News*
4. Improve quality of nursing care	• High patient evaluations in survey • New director of nursing recruited
5. Organize department of emergency medicine	• Department organized and Dr. George Simba recruited as chief
6. Establish effective management information and control system	• Implemented auditors' recommendation • Evaluating new data processing alternatives
7. Increase communication with Spanish-speaking community	• Several meetings held with Hispanic leaders • Increased Hispanic staff in patient areas, including social services
8. Increase accountability of medical departments for quality assurance	• Board resolution requiring annual reports • Joint conference committee and trustee seminar for better communication between medical staff and trustees
9. Increase community participation in long-range planning	• Four community members added to long-range planning committee • Wide distribution of annual report with attendance encouraged at annual meeting
10. On-schedule, on-budget, fully accredited new wing	• New wing scheduled to open in April 1979 • Building roughly within budget and on schedule

1. Stabilize hospital finances and improve cash flow
2. Improve board, administration, and medical staff communication
3. Increase hospital involvement of Spanish-speaking community
4. Fill administrative vacancies and recruit needed medical staff
5. Increase pediatric and obstetrical inpatient occupancy
6. Accomplish complete availability of new wing by April and obtain full hospital accreditation
7. Establish quality assurance programs for all professional departments
8. Establish productivity and efficiency goals for all hospital departments
9. Develop an operational long-range plan, including time and dollar estimates for new programs
10. Continue to contain increases in hospital costs

patients made complaints about doctors I took these up with the respective chiefs of departments. I investigated the assertion by a lab technician that tests were being reported and not done by the laboratory. I questioned and had to renegotiate remuneration of pathologists and radiologists, all with knowledge of the president of the board, Mr. DeFalco, and I have done nothing without involving the medical executive committee.

I have been involved in the lengthy and frustrating process of getting support from other hospitals for a CT scanner and in justifying financial feasibility of the CT scanner at this hospital. I have suggested ways to recruit needed physicians into Lockhart and have shared with the staff other approaches used by East State hospitals, such as a guaranteed income for the first year. I followed up a trustee's question about the appropriateness of fetal monitoring with the chief of obstetrics and gynecology, and worked out a satisfactory response to poor ophthalmology coverage in the emergency room with the chief of ophthalmology. I became involved in trying to convince one of our three pathologists not to resign because of a run-in with the chief of pathology. I have to get after physicians who do not indicate final diagnosis or complete their charts on time, because this delays needed cash flow for the hospital. I suggested that the hospital develop a model program for providing day hospital and other care to the elderly and chronically ill, and sought the cooperation of State University in designing a research protocol to measure the need for such services. This action was resented by several members of the staff, although we have not gone ahead with the state research program pending staff approval, and, if they disapprove, I said we would not go ahead with it.

I initiated a study of how we can prevent malpractice at the hospital and conveyed board disapproval of radiology equipment, which we had scheduled to buy but couldn't afford because other radiology equipment broke down in an unforeseen way. There are several very difficult physicians on the medical executive committee who have never gotten along with any administrator or with other physicians. I am the one who has to discuss with the surgeons and the radiologists ways to decrease costs in their units when these costs are way above the state medians, and we have to reduce them or face financial penalties.

As far as nursing goes, here is a list of what I have done: I have met with all shifts, with head nurses, with supervisors, and regularly with the director and assistant directors. I hired a new director and fired an old assistant director whom the nurses said showed favoritism, lied to them, and overpromised. This was opposed, by the way, by Dr. Fanchini, former director of obstetrics and gynecology. I hired an expert nursing consultant to help us develop appropriate goals and ways of meeting these goals. I was in the process of obtaining the services of an operations research consultant, at no cost to the hospital, to help us with our scheduling problems. We implemented a study done by an administrative resident on improved staffing and scheduling. I pointed out all the problems of authoritarian leadership, lack of adequate quality assurance programs, and lack of appropriate scheduling and budgeting to the previous nursing director, which is why she had to be demoted. Mrs. Shaw always tried to do her best, but she lacked the proper education and skills. I obtained 15 additional approved nursing positions, including one additional full-time RN in in-service and an additional $80,000 for in-service, from the state rate-setters, something that no one has been able to do at this hospital for the past eight years. Our expenditures in nursing are already above the state median. I obtained a staffing plan from another hospital for the director of nursing and influenced her to distribute a questionnaire to all nurses to better find out their feelings and ideas.

I could go through each of the charges made by the people assembled here, but it won't really prove anything. Yes, I did call a doctor a . . . in my office. Yes, I did leave the hospital after the bomb scare before the police came, but only after I was convinced that it was a scare. I had a meeting to go to in Urban City, and I called one hour later to see that everything was all right. I think it is significant that none of the department heads supposedly humiliated by me showed up at this meeting. You have asked me to resign, but I'm not going to resign. That would not solve the hospital's problems. Firing me will not solve the bad nursing morale here or the doctor distrust. It will show the doctors and nurses and the community who runs this hospital. Is it the board of trustees or some doctors and nurses (the nurses are mainly being used by the doctors)? Whose head will these doctors be asking for the next time they want to get rid of somebody? The bond issue set for next month that could refinance our debt on the new wing will not go through if you fire me. And we shall have a $355,000 payment to make in August, which will be difficult to meet.

"Does anybody have any questions?" DeFalco asked the other trustees. There were a few questions, but nothing significant, no major contradictions of anything Wherry had said. A vote was taken to clear Wherry of the charges without rebuttal, and this passed 7 in favor, 5 against, with 4 abstentions. Then the trustees asked Wherry to leave the room and told him that they would make a decision.

That evening, after dinner with his wife and teenagers, DeFalco watched a baseball game on television. He couldn't get his mind off that Friday night board meeting, the vote 10 to 6 against Wherry, and the ultimate unanimous vote to dismiss him with two months' severance. During the previous week, DeFalco had made it his business to discuss the Don Wherry situation with the other 16 trustees (Wherry and he made 18). As best as he could recollect, the following was the essence of their comments to him.

Board Comments

Clock (age 55, life insurance salesman, first vice president of the board, former mayor, and DeFalco's long-time confidant): I have been one of Don Wherry's strongest supporters since he got here and before he got here. I was a member of the search committee that selected Don, as you remember. I still like Don personally, really I do, but it has become obvious to me, at least, that Don can no longer manage the hospital. Whether Don is right or wrong, the docs don't like him. [Wherry told DeFalco that Clock sold a lot of life insurance to a lot of doctors.] Don's biggest mistakes have been in not firing Mel Queen, the associate administrator, who never has supported him properly, and Winnie Shaw, the ex-director of nursing, whom he should never have kept around and I told him so.

Gotthuld (age 50, second vice president of the hospital board, president of the board of Preston College, and wife of a beer distributor): I have been spending one or two weeks out of every month in Vermont, you know, George, where we bought a distributorship, and last year Sam and I spent six months on a luxury liner trip around the world. So I really don't know what's going on that well. As chairman of the executive committee, I know we gave Don a good evaluation and if he isn't acting properly as chief executive officer, then at least part of the fault is ours. I see no reason to fire Don abruptly because of these alleged charges.

Lance (age 45, president of a local lumber company, treasurer of the hospital, and chairman of the buildings and grounds committee): I have always been one of Don Wherry's closest friends, although he may not admit it now. I think Don could do an excellent job managing a university hospital, but he definitely cannot do the job here at Brendan and we should get rid of him now. Don might care more than anyone else, certainly more than I do, about the welfare of the hospital employees, but he just hasn't communicated that to them.

Gonce (65 years old, RN, secretary of the hospital, recently returned for the board meeting from University Hospital in Urban City where she was recovering from a heart attack): Tony, you know I fought bitterly against Don Wherry's coming to Brendan in the first place, voted then for Mel Queen, the associate administrator, to do the job, and I vote for him now to do a better job than Don Wherry. Don should be working for the government somewhere, not in a small town. Mel Queen will make an excellent administrator of Brendan Hospital. We should have given it to him in the first place.

Giancarlo (age 60, president of a local canning firm, newly elected to the board in January): I don't know much about the facts of the situation, Tony; I like Don Wherry personally, but obviously the doctors and many of the employees are unhappy with him. They must be listened to. It doesn't seem that anything they are complaining about is new or isolated.

Gonzales (age 40, secondary school teacher, was one of Don Wherry's strongest supporters): I see what Don has done to meet with all the Latino leaders without any crisis, to hear out our problems and respond to us. Don has reorganized and improved services in the emergency room, hired a Spanish-speaking social work assistant, and increased the number of minority supervisors. I am not that impressed, really, by these charges. There's no meat to them. I think this is just a bunch of doctors trying to get rid of Don as they got rid of Mr. Drew, the last CEO, and I do not think the board should bow down to them this time.

Peppino (age 34, senior bank vice president): Knowing Don Wherry as I do, I can understand a lot of the charges and sympathize with those making the complaints. Don Wherry is cold and authoritative, and if he knows so much, maybe that isn't what the job needs anyway. Mel Queen can run the hospital perfectly well, I'm convinced of that. And if the doctors are going to stop admitting patients as they threaten to do, they must feel very strongly about Don Wherry. It's important to calm the doctors down and get on with business as usual, and the sooner the better. Don Wherry will have no problem finding a job somewhere else. Maybe he was going to leave Lockhart anyway after a few more years.

Black (age 45, president of the medical staff): We have to get rid of this guy. He's nothing but trouble. I tried to work with him, but the guys don't like him. Maybe it's because he went to Princeton or something. He gives the guys this feeling that he feels superior to us. He's the big-time administrator and we're the lowly doctors. We'd much prefer Mel Queen running the hospital. We don't have to put up with this Wherry guy, and now's the time to get rid of him.

Romano (age 50, president of a lumber company, newly elected to the board in January): I feel the way Lew Giancarlo does. I never thought being elected to this board would involve all these problems, and I'm certainly spending more time on this darn hospital than I would like to be spending. It's a tough thing for this Wherry guy. I like Don personally, but I really think we're going to have more problems with him than without him.

Levine (age 45, attorney, newly elected to the board in January): I think this is disgraceful what we're doing to Don. I don't like the way the whole thing was done, even if Don has made mistakes. You don't treat an employee this way, certainly not the chief executive officer. But I don't think that Don has handled it right, either. He should have gone to the mass meeting and defended himself. He should have organized people to speak on his behalf. That's the advice I would have given Don as a lawyer. And I think it's a darn shame this has to happen. It doesn't have to happen, really, if someone would only stand up and fight for Don and his cause. I'm doing the best that I can, but I've only been on the board a short time, and I feel I'm therefore limited in what I can do.

Morrissey (age 47, housewife): Don and his wife Sue are personal friends of mine, but I can't let that get in the way of making the right decision for the hospital. Don is certainly a brilliant guy who cares about people and doesn't want to see the patient or the consumer taken advantage of. He wants to do all the right things and he has done a lot of the right things. The hospital is a safer, warmer, financially sounder place than it was when Don took over. I'm certainly going to vote for Don. I'm sorry, but I don't feel I know enough to be really energetic about this.

Viggiani (age 60, owner of a large real estate firm and chairman of the county Democratic Party): I think it's a terrible thing what they're doing to Don. It's just like with the other guy, Phil Drew. This guy has always been there when we needed him. He works night and day. If anything's the matter, then it must be our fault because this guy has been doing what we've been telling him to do. He hasn't done anything without telling the doctors and us first. I think it's a disgrace.

Asselta (age 70, general practitioner): The staff just doesn't like him. I like Don Wherry. I know he's been trying to do the right thing. I've tried to help Don, after I made sure of him, every way I can. You know my wife has been very sick and I haven't been able to attend to hospital affairs lately as I would like. I guess I'll go along with the majority, either way.

Goldman (age 61, chief of ob-gyn, newly elected to the board in January): I don't think the man knows how to manage the hospital, asking the employees to come up with the solutions to their own problems. That's bad management. Our group is against him.

Catrambone (age 50, director of a large funeral home): Tony, I'm only sorry I won't be at the meeting to speak for Don. There's a right and a wrong, and I can tell the difference. Ask yourself who is right and who is wrong, and you've got to vote for Don Wherry. I happen to think he's a pretty fair manager to boot. I wish you would count my vote. Since my open heart surgery, I've got to be in Rochester, Minnesota, for my annual heart examination.

Stuart (age 41, senior vice president of the same bank of which Mrs. Peppino is assistant vice president): [Don Wherry had told DeFalco that Stuart and Peppino were against him because he gave all the bank business, per finance committee recommendation, to a competing bank.] I don't like Don Wherry. I never have. I served with him on the personnel committee and we were usually in disagreement. Don always made me feel somehow that I was ignorant, that he felt himself superior to me. This is not how he should have acted. And I'm sure a lot of the employees feel the same way about Don that I do.

	Rating 1–5 (1 is high, 5 is low)	
	Self	**Avg. Trustee**
I. Goal Achievement		
1. Stabilize hospital finances	1	2.7
2. Increase fund-raising	3	3.6
3. Improve hospital morale	3	4.9
4. Improve quality of nursing care	1	3.7
5. Organize emergency room department	1	2.9

APPENDIX VI.1

Summary of CEO Evaluation (November 25, 1978)

(continued on next page)

6.	Establish an effective management information and control system	2	2.1
7.	Maintain on-schedule, on-budget west wing building program	3	2.3
8.	Establish plan for utilization of west wing and integration with total hospital operations	3	2.1
9.	Increase communications with the growing Spanish-speaking community	1	3.1
10.	Increase accountability of medical departments for quality assurance	1	3.1
11.	Prepare to obtain three-year hospital accreditation upon completion of west wing	3	1.9
12.	Increase community participation in hospital long-range planning	1	2.2

CEO Remarks:
1. CEO is goal-oriented.
2. He needs to spend yet more time developing consensus and persuading key stakeholders and earning their respect.

Trustee Remarks:
1. Many of these "specifics" are difficult for an outside director to judge.
2. I think CEO's contributions are acceptable except in items 3 and 4, where they should have been significantly greater.
3. Morale is a question.
4. CEO is doing a fine job for Brendan.
5. CEO's capability is great for achieving all goals. Sometimes his motives are not understood, and some obstacles are not of his doing.
6. The answers to some of these questions are based more on perceptions than actual knowledge.

President's Remarks:
I agree that the CEO is goal-oriented. He has attained goals we have given him about as well as anyone could reasonably expect.

II. System Maintenance	2	3.5

CEO Remarks:
1. Given what the CEO was hired to do, a certain amount of distrust is inevitable.
2. The CEO tries diligently to establish regular and continuing dialogue with all key hospital groups and individuals.

Trustee Remarks:

1. Greatest weaknesses in this category are in maintaining adequate commitment of employees to organizational goals and developing adequate trust between management and medical staff.
2. The board is not made aware of exactly the number of employees needed and the department that has this need. There seems to be a feeling of unrest among the administrative staff (department heads). Trust between management and medical staff is currently very poor.
3. CEO's capabilities are limitless, but I feel he has developed a schism between himself and the medical staff.
4. Small areas of difference need to be cleared by better communication and understanding of mutual problems. Main problem area is with doctor contracts.
5. I suspect that the only positive factor in the above list would be "maintaining adequate administrative and control systems."

President's Remarks:

1. Our "hospital system" has undoubtedly provided sufficient patient care of adequate quality at reasonable cost. I therefore believe the trustee evaluation to be too low in this area.
2. A mistrust of the administration by the medical staff does exist. I am also apprehensive about the "team play" of the administrative staff. We must address these problems in 1979.

III. Relationships with Important External Publics 1   2.1

CEO Remarks:

The hospital has done well with licensing, regulatory, and reimbursement agencies, and with other provider agencies during 1978. The CEO speaks frequently to consumer organizations and volunteer groups as well and has been well received.

Trustee Remarks:

1. The CEO has done an especially good job with third-party payers.
2. This is definitely the CEO's strongest area.

(*continued on next page*)

3. Excellent record.

President's Remarks:
    I am pleased with the CEO's
    accomplishments in this area.

IV. Management Roles

1. Interpersonal	3	3.6
2. Informational	1	2.4
3. Decisional	1	2.8

CEO's Remarks:
    The CEO is intelligent and quick. He works
    long hours and is subject to constant
    pressures. He cannot possibly talk at length
    continuously with 18 trustees, 40 key doctors,
    20 department heads, and other key personnel
    outside the hospital. He must try harder to be
    cheerful, quiet, friendly, and low-key.

Trustee Remarks:
1. I think the CEO has done a good job in 1978, especially in view of what he walked into.
2. The CEO has weakness in providing motivation, also in recognizing disturbances of uneasiness within the hospital personnel, and in dealing with incompetent or unproductive personnel.
3. The CEO seems to be seeking many changes. His method for achieving this isn't always productive. The CEO has great potential but doesn't seem to implement it well.
4. I'm not too sure if the CEO is handling personnel adequately. Morale has not improved within the hospital.
5. The CEO has done and is doing an outstanding job. I am proud to work with him and would give him even higher marks if possible.
6. The CEO is excellent on a one-to-one basis. He handles groups well. He is anxious to please and to get cooperation.

President's Remarks:
1. Changes in staff personnel in 1978 have hampered the efficiency and effectiveness of this group. When stability of this group occurs, provided the right group has been chosen, improvement in hospital management will be most evident.
2. The dissemination of information is exceptional.

3. I have confidence in the decisions that are being made. I am not sure about their method of implementation.

V. President's Summary
1. Areas of evaluation:
   The CEO has exceeded my expectations. In sum total, I am extremely pleased with his accomplishments.
2. Strengths:
   Planning, establishing priorities, dealing with regulatory agencies, understanding and articulating hospital organization, financial management, intelligence, creativity, ability to negotiate, potential, sincerity, and directness.
3. Weaknesses:
   Impatience and aloofness (coldness).
4. Uncertainties:
   Evaluation of personnel, evaluation of situations, employee motivation, and nonpeer and subordinate relationships.
5. Recommendations:
   Attempt to gain trust and respect of medical staff.
   Improve trust and respect of employees in presence of others.
   Refrain from reprimanding employees in the presence of others.
   Work toward having assistant responsible for day-to-day operation of hospital.
   Continue to attempt to improve morale.
   Improve patience; realize that few people can match intelligence quotient.
   Continue to develop administrative staff.
6. Conclusion:
   The CEO has performed well in 1978. He has acceptably attained his goals. As a new manager, he has been severely tested by the board of trustees, medical staff, and employees and has withstood their challenge. I believe his inherent intelligence will allow him to correct any and all identifiable deficiencies.
   The CEO's self-evaluation was extremely accurate. It is comforting to know that he has the ability to correctly assess his strengths and weaknesses.
   The following elements will be necessary for his continued success:

(*continued on next page*)

APPENDIX VI.1
(*continued*)

a. Constructive advice and support by board of trustees
b. Trust of medical staff
c. Melding of administrative staff into stable, competent, and qualified team with common objectives

APPENDIX VI.2
Letter from
Tony DeFalco
to Don Wherry
on January 10,
1979

Personal and Confidential

Mr. Don Wherry   January 10, 1979
Brendan Hospital
Lockhart, East State

Dear Don,

The Board of Trustees of Brendan Hospital, on January 8, 1979, unanimously approved a 10 percent increase in your annual salary along with a $500 increase in automobile allowance for 1979. The above increases will result in a per annum salary of $57,750 and an automobile allowance of $2,300. Your receipt of this letter provides you with the authority to make the stipulated adjustments effective January 1, 1979.

Our board believes that you have done an outstanding job as our chief executive officer and hopes that the above increases have fairly rewarded your effort.

Very truly yours,

Tony DeFalco, President
Brendan Hospital, Board of Trustees

Case Questions

1. How do you feel about what happened to Don Wherry?
2. Do you feel the board was justified in acting as it did?
3. What could Wherry have done to prevent being fired? What could the board have done to have prevented this? Should the medical board have acted any differently?
4. Should Wherry have resigned as the board wished him to?
5. Whose hospital is Brendan Hospital? What are the consequences of this being the case—for consumers, patients, managers, physicians, and trustees?

Case R
What More Evidence Do You Need?

Anthony R. Kovner
(Reprinted with permission from *Harvard Business Review*, May 1, 2010)

Sally Randolph rose from her swivel chair and walked over to the Norman Rockwell print hanging on her wall. A remnant from the days when she and Mark Wiley worked together as resident physicians, it showed a concerned young girl holding up her doll to a white-haired doctor, who was kindly "listening" to its heart.

She loved this image and what it stood for: medicine focused on people. Mark had caught a glimpse of the print in her locker back then, and he had liked it. She wondered what he'd think of it now.

They both still worked at American Medical Center (AMC), a $2 billion institution, but Mark was now CEO and Sally chief medical officer. The image of the e-mail he'd just sent—marked urgent with a red exclamation point and the subject line "Evidence-Based Management Seminar Cancelled"—blurred her vision. Apparently Mark's focus had shifted from patient care to profits.

Middle Managers Versus Chiefs

"Hi, Dr. Randolph. Are you interruptible?"

Richard Lee stood with his fist against the door frame, as if he'd been knocking. She wondered how long he'd been there.

"Oh, sorry, Richard! Yes, of course. Come in."

She walked back behind her desk and motioned for Richard to take the seat across from her. "What's up?"

Richard was one of 36 participants in the Evidence-Based Management (EBMgmt) seminar Sally had run for the past year with Harry Bradshaw, a professor at Lucas Business School. Every other month, clinicians and managers had met in teams of six and used EBMgmt to tackle the management challenges facing AMC.

Last month, Sally had presented a series of recommendations from the seminar, including those from Richard's team, to Mark and the medical chiefs. AMC clearly needed to improve the delivery and coordination of patient care, and the seminar participants had identified a structural reorganization as the best way to accomplish this. Despite all the proof, though, the chiefs didn't think that pursuing these improvements was as important as their research and teaching. Without their support—or Mark's—the recommendations never got off the ground.

Now Mark was asking seminar participants to serve as middle managers on task forces he was creating to carry out a new strategic plan. Everyone at AMC, he had written in the e-mail, could learn a lot from the participants about the importance of basing decisions on sound evidence. Sally couldn't help thinking, though, that Mark didn't really seem to respect EBMgmt when he rejected the recommendations that resulted from it.

"I just read the e-mail from Mark, and I'm really frustrated," Richard said. "Making us middle managers on these task forces won't change how anyone works. The medical chiefs weren't receptive to our recommendations, and they certainly won't like it if we start telling them how to make decisions. It seems like we can't get anywhere with evidence-based management in this organization."

Sally couldn't argue with him. Richard's team had tirelessly followed the evidence-based approach: translating management challenges into research questions, answering those questions with the best literature out there, and conducting pilot studies to support the interventions they proposed to senior management.

"I know, Richard," Sally sighed. "It's hard to imagine decisions ever getting made differently around here. If the chiefs weren't wowed by evidence-based management when Harry and I were selling it, all of you middle managers on the task forces will have an even harder time getting them on board. I'll talk to Mark, but I can't make any promises."

She thought of Mark's e-mail and how it seemed his focus had shifted from EBMgmt to Centers of Excellence, which he clearly considered to be the centerpiece of his new strategic plan. These would be run by the chiefs, and with this new responsibility—and power—Sally worried they'd have even less tolerance for change.

"Thanks, Sally. I appreciate it," Richard said as he stood to leave.

"We'll see how it goes," Sally said. She thought to herself, "Don't thank me yet."

Running Out of Options

Deciding to make her morning run six miles instead of three, Sally began a second loop around the lake. She always entered a sort of Zen state after 30 minutes, and today she needed all the clarity she could get.

She knew AMC historically broke even financially, and chatter among senior management was that Mark had received clear direction from the board to focus on "not losing money." One way to boost the center's financial results was to increase patient volume, which surely was behind Mark's new strategic plan.

Centers of Excellence attracted more patients, and more patients equaled bigger profits—in most circumstances. Sally couldn't help but think that Mark had missed one crucial fact: 90% of AMC's current patients were low income, and their health care was paid for by Medicare or Medicaid. The chances of the new centers attracting enough higher-income patients to make up for the no-pay patients were slim, especially considering the nicer facilities that already existed in wealthier neighborhoods.

Shaking out her arms on a downhill stretch, she wondered if it was possible to salvage the situation. Perhaps if evidence-based management were part of the new strategic plan, the data would eventually tell the story the EBMgmt team had been trying to tell for some time.

Before she approached Mark, she decided, she'd check in with Harry. He had co-run the seminar, after all, and might have ideas of his own.

A Patient Approach

"Have you tried the stir fry?" Sally asked.

Sally and Harry maneuvered around the Lucas Business students in the dining hall. It was a beautiful day—April like it is only in Virginia—and many students were taking their lunches out to the quad. One of them recognized Harry as her professor, giving him a polite smile as she passed with her cell pressed to her ear.

"The stir fry is good, but beware the hot sauce," Harry responded.

They found a seat at a corner table, and Sally laid out the situation, emphasizing her worry about Mark's new direction, which left the fate of EBMgmt in the hands of a few relatively junior managers.

"Sally," he went on, "I've worked with Mark for 16 years. I know him, and I know AMC. My advice is to start small. There's no proof that evidence-based management has a high ROI. Limit your efforts to your jurisdiction, to quality and safety, and prove the effectiveness of the approach there before trying to sell Mark on structural change."

"But, Harry, Mark's focus on Centers of Excellence is a big step in the wrong direction," Sally said.

"Believe me, I wish the seminar hadn't been cancelled. And I completely agree it's a bad idea to leave it to the middle managers to enlighten the chiefs. At this point, though, there's not enough support for restructuring."

Back in her office, Sally pondered Harry's advice. Trying to show modest results in her own area would take months or years, and all the while AMC would be pouring resources into a misguided plan to increase profits and moving further away from better patient care.

True, the consequences of not having a seamless delivery system weren't always dire—one patient receiving a cold meal wasn't the end of the world. But it was unacceptable when a high-risk patient had trouble scheduling a crucial follow-up visit or when a patient missed several doses of medication because of miscommunication.

Doing what was right to improve the patient experience was increasingly complex, but every indicator suggested a seamless delivery system was the solution. If the organization seriously committed to using evidence for making better managements decisions, maybe everything else would fall into place. Fostering that sort of commitment would require leadership from the top. And what better way to begin that process than as part of a new strategic plan?

Proof of Evidence

Back home, Sally plopped down on the couch, mentally exhausted. Her husband walked in minutes later with their small dog, Penny, who was excited and straining to be let off her leash.

"How's it going?" Joe asked.

She let out a big sigh and recapped her conversation with Harry.

"I can accept that there's no appetite for a restructuring, but creating these Centers of Excellence shows a complete lack of interest in using evidence to make smart decisions. Mark needs to do more than pay lip service to promoting the 'great skills' we learned in the seminar."

"Well, maybe Harry has a point," Joe said, unlacing his shoes. "We have all the evidence we need that the U.S. health care system is not sustainable. Our costs are too high, quality is too uneven, and millions of people can't even get care. Still, that hasn't resulted in the right changes. Proving the value of evidence-based management is going to be tough."

Sally's look told him that wasn't the reaction she wanted.

"But why do I need to prove its value first?" she asked. "Is there a known positive ROI for top-down decision making? For decisions based on anecdotes and gut reactions?"

Joe didn't have the answers, but he did have the ingredients to make a killer baked ziti. As Sally watched him walk to the kitchen, Penny pitter-pattering behind, she thought about the odds of changing Mark's mind. At most institutions, it would be career suicide to confront the CEO about flaws in his strategic plan. But Mark had recruited Sally for this position. If she played up the potential cost savings of EBMgmt, she might have a chance.

Unfortunately, as Harry pointed out, scientific proof of evidence-based management's positive ROI did not exist—yet. She'd be taking a gamble by advocating for it so strongly. On the other hand, if they committed to Mark's plan as is, they might never make any improvements at all in patient care.

Commentaries

1. Sally needs to argue for using data to make every decision at AMC.

Jeffrey Pfeffer, professor at the Stanford Graduate School of Business

Sally Randolph hasn't done the best job promoting organizational change, but it's not too late. First, she needs to create a much greater sense of urgency. Slow change often equals no change. That's because "slow" gives people the opportunity to put off action. It's the deadline effect (people work harder as a deadline approaches) in reverse. The fact that the EBMgmt seminar produced nothing tangible after one year means that talk has substituted for action.

Second, she must help the medical chiefs understand what's in it for them. If American Medical Center is like most other hospitals, it suffers from quality problems that expose it to financial difficulties, because Medicare and private insurers won't pay for care necessitated by treatment-induced issues such as infections. The medical chiefs should be alerted to initiatives such as the Institute for Healthcare Improvement's 5 Million Lives project, intended to reduce incidents of medical harm, and they need to see data on preventable deaths from the Institute of Medicine. The medical chiefs also need updates on AMC's own cost and medical outcomes performance, which Sally can assemble in frequent reports distributed widely throughout the medical center. In short, Sally needs to remind the chiefs that they have obligations to patients, not just to research and teaching—something that is easy to lose sight of in an academic medical center.

Third, Sally needs to spend much more time with Mark Wiley. He suffers from the "program du jour" disease—going from one thing, evidence-based management, to another, Centers of Excellence, apparently just to try something new. Quality and other organizational change initiatives often fail because of the short attention spans of senior leaders and the consequent tendency of people further down the ranks to wait until the latest program passes. Sally needs to explain that her work can yield improvements that will enhance not only AMC's financial results but also Wiley's stature as a hospital administrator.

Fourth, Sally needs to argue for using data to make every decision at AMC—even for creating Centers of Excellence. It sounds as if the incremental increase in patients may not be profitable, and the concept can easily be imitated. In contrast, evidence-based management results in process improvements that provide an enduring advantage. The value of EBMgmt doesn't need to be proven—its effects are in the studies on which it relies. Just as in medicine, if an organization implements something that has been shown to work, it will work in that organization, too.

Sally confronts the political realities of accomplishing organizational change. But she should be on her way to success if she shows people what's in it for them, provides information that builds a compelling case, creates a sense of urgency, highlights what other hospitals have done to improve, and argues that evidence should be used for guiding not just medical practice but administrative practice as well.

2. Managers could pilot the approach in pockets of the organization.

David Fine, CEO of St. Luke's Episcopal Health System

Mark Wiley's strategy to address profitability on the revenue side, through increased clinical volumes in Centers of Excellence, is commonplace. But this approach is not likely to generate the margins Wiley is hoping for unless the new centers radically change AMC's distribution of patients. AMC's Medicare and Medicaid payer mix is reported to be 90% of current patients. According to published reports from the American Hospital Association, 53% of hospitals receive Medicare payments less than cost, and 56% of hospitals receive Medicaid payments less than cost.

A more effective approach would be to focus on reducing costs associated with specific clinical outcomes through treatment protocols driven by best practices, supply chain standardization, simple strategies that decrease patient falls and reduce hospital-acquired infections, and other process improvements. The literature is replete with studies documenting the cost improvements that follow such interventions, all of which are illustrative of evidence-based management.

EBMgmt is a commitment to the use of informed decision making rather than instinct or precedent. Sally Randolph and at least one middle manager, Richard Lee, see the Centers of Excellence strategy as contrary to the culture promoted in the EBMgmt seminar. But there is little reason to conclude that evidence can play no role in establishing the centers. The EBMgmt partisans at AMC, acting through Sally, can help ensure that the centers are chosen and then financed on the basis of a realistic view of profit potential, ROI, community need, or other objective criteria.

Harry Bradshaw's encouragement of an incremental approach is wise. I have had the opportunity to manage as a disruptive innovator; this is easier from the CEO chair than from other places in the enterprise. If AMC is not ready to absorb EBMgmt across the board, some executives and middle managers could pilot the approach in pockets of the organization. Organizational politics at AMC need not impede the use of the best available scientific evidence. Those who aspire to adopt potentially transforming approaches don't have to wait until Mark designates lean management, Six Sigma, evidence-based management, or some other "state religion." I think a Randolph and Lee skunk works could do some good and certainly, in the spirit of Hippocrates, would do no harm.

Short Case 26
The Conflicted HMO Manager

Anthony R. Kovner

Bill Brown had built up University Hospital's HMO over the past ten years so that now it had 100,000 members. His boss, Jim Edgar, had decided to sell the insurance part of the business (retaining the medical groups) because University wasn't in the insurance business. Brown was asked to recruit some bidders, one of whom, Liberty National, Edgar came to prefer because of its financial strength and excellent reputation. In the process of working with Liberty National, Brown learned that it wanted to hire him, after the sale, to be the president of its regional HMO activities. Brown told Edgar what was likely to happen in this regard. The deal was subsequently approved by Brown's board (of the HMO) and by Edgar's board (of the hospital). Two years after the sale, Brown works for Liberty and is making $5 million a year, while University is losing $5 million a year. Joe Kelly, University's new CEO, figures out that the contract that Brown negotiated for University was highly favorable to Liberty and now University can't get out of it for another nine years.

Case Questions

1. Did Brown act unethically? If so, how? What should Brown have done? Why didn't he do it?
2. Did Edgar act competently? If not, what should he have done differently? Why didn't he do it?
3. What should the University CEO, Joe Kelly, do now?

Short Case 27
What Benefits the Community?

Paula H. Song and Ann Scheck McAlearney

Barney Wiseman looked at his hospital's most recent community benefit report. His hospital has been reporting its community benefit activities for years, well before the state required all not-for-profit hospitals to report their activities annually to the state attorney general's office. Year after year, Wiseman's department submitted the report, but there had never been any feedback from the state about his hospital's level of community benefit or activities.

But today the community benefit report took on new significance. The big news of the week was the neighboring state of Illinois' move to revoke the property tax-exemption status of three hospitals. If the state of Illinois succeeded, these three hospitals would then be responsible for property taxes, which could translate into a new financial burden that could involve millions of dollars for these hospitals.

The state had identified these hospitals when it had reviewed the levels of charity care hospitals in Illinois provided. These three hospitals had been singled out because they were deemed to be providing only "low" levels of charity care, ranging from 0.96 percent to 1.85 percent of patient-care revenue, according to the Illinois Department of Revenue (Japsen 2011).

However, as Wiseman knew, the "appropriate" level of charity care that a not-for-profit hospital should provide had not yet been defined. Hospitals typically provide a host of services that could be considered community benefits, including hosting community health fairs and providing health services that are often unprofitable, such as emergency department services, burn units, and counseling services. In addition, many hospitals are reimbursed by Medicare and Medicaid at levels below the cost of the services they deliver; thus, these unreimbursed costs could be seen as part of a benefit to the community. Other activities, such as providing graduate medical education and performing unfunded research, are also typically understood to benefit the broader community hospitals serve, but again, whether and how to count these activities when evaluating a hospital's community benefits are still unclear.

Wiseman had always thought that his hospital provided care and services well above the "acceptable" level for community benefits, but the situation in Illinois has made him wonder whether this was really the case. Moreover, Wiseman wondered if his current community benefit report adequately accounted for all of the community benefits the hospital did provide, well beyond charity care.

Case Questions

1. Who should benefit from a hospital's community benefits? (Who are the hospital's stakeholders, and how do they benefit?)
2. How much community benefit should not-for-profit hospitals provide?
3. What activities, other than charity care, should be counted as community benefits?
4. What are the implications if a not-for-profit hospital's tax-exempt status is revoked?

Reference

Japsen, B. 2011. "State Challenging Hospitals' Tax Exemptions." *New York Times.* Accessed August 7, 2012. www.nytimes.com/2011/09/11/us/11cnchospitals .html?pagewanted=all.

Short Case 28
CEO Compensation: How Much Is Too Much?

Paula H. Song

"Hospital CEO Pulls in $1 Million in Compensation" read the headline in big, bold letters on the front page of the local newspaper this morning. Alicia Cooper, CEO of Golden Valley Health System (GVHS), sighed when she saw the headline. Every year, the local newspaper reports on compensation for the five hospital CEOs in the local market. The newspaper uses the information that is reported in the each hospital's IRS 990 form, the annual tax return filed by all not-for-profit hospitals.

Cooper is the third-highest-paid CEO on the list, despite the fact that GVHS is the largest not-for-profit hospital system in the local market, comprising three hospitals, one large outpatient surgery center, and comprehensive rehabilitation services. GVHS represents approximately $800 billion in revenues each year. Although GVHS has experienced a 3 percent increase in admissions and overall patient visits, it reported a loss of $5 million last year, and a $3 million loss the prior year. While GVHS typically budgets a 3.5 percent total profit margin, the losses incurred over the past few years were not atypical given the weak economy, high unemployment rates, and the corresponding increase in the number of uninsured patients and escalating costs of healthcare delivery.

Nonetheless, executive compensation has grown significantly in recent years, particularly in the healthcare industry. This growth, coupled with the recent federal government bank bailout, has raised national criticism about "excessive" executive compensation. CEOs of multimillion-dollar not-for-profit health institutions are not immune to this criticism, as the charitable mission of not-for-profit HCOs exempts them from all federal—and most state and local—taxes. The benefit of tax-exemption is substantial, and critics argue that the public subsidizes not-for-profit hospitals (and therefore "excessive" CEO compensation) by forgoing this tax revenue. Still, not-for-profit hospital CEOs are, on average, compensated at lower levels than their CEO counterparts at similarly sized for-profit hospitals.

Cooper knows this new newspaper story will reignite conversation among members of the board of trustees, and they ultimately determine her salary. Until then, she wonders how she will respond to the criticism she expects to follow this story—criticism from the board, from hospital staff, and likely from the media.

Case Questions

1. How should CEO compensation for not-for-profit hospitals be determined?
2. How should compensation of CEOs of not-for-profit hospitals and for-profit hospitals be compared?

Short Case 29
A Real Story of a Patient's Experience in Vancouver

Caroline Wang

This case relates the personal experience of a Canadian physician navigating the Canadian healthcare system. She writes from her own perspective, based on her experience helping her mother resolve a health problem. The opinions stated here are her own.

On New Year's Eve in 2010, I brought my 76-year-old mother to the emergency department (ED) of a Vancouver hospital after she mentioned having blurred vision and redness in her one good eye (the other eye had been blinded in a traumatic accident during childhood). The ED physician promptly referred her to the ophthalmology service, and my mother was given an urgent appointment for the following morning.

When we arrived at the eye care center at 9:30 a.m. on January 1, the front door to the concrete building was locked. We could not see anyone inside, and the building had no sign or intercom, so we worriedly returned to the ED to ask what we should do. After we received an initial response of "this isn't my job," the ED triage nurse at the window told us to go back and just wait in front of the building for someone to open the door. "But how does anyone know we are there?" I asked. "My mother is elderly, and this is the middle of winter." I made the gentle suggestion to the ED triage nurse to call someone to come and open the door for us. Then we walked several blocks down the street back to the eye care center and waited outside, shivering in the cold. After about 15 minutes that felt like an eternity, a patient's family member pushing a baby stroller inside the building saw us and let us in.

Inside the dark building, we saw several patients sitting in the waiting area but found no clerk to receive patients or record their information. After a while, a harried young resident doctor wearing a shirt and jeans emerged from one of the examining rooms in the back. He was very polite and apologized for the situation that was not of his doing. Being the only on-call doctor working in the building, it was clearly impossible for him to see patients in the back, answer his pager, and constantly check whether there were any patients waiting outside the building. The resident then added in a hushed tone, "because security personnel are in only from 1:00 p.m. to 5:00 p.m., and things have been stolen in the past."

Throughout the rest of the morning, we observed that a few patients would occasionally let other patients into the building. One woman in the common waiting area remarked that she had to travel here from Vancouver Island because "the only retinal surgeon in Victoria is on vacation in Mexico." However, because the waiting room is located behind a long hallway and the building has no buzzer or intercom system, knowing whether someone was waiting outside was impossible. Moreover, anybody can let anyone else inside the building by stepping on the door sensor on the floor.

After three hours, my mother was seen, and we were on our way. We then left that cold and dark building—the tertiary eye care referral center in one of the largest urban centers in Canada.

The Vancouver Coastal Health Authority may be trying to save money. However, having no security personnel or administrative staff in the eye care center building on a holiday weekend, while leaving a single doctor on call to handle all the patients, is not only substandard care, it is also unsafe.

I wondered about how other patients, especially those who are vulnerable and lack resources, might cope under such circumstances. What about the frail elderly patient needing emergency eye treatment (thus visually impaired) who is unfamiliar with the hospital, and who may lack facility with the English language (especially in view of the large immigrant population in the region)? Or those patients who have difficulty with mobility or cognition? What will happen to those patients? The chances of people falling through the cracks are so high that it is only a matter of time for preventable disasters to happen, and they may then go unreported.

This experience in the largest referral center in the province may just be the tip of an iceberg. But as a sign of how our hospitals are being run, what message does it send to patients? More important, how can we have confidence that our serious medical care needs will be properly attended to when it is our turn to depend on the system?

Case Questions

1. What are the problems in this story, and what are the causes of these problems?
2. What are alternative solutions for these problems, and what are their pros and cons?
3. How would you begin to address these problems within this hospital? (How would you figure out who is responsible and where you might go to find some answers?)

Short Case 30
What's in a Name?

Ann Scheck McAlearney and Sarah M. Roesch

Donna Taylor was on her way to the mall to pick up an item donated to the carnival silent auction benefiting her daughter's school. In her head, she was going over the last-minute list of things she had to do to get ready for that night's carnival. Taylor really didn't have anything to worry about, because she was a master planner of fund-raisers and community service events. Ten years ago, Taylor had worked in the insurance industry, but left to stay home with her kids after her third child. Taylor enjoyed staying home with her children, but soon realized she needed more responsibilities than monitoring her children's nap schedules and play dates to make her feel useful. As a result, Taylor became active in the community through volunteerism, and participated in many service projects offered by the Junior League, YWCA Women's Board, and Children's Hospital Auxiliary. Taylor also participated in various capital campaigns and was a natural fund-raiser. Taylor was an organized, creative, and capable volunteer who quickly climbed the volunteer hierarchy and became a leader of these organizations. As her three daughters each entered school, she also became active in their school's PTA, and this involvement had led to her current run to the mall to pick up a donated auction item.

Taylor sprinted into the mall to gather her item and let out a deep sigh as she passed the Ashley and Mitch store. Taylor's oldest daughter, Stella, was in the sixth grade and just getting interested in fashion. A pair of Ashley and Mitch jeans was at the top of Stella's birthday list. Taylor shook her head at the large poster in Ashley and Mitch's window. Taylor was no prude, but she didn't quite agree with the photo of three scantily clothed teenage models. Ashley and Mitch was infamous for its risqué promotional material and sexual imagery enticing preteens and teens to buy its clothing. She did not think it was appropriate to entice teenage consumers with this type of marketing. However, it certainly seemed to work, since most preteens she knew were very interested in Ashley and Mitch's clothing. Taylor personally believed this type of advertising was sleazy and demeaning to young people. Even though she was able to shrug her shoulders at the poster with a mental note that "it's only clothes," she knew her daughter would not be getting those jeans for her birthday.

Taylor hurried to pick up her donation. Back in the car, she again went over her mental list for the fund-raiser, and decided she had everything covered. She was just beginning to relax when the news came on the radio. The reporter was relating a story about the local Children's Hospital renaming its emergency room "The Ashley and Mitch Emergency Department and Trauma Center" in exchange for a $10 million donation. With this new information, Taylor was struck by the realization that maybe this wasn't "only clothes." Taylor thought back to several middle-of-the-night trips to Children's Hospital and how thankful she was that her children had such a good place to go in an emergency situation. She also thought about the hours she spent volunteering at Children's Hospital, pushing a book cart and delivering books to patients. Taylor knew what $10 million could do for a children's hospital. Yet to name an emergency room after a company with a reputation for relying on sexual image marketing to target preteens and teens? She wasn't convinced. As the mother of three preteen girls, Taylor knew how insecurities about image can damage self-esteem. She was confused about the apparent inconsistency with Ashley and Mitch's message and Children's Hospital's mission of "protection and caring for children." As she approached the school for the carnival fund-raiser, Taylor's confusion had changed to anger at Children's Hospital for deciding to associate with a company notorious for egregious advertising.

Arriving at the school, the first person Taylor ran into was her fund-raising co-chair, Meg Flynn. After telling Flynn about the new partnership between

Ashley and Mitch and Children's Hospital, she was amazed that Flynn appeared ambivalent. Flynn's first response was to ask, "Why would Children's turn down such a large donation? They would be crazy to turn down that kind of money for all it could do to improve healthcare for children." Further, Flynn argued, despite the advertising, the consumer is the one with the true power. "No one is forced to buy Ashley and Mitch clothing. People can choose to look away." Flynn also suggested that maybe Ashley and Mitch owes something to the consumer, and *should* give back to children. Since it makes millions of dollars each year selling its inappropriate clothing, giving back some money to help children makes a lot of sense. While Taylor saw Flynn's points, she didn't think she could actually look the other way. Even though she knew how hard it is to raise money and realized that $10 million is a sizeable donation, Taylor thought Ashley and Mitch should donate the money, but not get naming rights. She remained unconvinced that this was a good trend for an industry focused on health and well-being.

Case Questions

1. What are the pros and cons for Children's Hospital in accepting the donation from Ashley and Mitch in exchange for naming rights?
2. Are there alternatives, such as a donation without naming rights, that you might propose?
3. Given the sentiments among community members, are there steps the hospital should take to work with the community to establish donation guidelines, or are such decisions only relevant to the hospital itself?
4. Should guidelines be established about which companies or industries should be allowed to donate money?

Short Case 31
Patient Satisfaction in an Inner-City Hospital

Claudia Caine and Anthony R. Kovner

Lutheran Medical Center is a 400-bed, inner-city, community teaching hospital located in Southwest Brooklyn. It is also one of only two Level I trauma centers in the borough of Brooklyn. Three major competing hospitals are located within five miles of the hospital, and this competition continually challenges the hospital's efforts to grow and gain market share. Lutheran's community is made up mainly of immigrants and blue-collar wage earners.

The payer mix is 75 percent Medicare and Medicaid. Recent efforts, therefore, have focused on reaching out to the neighboring community of Bay Ridge where the population is dense, better insured, and facing the closure of its only hospital (one of the aforementioned three hospitals).

With low New York State reimbursement rates and the high cost of New York healthcare (wages, malpractice, benefits, etc.), the hospital must keep 90 percent of its beds filled to break even. Lutheran is already known as a low-cost provider, so growth is its only real option.

Most hospital administrators know that having a hospital routinely filled at more than 85 percent creates many challenges. Safety, quality of care, and patient satisfaction must be emphasized more than at hospitals at lower, more comfortable occupancy rates.

In response to its primary objective (i.e., growth and maintenance of high census while still improving quality of care, safety, and patient satisfaction levels), the hospital embarked upon an effort to dramatically improve its emergency department (ED). Generally known to be the hospital's "front door" to the community, more than 70 percent of Lutheran's admissions come from the ED. Lutheran's thinking about the ED is that if it works beautifully, patient satisfaction will go up, first impressions will be positive, quality of care and patient safety will be improved, and more and more residents of the community, and beyond, will choose the hospital for care.

The hospital did three main things to address the goal of becoming the ED of choice in Brooklyn:

1. Replaced the leadership of the ED
2. Expanded the ED's space by 60 percent and modernized it
3. Redesigned all ED systems and processes

The specific measurable goals for this redesign project were:

1. Increase the percentage of patients reporting being "satisfied" or "very satisfied" from 52 to 70 percent.
2. Increase visits from 147 per day to 175 per day.
3. Have a provider see every patient within 30 minutes of arrival in the ED.
4. Have fewer than 2 percent of patients return to the ED for a second visit within 48 hours of their first visit.
5. Hire 100 percent ED-trained physicians in the ED.

The project began in 2002 and was completed in 2006. The first step was to replace the leadership. The leaders, at that time, were reluctant to change and were not familiar with national best-practice models in ED care. Also, 80 percent of the physicians were non-ED-trained. Replacing the chairman and the vice president of nursing for the ED took one year to accomplish. Turning over the staff to have 100 percent ED-trained physicians took three and a half years.

Next, in 2005, the hospital formed an ED Process Redesign Task Force. Previous leadership had attempted a redesign in 2002, but it failed. A major lesson learned was that redesign and "overhaul" are impossible without the right leadership in place.

This effort was led by the hospital chief operating officer and the new chairman of the ED. The other members of the team included the chief nursing officer, the vice president of nursing for the ED, the nurse manager for the ED, the ED educator, and the VP of operations responsible for the ED.

The process redesign had seven main results:

1. A care team model for the ED was created, allowing small groupings of patients to be treated by a team that included an MD, RN, and aide.
2. A position called *ED patient navigator* was created. This person was available to communicate with referring physicians about their patients and serve as a case manager for ED patients.
3. The role of the ED nursing care coordinator/charge nurse was redefined to be the daily "director" of movement, operations, and oversight of the entire ED.
4. The traditional nursing triage model was replaced with a combined triage/fast-track model. Physician assistants (PAs) replaced nurses at triage and triaged, treated, and released (when appropriate), or triaged and moved patients to the main ED when appropriate.
5. All ED staff were given portable internal zone phones to increase communications and reduce the noise level.
6. Paper charts were replaced with a fully automated medical record and tracking system.
7. Bedside registration was implemented, so patients go directly from triage to an ED bed without stopping to be registered.

Within 18 months of introducing the process redesign team, the following occurred:

- Patient visits went from 147 per day to 172 per day.
- The average door-to-provider (MD or PA) time went from 90 minutes to 30 minutes.
- One hundred percent of MDs were ED-trained.
- Two percent of patients needed to return to the ED within 48 hours of their initial visit.

- ED patient satisfaction went from 52 to 66 percent (still four percentage points short of the goal).

Clearly the team was disappointed by the lack of progress in patient satisfaction, but they were not confused by it. The reason was that as patient volume increased, the number of available hospital beds remained fixed, so patients waited longer as more time was needed to move patients from the ED to a hospital bed. Because the hospital must remain at over 90 percent occupancy to break even, adding beds would have created operating losses for the institution—an option the team did not have available.

The new challenge became improving patient satisfaction given the increasing wait times for hospital beds. The team took the following eight actions:

1. Added a team of physicians to the ED to provide care to admitted patients as they awaited beds
2. Created a labor-management joint team to improve patient flow on the inpatient units (with a goal of discharging patients within four hours of a discharge clearance note being written by a physician)
3. Created the ED Diplomat program, which is a daily 2:00 p.m. to 8:00 p.m. rotation of senior hospital leaders who meet each ED patient with a long stay, explain the wait, manage expectations, and give free hospital TV services and free parking when necessary
4. Increased nurse and nurse aide staffing in the ED
5. Ordered hospital beds to move patients from stretchers to more comfortable beds while they wait
6. Began a program to provide food and telephones for patients in the ED
7. Opened a discharge lounge for patients awaiting discharge to open up beds sooner
8. Created housekeeping and transport "SWAT" teams to facilitate room turnovers on inpatient floors

Most recent measurements show patient satisfaction in the ED has increased to 75 percent. However, calling this an upward trend is premature.

Discussion Question

What more can this hospital do to address this problem—understanding that opening more inpatient beds would cost upwards of $1.5 million and put the already ailing institution into a negative financial position?

INDEX

ABOUT THE EDITORS

Ann Scheck McAlearney, ScD, MS, is professor of family medicine and vice chair for research in the Department of Family Medicine in The Ohio State University College of Medicine. She also holds courtesy appointments as professor in the Division of Health Services Management and Policy in the College of Public Health and as professor of pediatrics, both at The Ohio State University. She has taught for 14 years at The Ohio State University, including courses in organizational management, leadership, and strategic management for master's and doctoral-level students and a course on healthcare organization and financing for medical students. Dr. McAlearney has more than 20 years of health services research experience and has authored 88 peer-reviewed publications, seven monographs, and 32 book chapters. Dr. McAlearney is currently principal investigator (PI) in a study of the use of strategic human resources practices to improve quality of care and prevent healthcare-associated infections, funded by the Agency for Healthcare Research and Quality. She is also the local PI for two National Institutes of Health–funded studies on receipt of adjuvant therapies by breast cancer patients, exploring ways to create organizational and systems solutions to care delivery problems. Her research interests also include the areas of primary care quality improvement, information technology innovations in healthcare, and organizational development. Dr. McAlearney's book, *Population Health Management: Strategies to Improve Outcomes*, was published by Health Administration Press. Prior to returning to academics, Dr. McAlearney held positions and had consulting arrangements with various organizations, including UniHealth, Monsanto Health Solutions, PacifiCare Health Systems, Merck & Co., Massachusetts General Hospital, UCLA Medical Center, Arthur Young & Company, the Congressional Budget Office, and the World Health Organization. Dr. McAlearney received her bachelor of arts and sciences (BAS) degree in English and biological sciences from Stanford University, her MS in biological sciences from Stanford University, and her ScD in health policy and management from the Harvard School of Public Health.

Anthony R. Kovner, PhD, is professor of public and health management at the Robert F. Wagner Graduate School of Public Service at New York University and director of the executive master of science program for nurse leaders. An organizational theorist by training, Dr. Kovner's research interests include evidence-based management and nonprofit governance. He has been a senior manager in two hospitals, a nursing home, a group practice, and a neighborhood health center, and a senior healthcare consultant for a large industrial union. His other books include *Evidence-Based Management in Healthcare*, with David J. Fine and Richard D'Aquila (Health Administration Press 2009); *Healthcare Management in Mind: 8 Careers* (Springer 2000); and *Health Care Delivery in the United States*, 10th edition, with James Knickman (Springer 2011). Dr. Kovner has served as a consultant to the NewYork–Presbyterian Hospital, the Robert Wood Johnson Foundation, the W. K. Kellogg Foundation, Montefiore Medical Center, and the American Academy of Orthopedic Surgeons. He served on the board of the Lutheran Medical Center for 26 years and as director of NYU/Wagner's program in health policy and management for more than 20 years. In 1999, Dr. Kovner was awarded the Gary L. Filerman Prize for Educational Leadership from the Association of University Programs in Health Administration. He received his PhD in public administration from the University of Pittsburgh.

ABOUT THE CONTRIBUTORS

Sofia V. Agoritsas, FACHE, is the director for the Kidney and Pelvic Health Service Line at North Shore LIJ Health System and is a doctoral student in healthcare management at the New York University Robert F. Wagner School of Public Service.

Emily Allinder is the program director of strategic business development at Saint Luke's Hospital in Kansas City, Missouri.

James W. Begun, PhD, is the James A. Hamilton Professor of Healthcare Management in the Division of Health Policy and Management, School of Public Health, University of Minnesota.

Nathan Burt is the system director of facilities management at Ohio Health in Columbus.

Claudia Caine is the executive vice president and hospital director/chief operating officer of Lutheran Medical Center in Brooklyn, New York.

J. Mac Crawford, PhD, is an occupational epidemiologist and an associate professor of Clinical Public Health at The Ohio State University in the College of Public Health, Division of Environmental Health Sciences.

Richard D'Aquila, FACHE, is the president and chief operating officer at Yale–New Haven Hospital and executive vice president of Yale–New Haven Health System in New Haven, Connecticut.

Jason Dopoulos is a vice president with Lancaster Pollard, a financial services firm based in Columbus, Ohio.

Peter Follows is the cofounder of Carpedia International.

Kathleen Heatwole, PhD, is the vice president of planning and development at Augusta Health in Augusta County, Virginia.

Brian Hilligoss, PhD, is an assistant professor of health services management and policy in The Ohio State University College of Public Health.

Maria Jorina is a PhD candidate and a graduate research assistant in the division of health services management and policy, College of Public Health, The Ohio State University.

David M. Kaplan is the vice chairman for administration and finance for the Department of Surgery of The Mount Sinai Medical Center in New York City.

Wilhelmina Manzano, RN, NEA-BC, is senior vice president and chief nursing officer for New York–Presbyterian Hospital and chief operating officer for the Allen Hospital.

David G. Melman, JD, is the chief legal officer at The First Rehabilitation Life Insurance Company of America.

David Muhlestein, JD, is as a healthcare consultant for Leavitt Partners and is completing his doctorate in health services management and policy at The Ohio State University College of Public Health.

Duncan Neuhauser, PhD, is the Charles Elton Blanchard MD Professor of Health Management Emeritus, Medical School, at Case Western Reserve University in Cleveland, Ohio.

Ramya Roa, RHIA, is an administrative fellow at OhioHealth.

Julie Robbins has worked in the healthcare field for more than 15 years, focused primarily on strategy and program development. She is a PhD candidate at The Ohio State University.

Sarah Mathews Roesch is employed at The Ohio State University College of Public Health.

Thomas G. Rundall is the Henry J. Kaiser Emeritus Professor of Organized Health Systems at the University of California, Berkeley, and serves on the boards of directors for John Muir Health and On Lok.

Rebecca Schmale is an administrator of human resources at the University of Virginia Health System in Charlottesville.

Paula H. Song, PhD, is an assistant professor in the Division of Health Services Management and Policy in the College of Public Health at The Ohio State University.

Breanne Taylor is the site director for six ambulatory care facilities in the Dublin and Hilliard markets at Nationwide Children's Hospital.

Jacob Victory is vice president of performance management projects at the Visiting Nurse Service of New York.

Erick Vidmar is the administrator of Stephanie Tubbs Jones Health Center of Cleveland Clinic located in East Cleveland, Ohio.

Jason Waibel is the director of therapy operations for HealthSouth Rehabilitation Hospital of Northern Virginia.

Dr. Caroline Wang is a Canadian family physician and student of public administration at the Robert F. Wagner Graduate School of Public Service, New York University.

Karen Weingrod is the manager of the Partnership for Breast Care, Hartford Hospital's comprehensive breast care program.

Michael J. Zaccagnino is the president of Lucania Partners, a New York City–based consultancy, and an advisor at Carpedia International.